WHAT TO EXPECT WHEN YOU'RE EXPECTING

❖ ❖ ❖ ❖

Arlene Eisenberg

Heidi Eisenberg Murkoff

Sandee Eisenberg Hathaway, R.N., B.S.N.

With a foreword by Dr. Richard Aubry,
Director of Obstetrics, Upstate Medical Center,
Syracuse, New York

WORKMAN PUBLISHING, NEW YORK

To Emma, who inspired this book while still in the womb, who did her best to keep us from writing it once she was out, and who, we trust, will put it to good use one day.

To Howard, Erik, and Tim, without whom this book would not have been possible—in more ways than one.

Copyright © 1984, 1988 by Arlene Eisenberg,
Heidi Eisenberg Murkoff, and Sandee Eisenberg Hathaway

Library of Congress Cataloging in Publication Data
Eisenberg, Arlene.   What to expect when you're expecting.
Includes index. 1. Pregnancy. 2. Childbirth. 3. Postnatal care.
I. Murkoff, Heidi Eisenberg. II. Hathaway, Sandee Eisenberg. III. Title.
RG525.E36 1984   618.2′4   84-40315   ISBN 0-89480-769-2

Art Director: Paul Hanson
Book Design: Susan Aronson Stirling
Cover Illustration: Judith Cheng
Book Illustration: Carol Donner

Workman Publishing Company, Inc.
708 Broadway
New York, N.Y. 10003

Manufactured in the United States of America
First printing October 1984

35 34 33 32 31 30 29

ACKNOWLEDGMENTS

Books and babies have a lot in common. Both take plenty of time, hard work, dedication, and care (not to mention a healthy dose of worry) to turn out the best possible product. Both also require the cooperation of a team of concerned people. We've been lucky to have a fine team involved in the creation of our book, all of whom we gratefully thank:

Elise and Arnold Goodman, our agents, for their confidence, advice, support, and friendship.

Suzanne Rafer, our editor at Workman, for her perceptive suggestions, her patience, her sense of humor (she needed it), and her endless capacity for what sometimes seemed endless work.

Susan Aronson Stirling, designer, who fit together the pieces (which would have left others, including us, puzzled) and supervised the illustrations, with skill and sensitivity.

Ann Appelbaum (who read our chapters-in-progress during her pregnancy-in-progress and insists that credit for her beautiful end product, Abby, goes at least partially to the Best-Odds Diet), for her practical and thoughtful suggestions, particularly on the cesarean section material. Beth Falk, another encouraging reader whose nine months paralleled ours. And the hundreds of expectant parents who shared their concerns with us.

Richard Aubrey, M.D., Professor of Obstetrics and Gynecology and Director of the Division of Obstetrics: Maternal-Fetal Medicine at The Upstate Medical Center (Syracuse, NY), and Henry Eisenberg, M.D., Assistant Clinical Professor at Upstate, who reviewed the book, for their invaluable critiques, suggestions, and fact-checking. We feel privileged to have worked with two such remarkable physicians.

Howard Eisenberg, husband and father, who understood the importance of the father in pregnancy and childrearing long before it was the vogue, who taught all of us all we know about writing, and who gave us unfailing support and counsel every step of the way.

Erik Murkoff, whose worries during Heidi's pregnancy served as an inspiration to the project.

Tim Hathaway, who, though only father-come-lately to the project, has contributed much, and who spent many lonely days in Boston while his wife helped complete the book in New York.

The women who allowed us to "shoot" their bellies, so our artist could have photographs of real pregnant woman to work from; and Peggy Levine of Great Shapes, in Manhattan, who permitted us to attend exercise classes to photograph her students.

CONTENTS

--------- *Part 1* ---------

IN THE BEGINNING

Chapter 1: Are You Pregnant? 18

WHAT YOU MAY BE CONCERNED ABOUT 18

Signs of Pregnancy ♦ Pregnancy Tests ♦ *Possible Signs of Pregnancy* ♦ *Probable Signs of Pregnancy* ♦ *Positive Signs of Pregnancy* ♦ Due Date

WHAT IT'S IMPORTANT TO KNOW: CHOOSING (AND WORKING WITH) YOUR PRACTITIONER 23

What Kind of Patient Are You? ♦ Obstetrician? Family Practitioner? Nurse-Midwife? ♦ Type of Practice ♦ Finding a Candidate ♦ Make the Most of the Patient-Practitioner Partnership

Chapter 2: Now That You Are Pregnant 30

WHAT YOU MAY BE CONCERNED ABOUT 30

Your Gynecological History ♦ Your Obstetrical History Repeating Itself ♦ Repeat Cesareans ♦ Pregnancies Too Close Together ♦ Tempting Fate the Second Time Around ♦ Having a Baby After 35 ♦ The Father's Age ♦ Chronic Health Problems: Diabetes ♦ Chronic Health Problems: Asthma ♦ Rh Incompatibility ♦ Herpes ♦ Other STDs (Sexually Transmitted Diseases) ♦ An IUD Still in Place ♦ Birth Control Pills in Pregnancy ♦ Spermicides ♦ Provera ♦ DES ♦ Genetic Problems

—————— *Part 3* ——————
LAST BUT NOT LEAST:
Postpartum, Fathers, and the Next Baby

A Word From the Doctor

The 1980s are the best years in history to be expecting a baby. In recent decades, there has been a remarkable improvement in the outcome of human pregnancy—for mothers as well as for infants. Women enter pregnancy healthier; they get better, more complete prenatal care; and the hospital maternity wing has replaced the kitchen table and the four-poster as the place to have a baby.

Yet more can be done. To those of us in academic medicine it is becoming increasingly clear that superior doctors and superior equipment aren't enough. Further reductions in pregnancy and childbirth risks will require actively participating expectant couples as well. In order to participate more, couples will have to be more completely and accurately informed, not just about the climactic birth experience, but about the all-important nine months that precede it, not just about the risks that pregnancy presents, but about the steps parents can take to minimize and eliminate risks; not just about the medical aspects of pregnancy, but about psychosocial and lifestyle factors as well.

How can parents become so informed? High schools and colleges have no time or place in their curricula for Babymaking 101. Professionals who provide obstetrical care have a time problem, too. And they are sometimes overly scientific in their explanations and insufficiently sensitive to the psychological and emotional needs of expectant parents.

Consumer advocates have vaulted into the void with books, magazine articles, and classroom instruction. They are often tremendously helpful, but almost as often they're medically inaccurate, unnecessarily alarming, and/or disproportionately focused on the inadequacies of the health care profession, driving a wedge of suspicion and doubt between parents and their obstetrical caregivers.

The need for a book that provides accurate, up-to-date, and medically sound information with proper emphasis on nutrition, lifestyle, and the emotional aspects of pregnancy has long been apparent. Now, I believe, that need has been met in a highly readable and eminently practical month-by-month format.

The three authors—each an experienced "consumer" of maternity care—have given us that essential consumer perspective. They have wisely concentrated on giving expectant parents the information that will allow them to intelligently play their central role in the entire process, without threatening the doctors and nurse-midwives with whom they must work closely and congenially.

What to Expect When You're Expecting is lively in style, accurate, current, and well-balanced overall. But four aspects of its structure and content deserve special comment:

❖ The book's thoughtful family-centered approach to childbearing—with involvement of the husband throughout the pregnancy process and with a chapter responding to his special needs and problems—is excellent and important.

❖ Its practical chronological arrangement—sensibly answering all the big and little, trying and troubling questions that come up month after month—makes for timely reassurance and easy bedside-table reference.

❖ The book's emphasis on pre-pregnancy and pregnancy nutrition and lifestyle, and its common-sense approaches to lactation and the psychosocial dimensions of motherhood, make it particularly valuable and unique.

❖ Its accurate and up-to-the-minute medical detail—particularly the clarity of its sections on genetics, teratology, preterm labor, delivery, cesarean section, and again, lactation—is outstanding.

All in all, I believe that this excellent book should be *required reading* not only for expectant parents, but for doctors and nurses who are training to provide obstetrical care and for professionals already providing it. That is, I know, a long way out on a limb for a generally cautious medical school professor to go. But I say it out of strong conviction: the belief that only with properly informed and responsible consumers and providers working together can we draw near our common goal—healthy babies, mothers, and families. And, ultimately, society.

Richard Aubry, M.D., F.A.C.O.G.
Director of Obstetrics—Maternal-Fetal Medicine, SUNY, Upstate Medical Center, Syracuse, NY

How This Book Was Born

I was pregnant, which about one day out of three made me the happiest woman in the world. And for the remaining two, the most worried.

Worried about the wine I'd sipped nightly with dinner, and the gin and tonics I'd downed more than a few times before dinner in my first six weeks of pregnancy—after two gynecologists and a blood test convinced me that I wasn't pregnant.

Worried about the seven doses of Provera one of the doctors had prescribed to bring on what she was certain was just a tardy period, but which proved two weeks later to be a nearly two-month gestation.

Worried about the coffee I'd drunk, and the milk I *hadn't;* the sugar I'd eaten, and the protein I hadn't.

Worried about the cramps in my third month, and the four days in my fifth month when I felt not even a flicker of fetal movement.

Worried about the time I fainted while touring the hospital I was to deliver in (I never did get to see the nursery), my middle-of-the-street belly-flop in the eighth month, and a bloody vaginal discharge in the ninth.

Worried, even, about feeling *good* ("But I'm not constipated. . . . I don't have morning sickness. . . . I'm not urinating more frequently—something must be wrong!").

Worried that I wouldn't be able to tolerate the pain during labor, or stand the sight of blood at delivery. And worried that because I couldn't squeeze out a drop of the colostrum all my books told me should fill my breasts by the ninth month, I wouldn't be able to breastfeed.

Where could I turn to find reassurance that all would be well? Not to the ever-growing stack of pregnancy books piled high on my bedside table. As common and normal as a few days of no fetal activity is in the fifth month, I couldn't find a single reference to it. As often as pregnant women take a tumble—almost always without harming their babies—I could find no mention of accidental falls.

When my symptoms, problems, or fears *were* discussed, it was usually in an alarming way which only compounded my concern. *Never take Provera unless you would "absolutely abort,"* warned one volume—without adding that a woman who has taken the drug has so slight an increased risk of birth defects in her baby that an unwanted abortion need never be considered. "There is evidence that a single drinking 'binge' during pregnancy may affect some babies, depending on the stage of development they have reached," cautioned another book ominously—disregarding studies which show that a few drinking sprees in early pregnancy, when many women indulge unknowingly, appear to have no effect on a developing embryo.

I certainly couldn't find relief for my worries by opening a newspaper, flipping on the radio or television, or browsing through magazines. According to the media, threats to the pregnant lurked everywhere: in the air we breathed, in the food we ate, in the water we drank, at the dentist's office, in the drugstore, even at home.

My doctor offered some solace, of course, but only when I was able to summon up the courage to phone. (I was either afraid my worries would sound silly, or afraid of what I would hear. Besides, how could I spend two days out of three on the phone badgering her?)

Was I (and my husband, Erik—who worried about everything I worried about, and then some) alone in my fears? Far from it. Worry, according to one study, is one of the most common complaints of pregnancy, affecting more expectant women than morning sickness and food cravings combined. Ninety-four out of every hundred women worry about whether their babies will be normal, and 93% worry about whether they and their babies will come through delivery safely. More women worry about their figures (91%) than their health (81%) during pregnancy. And most worry that they worry too much.

But though a little worry is normal for pregnant women and their mates, a lot of worry is an unnecessary waste of what should be a blissfully happy time. Despite all that we hear, read, and worry about, never before in the history of reproduction has it been safer to have a baby—as Erik and I discovered some seven and a half months of worrying later, when I gave birth to a healthier and more beautiful baby girl than I'd dared to dream possible.

Thus, out of our concerns, *What to Expect When You're Expecting* was born. It is dedicated to expectant couples everywhere (especially to my co-author and sister, Sandee, and her husband, Tim, whose first baby will be in a tight race with this book for publication), and written with the hope that it will help fathers- and mothers-to-be worry less and enjoy their pregnancies more.

Heidi Eisenberg Murkoff
New York City

Part 1

IN THE BEGINNING

1
Are You Pregnant?

Am I really pregnant? This is the first preoccupation of the hopeful expectant parent, and it occurs the first moment one or another of the signs of pregnancy appears. Happily, it's one question that can very soon be answered, via the combination of a pregnancy test and a medical examination.

Some signs suggest the possibility you are pregnant, others the probability. *No* early signs are positive indications of pregnancy.

WHAT YOU MAY BE CONCERNED ABOUT

SIGNS OF PREGNANCY

"I only have some of the signs of pregnancy—can I still be pregnant?"

You can have all of the signs and symptoms of early pregnancy and not be pregnant. Or you can have only a few of them and be very definitely pregnant. The various signs and symptoms of pregnancy are only clues—important to pay attention to, but not to be relied upon for absolute confirmation. In fact the first sign that is proof positive of your pregnancy is your baby's heartbeat, which is audible at about 10, or more often 12, weeks with the sensitive ultrasound Doppler device, or with an ordinary stethoscope at 18 to 20 weeks.[1] Earlier signs only indicate the possibility or probability that you're carrying a child. Combined with a reliable pregnancy test and your doctor's examination, they can help provide an accurate diagnosis.

PREGNANCY TESTS

"My doctor said the exam and pregnancy test indicated I wasn't pregnant, but I really feel I am."

As remarkable as modern medical science is, when it comes to

---

1. Verification of a pregnancy can be made earlier through ultrasound or via a blood test, but these are not routine procedures.

pregnancy diagnosis, it still sometimes takes a backseat to a woman's intuition. The accuracy of the different pregnancy tests varies, and none are accurate as early as some women begin to "feel" that they are pregnant—sometimes within a few days after conception. There are basically three kinds of pregnancy tests available today—and a rabbit needn't give its life for any of them.

POSSIBLE SIGNS OF PREGNANCY

SIGN	WHEN IT APPEARS	OTHER POSSIBLE CAUSES
Amenorrhea (absence of menstruation)	Usually entire pregnancy	Travel, fatigue, stress, fear of pregnancy, hormonal problems or illness, extreme weight gain or loss
Morning sickness (any time of day)	2–7 weeks after conception	Food poisoning, tension, infection, and a variety of diseases
Frequent urination	Usually 6–12 weeks after conception	Urinary tract infection, diuretics, tension
Tingling, tender, swollen breasts	As early as a few days after conception	Birth control pills, menstruation
Changes in color of vaginal and cervical tissue as blood flow increases to area*	First trimester	Menstruation
Darkening of areola around nipple and elevation of tiny glands around nipple	First trimester	Hormonal imbalance
Blue and pink lines under skin on breasts and later on abdomen	First trimester	Hormonal imbalance
Food cravings	First trimester	Poor diet, imagination
Darkening of line from navel to pubis	4th or 5th month	Hormonal imbalance

The Home Pregnancy Test. This test is more accurate than in the past, but it is still less than a sure thing. Very much like the urine test done in the lab, it diagnoses pregnancy by detecting the presence of the hormone HCG (Human Chorionic Gonadotropin) in the urine. Some can tell you if you're pregnant as early as the first day of your missed menstrual period, or about 14 days after conception. If it's done correctly—and that's an important "if"—the at-home test is about as accurate as a urine test done in a doctor's office or laboratory, with a positive result more likely correct than a negative one. Home tests offer the advantage of privacy and on-the-spot results, but they can be expensive, and because you're less likely to feel confident in the results, you're more likely to want a retest, increasing the cost. (Some brands include a second test in the package.) The major drawback is that if your test is a false negative and you actually are pregnant, you may postpone seeing a doctor and taking good care of yourself. If you decide to use a home test, be sure to buy it the day before you plan to use it (tests require a first-of-the-morning urine sample).

The Lab Urine Test. Like the home test, this test can detect HCG in the urine with an accuracy of about 95%—and as early as 20 days after conception. Unlike the home test, it's performed by a professional, who is more likely to do it correctly. (Of course, labs have been known to make mistakes, too.) If you plan on taking the test, call the lab the day before and ask for instructions on collecting your urine. This test is sometimes the least expensive pregnancy test, but it is less reliable than a blood test.

The Blood Test. The serum pregnancy test can detect pregnancy with 95%-plus accuracy as early as

PROBABLE SIGNS OF PREGNANCY

SIGN	WHEN IT APPEARS	OTHER POSSIBLE CAUSES
Softening of uterus and cervix*	2–8 weeks after conception	A delayed menstrual period
Enlarging uterus* and abdomen	8–12 weeks	Tumor
Intermittent painless contractions	Early in pregnancy, increasing in frequency	Bowel contractions
Fetal movements	First noted 14–20 weeks of pregnancy	Gas, bowel contractions

POSITIVE SIGNS OF PREGNANCY

SIGN	WHEN IT APPEARS	OTHER POSSIBLE CAUSES
Visualization of fetus through ultrasound*	4–6 weeks after conception	None
Fetal heartbeat*	At 10–20 weeks**	None
Fetal movements felt through abdomen*	After 16 weeks	None

*Signs of pregnancy looked for in medical examination.

**Depending on device used.

8 to 10 days after conception, and with virtually 100% accuracy (barring lab error) six weeks after conception. Now that they're in common use, blood tests often cost no more than urine tests, and their accuracy renders the necessity of a retest less likely.

No matter which test you choose, the chances of your pregnancy being correctly diagnosed are enhanced when the test is followed up by a medical examination. The physical signs of pregnancy—an enlarging and softening of the uterus, and a change in the texture of the cervix—may be apparent to a doctor by the sixth week of pregnancy. False-negatives are more common than false-positives: The doctor is more likely to know for sure that you are pregnant than that you're not.

If you are experiencing the symptoms of early pregnancy (absent periods, full and tender breasts, morning sickness, frequent urination, fa-tigue) and feel, test or no test, exam or no exam, that you are pregnant, act as though you are until you find out definitely otherwise. Neither tests nor doctors are infallible. You know your own body—at least externally—better than your doctor does. Ask for a retest (preferably a blood test) and another exam a week later; it may just be too early for a correct diagnosis. We know of one baby girl born seven and a half months after two physicians and a blood test said her mother wasn't pregnant!

It is possible, of course, that you can experience all of the signs and symptoms of early pregnancy and not be pregnant. None of them alone are proof positive of pregnancy. After two pregnancy tests and a second exam determine that you are not pregnant, you must consider that the "pregnancy" may be psychological—possibly because you very strongly do, or don't, want to be pregnant. Or the symptoms may have some other biological cause, which should be investigated by your doctor. (See Signs of Pregnancy, page 18.)

DUE DATE

"My periods are irregular. How can I know if my due date is correct?"

Life would be a lot simpler if you knew from the onset of pregnancy the exact day you were going to give birth. But life isn't that simple very often. According to some studies only four women in a hundred give birth exactly on their due date. Most others, because a normal full-term pregnancy can last anywhere from 38 to 42 weeks, deliver within two weeks either way of that date.

That's why the medical term for "due date" is EDC, or the *estimated* date of confinement (or delivery). The date your practitioner gives you is only an educated estimate, calculated this way: Note the date of the first day of your last normal menstrual period (LMP), and add to it seven days. From that date, count back three months and you have your due date—one year later. (LMP + 7 days − 3 months + 1 year = EDC.) If your periods come every 28 days, you are more likely than most to deliver close to your estimated due date. If your cycles are longer than 28 days, you are more likely to deliver after the EDC, and if they are shorter, before it.

But if your cycle is irregular, this system may not work for you at all. Say you haven't had your period in three months and suddenly you are pregnant. When did you conceive? The only clue the doctor has to work with early in pregnancy, unless you can pinpoint the time of conception, is the size of your uterus. Later on there are other milestones that together can more accurately gauge just how pregnant you are: the first time the fetal heartbeat is heard (at about 10 to 12 weeks with a Doppler device, or at about 18 to 20 weeks with a stethoscope); the first flutter of life (at about 20 weeks with a first baby, or 16 to 18 with subsequent ones); the height of the fundus (the top of the uterus) at each visit (for example, it will reach the navel at the 20th week). If all of these indications seem to correspond to the due date you and your practitioner have calculated, you can be pretty sure that it is close to accurate—that is, that you are fairly likely to deliver within two weeks of that date. But if they don't correspond, the doctor may decide to do a sonogram, which can more closely pinpoint the gestational age of your fetus. (See page 49.)

As delivery nears, there will be other clues to the date of the big event: painless contractions will become more frequent (and possibly even uncomfortable), the fetus will move down into the pelvis (engagement), your cervix will begin to thin (effacement), and last of all, your cervix will begin to dilate. These clues will be helpful, but not definitive—only your baby knows for sure what his or her birthday will be. (For more information, see Lightening and Engagement, page 227; When You Will Deliver, page 228.)

WHAT IT'S IMPORTANT TO KNOW:
CHOOSING (AND WORKING WITH) YOUR PRACTITIONER

While it takes two to conceive a baby, it takes a minimum of three—mother, father, and at least one health care professional—to make that transition from fertilized egg to delivered infant a safe and successful one. Assuming you and your husband have already taken care of conception, the next challenge you face is selecting that third member of your pregnancy team. And making sure that it's a selection you can live with—and labor with.

The selection of a pregnancy caregiver wasn't a major consideration for mothers-to-be 30 years ago. Those were the days of no-questions-asked obstetrical care, when the few choices there were in childbirth were left up to the doctor. As far as selecting an obstetrician, one seemed pretty much like the next. And besides, since you were likely to be unconscious during delivery, it didn't ultimately matter whether you had rapport with your doctor. Instead of being a participating team member, the mother-to-be was more or less a spectator, sitting obediently on the bench while her obstetrical captain called the plays.

Today there are almost as many choices in childbirth—yours for the choosing—as there are doctors in the Yellow Pages. The trick is in matching yourself with a compatible practitioner.

WHAT KIND OF PATIENT ARE YOU?

Your first step in figuring out the kind of practitioner who is right for you is to give some thought to the kind of patient you are.

Do you believe that "doctor knows best" (after all, he or she's the one who went to medical school)? Would you prefer your physician to make all the decisions without consulting you, and do you feel safest when all the latest medical technology is being used in your care? In your medical fantasies, does the man in the white lab coat taking your pulse fit the description of Dr. Welby or Dr. Kildare? Then you probably will feel most comfortable with an obstetrician who has a traditional practice, a godlike aura, and an unswerving dedication to his or her own obstetrical philosophy.

Or do you believe that your body and your health are your business and no one else's? Do you have definite ideas about pregnancy and childbirth and feel you'd like to run the show, from conception to delivery, with minimal interference from your health professional? Then skip over the Welbys and Kildares, and look for a physician or a nurse-midwife who's willing to give up the starring role and serve as your consultant on the production of your baby. Someone who will step aside, though not entirely out of the picture, while you make as many of the childbirth decisions as is medically practical; who is dogmatic only when it comes to giving the patient a controlling vote. Don't assume, however, that a doctor who leans toward "New Wave" obstetrics is going to be any less doctrinaire in his or her beliefs than a traditional physician.

Or perhaps you'd prefer a practitioner who'll put you in the position of partner; that is, who will make decisions based on his or her experience and knowledge, but include you in the process. Who will keep, as the number one priority, your health and the health of your baby, not some inflexible medical gospel or your whims or wishes. Then the practitioner for you is probably a physician who sees his or her role in your pregnancy as somewhere *between* star and consultant. A doctor who is neither inflexible nor putty in your hands; who feels that either a natural delivery or a cesarean can be the best way, depending on the situation; who doesn't routinely withhold or order pain medication. He or she should see nothing incongruous in using a fetal monitor and a birthing room at the same time—if that is best for mother and child. The practitioner with your name on his or her shingle sees the doctor-patient relationship as an equal but definitely separate partnership, in which each partner contributes what he or she does best.

Whatever your patienting style, if you believe that the father-to-be should have equal billing in the pregnancy-childbirth drama, you'll

also need to make sure that the caregiver you've selected agrees with you. His or her attitude will be clearly apparent at the first visit, sometimes even when you make your first appointment. Is the father invited to participate in both the examination and consultation? Are his questions given full consideration? Is the discussion addressed to both expectant parents, not just to the mother? Is it clear that the father will be permitted to share in both labor and delivery?

OBSTETRICIAN? FAMILY PRACTITIONER? NURSE-MIDWIFE?

Narrowing your ideal practitioner down to one of three general personality types makes your job of finding him or her easier, but it doesn't mean your task is finished. Examination-table-side manner and philosophy are important, but they aren't everything. You'll also have to give some thought to the kind of medical credentials that would best meet your requirements.

The Obstetrician. If yours is a high-risk pregnancy,[2] then you will very likely want a specialist who is trained to handle every conceivable complication of pregnancy, labor, and delivery: an obstetrician. You

2. A high-risk pregnancy is one in which the expectant mother has had a problem pregnancy before; has a medical problem, such as diabetes or hypertension; has an Rh or other genetic problem; or is under 20 or over 35 (though not every study shows over-35 mothers to be high risk).

may even want to find a specialist's specialist, an obstetrician who specializes in high-risk pregnancies.

If your pregnancy looks pretty routine from an obstetrical point of view, you can still select an obstetrician (more than 8 out of 10 women do) or you can choose between a physician who is a family practice specialist (about 10% to 12% of women use one), and a certified nurse-midwife (selected by 1% to 2%).

The Family Physician. Family practice is a relatively new specialty, actually a throwback to the old-fashioned general practice, which once served as a one-stop medical center for every member of the family. The only major difference between the old-fashioned GP and the new-fangled family physician is training; the FP, unlike the GP, has had several years of special training in primary care, including obstetrics, after receiving an MD. If you decide on an FP, he or she can serve as your internist, obstetrician/gynecologist, and, when the time comes, pediatrician. An FP will become familiar with the dynamics of your family, will be interested in all aspects of your health, not just your pregnancy, and will give you the feeling that pregnancy is just a normal part of the life-cycle, not a medical condition. If complications occur, your FP may call in a specialist for consultation, but will often remain in charge of your case.

The Certified Nurse-Midwife. If you are anxious to have a practitioner whose emphasis is on you the person and not you the patient, who takes a great deal of time to talk with you about your feelings and problems, who will be very flexible and very oriented toward the "natural" in childbirth, then a certified nurse-midwife (CNM) may be right for you (though, of course, many physicians meet these requirements, too). Although a nurse-midwife is a medical professional, thoroughly trained to care for women with low-risk pregnancies and to attend uncomplicated births (having received not only a nursing degree but further training and certification in nurse-midwifery), she is more likely to treat your pregnancy as a human, rather than a medical, condition.

TYPE OF PRACTICE

You've decided on an obstetrician, a family practitioner, or a nurse-midwife. Next you've got to decide which kind of medical practice would make you most comfortable. The most common kinds of practices, and their possible advantages and disadvantages (though they will vary from one expectant couple to the next), are:

Solo Practice. A doctor works for him- or herself, using another doctor to cover when he or she is away or otherwise unavailable. An obstetrician or a family physician might be in solo practice; a nurse-midwife, in most states, cannot work alone. The major advantage of solo practice is that you see the same practitioner at each visit, and can get to know each other better and feel more comfortable. The major disadvantage is that if your doctor is not available, a physician you don't know may deliver your baby.[3] A solo practice may also be a problem if, midway during your pregnancy, you find you're not really crazy about the doctor. You're stuck unless you're rich enough to pick up and change to another without worrying about the investment you've already made.

Partnership or Group Practice.

Two or more doctors in the same specialty care jointly for patients, seeing them on a rotating basis. Again, you can find both obstetricians and family doctors in this type of practice—sometimes both in one group. The advantage of this arrangement is that by seeing a different doctor each time, you will get different points of view (though you may find that unsettling), and when those labor pains are coming strong and fast you know that there will be a familiar face in the room with you. The disadvantage is that you may not like all of the doctors in the practice equally, and you won't be able to choose the one who attends your birthing.

Combination Practice.

A group practice that includes one or more obstetricians and one or more nurse-midwives. The advantages and disadvantages are similar to those of any group practice. In addition, you have the advantage at many of your visits of seeing a nurse-midwife who may give you more time and atten-

tion, and at others, the security of having a physician's expertise for thorough checkups and answering tough questions. You can also have the benefits of a midwife-coached delivery, assured that if a problem develops, a physician you know is in the wings.

Maternity Centers.

These are nurse-midwife groups that have physicians on call as needed, and that operate either out of a separate facility or in a hospital. Their big advantage is that you are cared for by individuals who are sensitive to your needs and will usually take as much time as is needed to teach, answer your questions, make you feel comfortable. Disadvantages include the fact that if there's a complication you will have to switch practitioner midbirthing; the doctor-on-call will have to take over, since the nurse-midwife is only certified to attend at uncomplicated deliveries. If delivery begins in a maternity center, there is a 10% to 20% chance that you may have to be transported to a hospital in mid-labor. And if you become a high-risk patient in the course of your pregnancy, you will become disqualified for the midwifery program (which is for low-risk patients only) and will have to start afresh developing a relationship with a physician.

Independent Certified Nurse-Midwife.

(Not permitted to practice in all states.) These practitioners differ from old-fashioned midwives, who are still practicing (illegally) in some places, in that they are registered nurses with bachelors' degrees

---

3. You can remedy this by asking to meet the covering physician in advance.

in nursing and masters or other advanced degrees in maternal-child health. The kind of "natural"-oriented care they offer may be an advantage to some couples, especially those who want a home delivery with children, family, and friends present. But unless a nurse-midwife has an association with a physician, who can quickly step in in emergency situations and have emergency transport on call, the risk to mother and child can be significant.

FINDING A CANDIDATE

When you have a good idea of the kind of practitioner you are looking for and the type of obstetrical practice he or she should be in, you've got to find some possible candidates. The following are all good sources of names:

❖ Your gynecologist or family doctor (if he or she doesn't do deliveries) or your internist, assuming you're happy with his or her style of practice. (Doctors tend to recommend others with philosophies similar to their own.)

❖ Friends who have recently had babies and whose childbearing philosophies are similar to yours.

❖ An obstetrical nurse, if you're lucky enough to know one.

❖ The county medical society, which can give you a list of names but no other information about the individual doctors.

❖ The *Directory of the American Medical Association* or the *Directory of Medical Specialties,* often available at your public library or doctor's office (ask his assistant).

❖ The local La Leche League, if you're strongly interested in breastfeeding.

❖ A nearby hospital with facilities that appeal to you; for example, birthing rooms, rooming-in, father participation. They can give you the names of attending physicians.

❖ The International Childbirth Education Association, P.O. Box 20852, Milwaukee, WI 53220—if you are strongly interested in childbirth education. Or write the American Society of Prophylaxis in Obstetrics (ASPO)/Lamaze, 1411 K Street NW, Suite 200, Washington, DC 20005.

❖ A local maternity center, or the American College of Nurse-Midwives, 1522 K Street NW, Suite 1120, Washington, DC 20005, if you are looking for a CNM.

❖ The Yellow Pages, if all else fails, under Physicians—Obstetrics and Gynecology.

Once you've secured your prospective physician's or nurse-midwife's name, call and make an appointment for an introductory visit. Go armed with questions that will enable you to sense if your philosophies match, and if your personalities mesh comfortably. Don't expect that you and he or she will agree on everything—that doesn't happen in the happiest of marriages. If it's important that your doctor listen well or be good at explanations, does this one fulfill those requirements? If you're concerned with the emotional aspects of pregnancy, is this doctor, too? Ask about the practitioner's position on any of the following that you feel are important: natural childbirth vs. anesthetized childbirth vs. pain relief as needed in childbirth; breastfeeding; induction of labor; use of fetal monitoring; enemas; forceps; cesarean sections; home delivery; or anything else that concerns you. That way you won't have any unpleasant surprises when it's too late to make a change.

Perhaps the most important thing you can do at that first meeting is to let the practitioner know what kind of patient you are. You can judge from the response whether he or she will be comfortable with the kind of patient you are.

You will probably also want to know something about the hospital the doctor is affiliated with. Does it have features that are important to you, such as birthing rooms, rooming-in, a neonatal intensive care unit, the latest fetal monitoring equipment? Are they flexible about routines that concern you, such as shaving and enemas? Do they allow fathers in the labor, delivery, and operating room even during a cesarean? Will you have to be strapped to the delivery table?

Before you make your final decision, think about whether the practitioner inspires a feeling of trust. Pregnancy is one of the most important voyages you'll ever make—you'll want a skipper (or first mate) in whom you have complete faith.

MAKE THE MOST OF THE PATIENT-PRACTITIONER PARTNERSHIP

Choosing the right practitioner is only the first step. For the vast majority of women, who are ready neither to cede all responsibility to the physician nor to take over entirely themselves, the next step is nurturing a good working partnership with their professional. Here's how:

❖ When something you think worth mentioning crops up between visits, put it on a list that you take with you to your next appointment. (It helps to keep a few lists in convenient places—the refrigerator door, your purse, your desk at work, your bedside table—so that you'll always be within jotting distance of one.) That's the only way you can be sure that you won't forget to ask all your questions and report all your symptoms. And you won't be wasting your time, or your practitioner's, while you try to recall what it was you wanted to ask.

❖ Along with your questions list, bring a pen and pad to each office visit, so you can make a note of your practitioner's directions. Most people are too nervous in the presence of a physician to remember directions accurately. If your practitioner doesn't volunteer information, make inquiries before you leave, so there's no confusion once you get home. Ask about such things as side effects of treatments, how long to take a medication if one is prescribed, when to check back about a problem situation.

❖ Though you don't want to call your physician at every pelvic twinge, you shouldn't hesitate to call about worries that you can't resolve by checking in a book such as this one, and that you feel can't wait until the next visit. Don't be afraid that your concerns will sound silly. Unless your practitioner has just graduated from medical school, he or she's heard it all before. If you are having pain or bleeding, be very specific about location, duration, quantity (of bleeding), and quality (of pain), as well as about what makes it worse or better. Also report accompanying symptoms (such as fever, nausea, vomiting, chills, or diarrhea). (See When to Call the Practitioner, page 105.)

❖ When you read about something new in obstetrics, don't brandish the clipping in front of the practitioner saying, "I must have this." Instead, bring it in at your next visit, and ask your practitioner if he or she feels there is any value in this new procedure. Often the media report medical advances prematurely, before they are proven safe and effective through controlled studies. If indeed it is a worthwhile advance, your practitioner may already be aware of it.

If not, he or she may want to find out more.

❖ When you hear something which doesn't correspond with what your practitioner has told you, ask for his or her opinion on what you've heard. Not in a challenging way, just in order to get more information.

❖ If you suspect that the physician may be wrong about something (for example, okaying intercourse when you have a history of miscarriage), say so. Don't challenge, just open your suspicion to discussion. A doctor has many patients and may sometimes forget critical information about your particular obstetrical situation.

❖ If you have a gripe, tell your practitioner about it. Letting it fester jeopardizes your relationship.

❖ If your relationship with your practitioner breaks down irreparably, think about changing doctors. He or she probably doesn't enjoy the bad feelings any more than you do. Don't, however, expect to get good obstetrical care if you regularly switch from doctor to doctor trying to find one who will follow *your* orders. Consider, instead, that the problem with the care you've been receiving may originate with you.

2
Now That You Are Pregnant

WHAT YOU MAY BE CONCERNED ABOUT

Now that you no longer have to worry about whether or not the pregnancy test will be positive, you're sure to come up with a whole new set of concerns: What effect will my age or my husband's age have on my pregnancy and on our baby? How will chronic medical problems or family genetic problems affect him or her? Will our past lifestyles make a difference? Will my previous obstetrical history repeat? What can I do to lower any risks my history may present?

YOUR GYNECOLOGICAL HISTORY

"Several years ago I had fibroids removed. I've also had a couple of D and Cs. What effect could this have on my pregnancy?"

Your past gynecological history is important to your practitioner because it will provide clues to the cause of any problem that might come up. For the most part, however, you shouldn't expect surgery for the removal of small uterine fibroid tumors, or one or two dilatation and curettages (D and Cs) for spontaneous or therapeutic abortions, to affect your pregnancy— though unusually large fibroids that haven't been removed can keep a woman from conceiving or can cause miscarriage or preterm labor, and scarring from D and Cs can interfere with implantation.

It is possible that *deep* surgery for large fibroids could weaken the uterus enough so that it could not tolerate labor. If, on reviewing your surgical records, your physician decides this may be true of your uterus, he or she will plan a cesarean section for you. It is also possible (though evidence is contradictory) that *repeated* D and Cs could result in a weakening of the cervix (the opening of the uterus), which could lead to a midtrimester miscarriage or preterm labor. Should an incompetent cervix be suspected, or should your cervix begin to open prematurely, suturing (stitching) the cervix closed will probably allow the pregnancy to continue until the fetus is mature, when the stitches can be safely removed.

YOUR OBSTETRICAL HISTORY REPEATING ITSELF

"I had an easy first pregnancy. Can I expect this one to go well, too?"

In general, your first pregnancy is a pretty good predictor of future pregnancies, all things being equal. If it was uneventful, subsequent pregnancies probably will be, too. If, on the other hand, you had any kind of problem the first time around, it's a good idea to ask your doctor about the possibility of a repeat and to see what can be done to prevent it. For example, if you delivered prematurely there are a great many steps that can be taken to help you go to term (see page 190). Or if you developed gestational diabetes, you can take preventive measures before sugar shows up in your urine (see page 133). On the other hand, if your problem was caused by a one-time event (such as an infection or an accident), or by something you

did during your first pregnancy that you aren't doing in the second (such as smoking), then it isn't likely to recur.

Some problems may repeat no matter what you do. For example, if a first baby was in a breech position due to an irregularly shaped uterus, subsequent babies may be, too. Or if a baby was in an occiput posterior position (back of the head toward the mother's back) because of the shape of the mother's pelvis, any future brothers and sisters may be as well—which can mean uncomfortable back labor for mom. If, however, a specific reason for the fetus being in an unusual position was not identified, then the odds of the problem's repeating are probably not much greater than average.

REPEAT CESAREANS

"I can't have a vaginal delivery because my pelvis is abnormally shaped. I want to have six kids just like my mother did, but I understand three cesareans is the limit."

Tell that to Ethel Kennedy, the indomitable wife of Robert F. Kennedy, who is reported to have had 11 cesareans in an era when the procedure was neither as safe nor as easy as it is today. Of course, sometimes having numerous cesareans isn't possible. Much will depend upon the kind of incision that was made and the kind of scar that formed. Talk to your obstetrician about your concern, because only someone fully familiar with your case can tell you whether or not you can do an "Ethel Kennedy" (or even half an "Ethel Kennedy"). You may be pleasantly surprised.

Because of your scars, however, you should be alert for the signs of labor (contractions, bloody show, ruptured membranes; see page 233) in the final months of pregnancy. Should they occur, notify your doctor and go to the hospital immediately. You should also notify him or her at *any* time in your pregnancy if you have unexplained, persistent abdominal pain, or bleeding.

"I had my last baby by emergency cesarean. I'm pregnant again and have heard 'once a cesarean, always a cesarean.' "

"Once a cesarean always a cesarean" was, until very recently, an obstetrical edict engraved in stone, or rather in the uteruses of women who'd had at least one baby born through a classic vertical incision. Today, though many women who've had one cesarean delivery go on to have others, many other women, usually those who have had low-transverse incisions, are able to go through a vaginal delivery even after two cesarean sections.

Whether or not you can deliver vaginally will depend upon the reason for your first cesarean. If the reason was a one-time problem (fetal distress, premature separation of the placenta, faulty placement of the placenta, infection, breech, toxemia), it's very possible you can have a vaginal delivery this time. If it was a chronic disease (diabetes, high blood pressure, heart disease) or a permanent problem (an oddly shaped pelvis), you will certainly have a repeat cesarean. Don't rely on your recollection of the reason—check, or have your physician check, the medical records of the delivery. You will also probably have a repeat if the original incision was a vertical one, which is more likely to rupture than the low-transverse variety.

If you feel strongly about having a vaginal delivery with your next baby, then discuss the possibility with your physician now. Some doctors still cling to the old adage and will not permit a woman with a cesarean-scarred uterus to labor, fearing a rupture (which, however, is very rare with low-transverse incisions). In addition to finding an amenable doctor who is willing to be with you from the very beginning of labor through delivery, you must plan to be delivered in a fully equipped hospital with round-the-clock operating facilities in case problems develop.

Your role is as important as the doctor's in assuring a safe vaginal delivery. You should:

❖ Take childbirth education classes, and take them seriously, so that you will be able to labor as efficiently as possible.

❖ Notify your doctor the moment signs of labor, such as contractions, bloody show, ruptured membranes, occur.

❖ Expect to use little or no medication (which might mask signs of impending problems).

❖ If you notice any unusual pain or tenderness *between* contractions, tell your doctor immediately.

Though your chances of a normal vaginal delivery are good, even the woman who has never had a cesarean has a 10% to 20% chance of needing one. So don't be disappointed if you end up needing a repeat. The safest possible birth of that wonderful baby of yours is what this is all about, after all.

PREGNANCIES TOO CLOSE TOGETHER

"I became pregnant with a second child just 10 weeks after I delivered my first. I'm worried about what effect this might have on my health and on the baby I'm carrying."

Conceiving again before you've fully recovered from a recent pregnancy and delivery puts enough strain on your body without adding the debilitating effects of worry. So first of all, *relax.* Though conception in the first three postpartum months is rare (almost a miracle if the new baby is exclusively breastfed), it's taken other women by surprise, too. And most have delivered normal, healthy infants, little the worse for wear themselves.

However, it's essential to be aware of the toll two quickly consecutive pregnancies can take, and to do everything possible to compensate. Conception within three months of delivery puts the new pregnancy in a high-risk category, which, in this case, isn't as ominous as it sounds, particularly with the proper care and precautions, including:

❖ The best prenatal care, starting as soon as you think you're pregnant. As with any high-risk pregnancy, you're probably best off with an obstetrician, or a nurse-midwife who practices with one. You should be scrupulous about following doctor's orders and not missing office visits.

❖ The Best-Odds Diet (see page 75), adhered to, if not religiously, at least faithfully. Your body may still be at a nutritional disadvantage, and you may need to overcompensate—particularly with protein (at least 100 grams a day), iron (you should take a supplement), and possibly calories (insufficient weight gain will be a clue that you need more food).

❖ Adequate weight gain. Your new fetus doesn't care whether or not you've yet shed the extra pounds his or her sibling put on you. The two of you need the same 20-to-30-pound gain this pregnancy. So don't even think about losing weight, not even early on. A carefully monitored gradual weight gain will be relatively easy to take off afterward—especially with two infants keeping you on the go.

❖ Weaning your older baby immediately, if you're nursing. He or she's already reaped many of the benefits of breastfeeding, and weaning at this age should be neither difficult nor traumatic. Some women do continue nursing, but trying to rally the nutritional forces for both nursing and pregnancy can be a losing battle for all concerned.

❖ Rest—more than is humanly (and new-motherly) possible. This will require not only your own determination, but help from your husband and possibly others as well. Let chores or other work go undone, and force yourself to lie down when your baby is napping. Have daddy take over as many nighttime feedings as he can rise to the occasion for, as well as much of the cooking, housework, and baby care (particularly tasks which involve a lot of baby-lifting).

❖ Exercise—just enough to keep you in shape, but not enough to overtax you. Ask your practitioner for guidelines.

❖ Eliminate or minimize all other risk factors, such as smoking and drinking. Your body doesn't need any additional strains. (See page 52.)

TEMPTING FATE THE SECOND TIME AROUND

"I had a perfect first baby. Now that I'm pregnant again, I can't get rid of the fear that I won't be so lucky this time."

A million-dollar lottery winner isn't likely to hit the jackpot twice, though his or her odds remain as good as any other player's. A mother who has had a "perfect" baby, however, is not only likely to win again, her odds are better than they were before—because she has now proven she can successfully complete a pregnancy. In addition, with each pregnancy she has the chance to improve her odds a little—by eliminating the negative (smoking, drinking, using drugs) and accentuating the positive (eating better, exercising, getting good medical care).

HAVING A BABY AFTER 35

"I'm 38 and pregnant with my first—and probably last—baby. It's so important that it be healthy, but I've read so much about the risks of pregnancy after 35."

Becoming pregnant after 35 puts you in good (and growing) company. While the pregnancy rate has been dropping among women in their 20s, it has been zooming among women over 35. These women are a new breed of mothers—better educated (more than half have gone to college), career oriented, and more settled. Some believe they make better parents because of their maturity and because they've already had their flings and don't resent being tied down by a baby. On the other hand, some find motherhood a strain because they are more set in their ways, have less physical stamina, and are separated by a wide generation gap from their children. Yet few regret having had their children.

If you've lived for more than 35 years, you know that nothing one does in life is completely free of risk. Pregnancy, at any age, certainly isn't. And the risks do increase somewhat as age advances. Most older mothers, however, feel that the benefits of starting a family at the time that is right for them far outweigh any risks. And they are buoyed by the fact that new medical discoveries are reducing these risks almost daily.

The most notorious risk faced by older mothers is that of having a child with Down's syndrome. The risk increases with each passing year: 1 in 10,000 for 20-year-old mothers, about 3 in 1,000 for 35-year-old mothers, and 1 in 100 for 40-year-old mothers. It's speculated that this and other chromosomal abnormalities, though still relatively rare, are more common in older women because their ova (every woman is born with a lifetime supply) are older, too, and have had more exposure to x-rays, drugs, infections, and so on. (It is now known, however, that the egg is not always responsible for such chromosomal abnormalities. An estimated minimum of 25% of Down's syndrome cases have been linked to a defect in the father's sperm. See page 36.)

While Down's syndrome (characterized by mental retardation, a flat face, and slanting eyes) isn't preventable at this time, it can, like many other genetic disorders, be diagnosed in utero, through amniocentesis (page 47). Such diagnostic testing is now routine for mothers over 35 and others in high-risk categories. Often, so is a sonogram (page 49). Should Down's syndrome or another abnormality show up, the parents then have the option of terminating the pregnancy and trying again. Or, if abortion is unacceptable, they can choose to continue the pregnancy, with the knowledge that children with Down's syndrome generally have the potential for living fulfilling, if somewhat suboptimal, lives. Not only are they very loving and lovable, they can often, with early training, learn to take care of themselves, even to read and write.

In addition to chromosomal aberrations like Down's syndrome, 35-plus mothers are also slightly more subject to high blood pressure and diabetes (which are more common in older groups in general), and to miscarriage, often because of a blighted embryo (one that is too defective to develop normally). Delivery may be more difficult because of a decrease in muscle tone and joint flexibility—though at least one study showed older mothers with an average rate of cesareans, a high percentage of unmedicated births, and a much lower need for forceps delivery than mothers of all ages.

In spite of the risks—which are actually far less threatening than the media make them seem—older mothers have a lot going for them. Medical science, for example. Screening for birth defects can be done in utero through amniocentesis, sonography, and newer procedures—fetoscopy and chorionic villi sampling (see About Prenatal Diagnosis, page 46). Drugs can forestall a preterm labor, a somewhat more common complication among both younger (under 17) and older (over 35) mothers. Electronic fetal monitoring during labor can warn of fetal distress, allowing speedy measures to be taken to protect the fetus from further trauma.

As successful as these advances have been in reducing the risks of pregnancy after 35, they pale next to the strides older mothers have taken—and can take—to improve the odds for themselves and their babies, through exercise, diet, and quality prenatal care. Advanced reproductive age alone does not necessarily put a mother in a high-risk category. But an accumulation of many individual risks can. When the older mother makes a concerted effort to eliminate or minimize as many risk factors as possible, she can take years off her pregnancy profile—making her chances of delivering a healthy baby virtually as good as those of a younger mother. (See Reducing Risk in Any Pregnancy, page 52.)

THE FATHER'S AGE

"I'm only 31, but my husband is over 50. Does advanced paternal age pose risks to a baby?"

Throughout most of history, it was believed that a father's responsibility in the reproductive process was limited to fertilization. Only during this century (too late to help those queens who'd lost their heads for failing to produce a male heir) was it discovered that a father's sperm held the deciding genetic vote in determining his child's sex. And only in the last few years has it begun to be postulated that an older father's sperm might contribute to birth defects such as Down's syndrome. Like the older mother's ova, the older father's primary oocytes

(undeveloped sperm) have had longer exposure to environmental hazards and might conceivably contain altered or damaged genes or chromosomes. And from the isolated studies that have been done, there is some evidence that in about 25% or 30% of Down's syndrome cases, the faulty chromosome can be traced to the father. It also appears that there is an increase in the risk of Down's syndrome when the father is over 50 (or 55, depending on the study), though the association is weaker than in the case of maternal age.

But the evidence remains inconclusive—mostly because of the inadequacy of the existing research. Setting up the kind of large-scale studies required for conclusive results has been difficult so far, for two reasons. First of all, Down's syndrome is relatively rare (about 1 or 2 in 1,000 live births). Second, in the majority of cases, an older father is married to an older mother, making it tricky to clarify the independent role of paternal age.

So the question of whether or not advanced paternal age is linked to Down's syndrome and other birth defects remains largely unanswered. Experts believe that there probably is some connection (although it's not clear at what age it begins), but that the risk is almost certainly very small. At this time, genetic counselors do not recommend amniocentesis on the basis of paternal age alone. If, however, you're going to spend the rest of your pregnancy worrying about the possible—though unlikely—effects of your husband's age on your baby, you might discuss your fears with your practitioner to see if amniocentesis is warranted.

CHRONIC HEALTH PROBLEMS: DIABETES

"I'm a diabetic, and I'm concerned about the effect of my condition on my baby."

Until recently, getting pregnant was a risky business for the diabetic woman, and an even riskier business for her unborn baby. Today, if she receives continuous expert medical care, the diabetic woman has just about as good a chance of having a successful pregnancy and a healthy baby as any other pregnant woman does. In fact, diabetic women in one study took such excellent care of themselves throughout their pregnancies that they and their babies had even *fewer* problems than their non-diabetic counterparts.

Making your diabetic pregnancy a success won't be effortless. It will be more stressful than a non-diabetic pregnancy (blood sugar must be continuously monitored and insulin doses adjusted accordingly), more costly (weekly trips to your internist and obstetrician may be necessary), and will require more self-discipline (diet must be scrupulously adhered to). But the reward for those extra efforts—a healthy baby—can make them well worthwhile.

Research has proved that the key to successfully managing a diabetic pregnancy is maintaining euglycemia (normal blood glucose levels, usually under 100 milligrams per deciliter). The availability in the past few years of home monitoring, split-dose administration of insulin, and insulin pumps has made this increasingly possible. A variety of other factors also contribute to a safe diabetic pregnancy.

Following Doctor's Orders. You'll have many more orders from your doctor than most pregnant women. And you'll have to be far more scrupulous in following them, too.

Good Diet. A diet geared to your personal needs should be carefully planned with your physician, a nutritionist, or a nurse-practitioner who specializes in diabetes education. It will probably be high in fiber, which recent studies show may reduce insulin requirements in pregnant diabetics. This is not a time to be lax about your diet, although (especially late in pregnancy) exhaustion may tempt you to be. It is, rather, an ideal time to get your dietary act together—for you and your baby. Perfecting dietary control is so important that many specialists recommend in-hospital training for diabetic mothers-to-be prior to conception, or early in pregnancy.

If morning sickness is a problem at any time during pregnancy, don't let it interfere with nourishing your baby and keeping your blood glucose level stable. Don't fast or skip meals. Eating regularly is essential. If you have trouble getting down three large meals, take six to eight small ones, regularly spaced and carefully planned. (See page 95 for some general tips on dealing with morning sickness.)

Sensible Weight Gain. The ideal approach is to attain desirable weight before conception—something to remember before your next pregnancy. Even if it's too late for that, weight gain should be kept within strict guidelines set by your physician. If you start your pregnancy overweight, don't use the gestational period for slimming down. Getting sufficient calories is vital to your baby's well-being.

Exercise. Your exercise program, too, should be planned with medical assistance and in conjunction with your medication schedule and diet plan. Exercise will give you more energy, aid in stabilizing your blood sugar, and help get you in shape for delivery.

Rest. Especially in the third trimester, adequate rest is very important. Avoid overtaxing your energies and try to take some time off during the middle of the day for relaxation or a nap. If you're working, your doctor may recommend beginning your maternity leave early.

Medication Regulation. Certain pregnancy hormones are antagonistic to (work against) insulin. That's the reason why your insulin dose may have to be adjusted upward during the second trimester, when the secretion of these placental hormones substantially increases. If you are taking oral hypoglycemic (blood-sugar-lowering) drugs, which cross the placenta readily, you may be switched to injected insulin during your pregnancy, which is less likely to affect your fetus.

Reduction of Other Risk Factors. Since risk in pregnancy is cumulative—the more risk factors, the higher the risk—you should endeavor to eliminate or minimize as many as possible. (See Reducing Risk in Any Pregnancy, page 52.)

Careful Monitoring. Don't be alarmed if your physician orders a great many tests for you (in and out of the hospital), especially during the final trimester, or even suggests hospitalization for the final weeks of pregnancy. This doesn't mean something is wrong, only that he or she wants to be sure that everything stays right. The tests will primarily be directed toward continual evaluation of your condition and that of your baby, in order to determine the optimal time for delivery. Your retinas and kidney function will be checked regularly. (Retinal and kidney problems tend to worsen during pregnancy, but usually return to pre-pregnancy states after delivery.) Dropping levels of estriol, an estrogenic hormone (often measured several times a week), and a positive stress or non-stress test would warn of any deterioration in the condition of the placenta or fetus. Examination of amniotic fluid (through amniocentesis) will assess the stage of maturity of the fetal lungs, and readiness for delivery. Sonography may be used to size up your baby so that delivery is accomplished before he or she's too big for vaginal delivery.

Don't fear complications, either, if your baby is placed in a neonatal intensive care unit immediately after delivery. This is routine procedure in most hospitals for infants of diabetic mothers. Your baby will be observed for respiratory problems (which are unlikely if his lungs were found to be mature before delivery) and for hypoglycemia (which, though more common, responds quickly and completely to treatment).

Elective Early Delivery. Because babies of diabetics tend to be too large for full-term vaginal delivery (particularly when euglycemia is not maintained throughout pregnancy); because their placentas tend to deteriorate early (often robbing the fetus of vital nutrients and oxygen during the last weeks); and because they are subject to acidosis (abnormal acid-base balance in the blood) and other problems, they are often delivered before term, generally at about 37 weeks. The various tests mentioned above help the physician to choose just the right time to induce labor or perform a cesarean— late enough so that the fetal lungs are sufficiently mature, not so late that the fetus is in jeopardy. Women with very mild diabetes, gestational diabetes, and even some with very well-controlled moderate disease can often carry to term safely.

CHRONIC HEALTH PROBLEMS: ASTHMA

"I've been an asthmatic since childhood. I'm concerned that the attacks and the drugs I take for them might harm my baby."

While it's true that a severe asthmatic condition does put a pregnancy at higher risk, studies have shown that this risk can be almost completely eliminated. Asthmatics who are under close, experienced medical supervision (preferably by their internist and/or allergist in collaboration with their obstetrician) throughout their pregnancies have as good a chance of having normal pregnancies and healthy babies as non-asthmatics. But though asthma, if treated, has only a minimal effect on pregnancy, pregnancy often has a considerable effect on asthma. With about one third of pregnant asthmatics, the effect is positive—their asthma improves. In another third, their condition remains about the same. In the final third (usually those with the most severe disease) the asthma worsens, generally after the fourth month.

No matter how mild or severe your condition, it will benefit from good care:

❖ Get your asthma under control before conception or, if that wasn't done, early in pregnancy.

❖ Identify possible triggering factors. The most common offenders are pollens, animal danders, dust, and molds. Tobacco smoke, household cleaning products, and perfumes can also provoke trouble and it's a good idea to steer clear of these irritants. (See Allergies, page 134, for tips on avoiding such allergens.) Attacks brought on by exercise can be prevented by taking the proper medicines, as prescribed by your doctor, prior to exerting yourself. If your doctor began immunotherapy (allergy shots) for your allergies before pregnancy, treatment will probably be continued. A new series, however, is not likely to be initiated during gestation.

❖ Try to avoid colds, flu, and other respiratory infections. (See page 63.)

❖ If you have an asthma attack, treat it immediately with prescribed medication, to avoid cutting off oxygen to the fetus.

❖ Take only drugs prescribed by your physician *during pregnancy,* and take them only as prescribed *for pregnancy use.* If your symptoms are mild, you may not require medication. If they are moderate to severe, there are several medications, both inhaled and ingested, that are considered to be "probably safe" for the fetus. The risks of taking these medications, if any, are quite small compared to the benefits of preventing fetal hypoxia (too little oxygen).

❖ Reduce other pregnancy risk factors. Since pregnancy risks are cumulative, you should endeavor to eliminate or minimize as many as possible. (See Reducing Risk in Any Pregnancy, page 52.)

The normal breathlessness that afflicts a majority of women in late pregnancy (see page 204) may be alarming to the asthmatic mother-to-be, but it is not dangerous. In the last trimester, as breathing becomes more labored because of the enlarged uterus crowding the lungs, pregnant asthmatics may notice a worsening of asthmatic flareups. Proper treatment is especially important during such attacks.

The tendency toward allergies and asthma is inherited, and so it is wise for asthmatics to breastfeed their newborns exclusively for at least six months to delay the onset of allergic sensitization in their children.

RH INCOMPATIBILITY

"My doctor said the blood tests show I am Rh negative and my husband is Rh positive. He said not to worry, but my mother lost her second child because of Rh disease."

Every pregnant woman is tested to determine whether her blood is Rh positive (has the dominant Rh factor) or negative (lacking the factor). These blood factors are inherited, and if a woman is Rh positive (85% are), or if both she and her husband are negative, there is no cause for further concern. If, however, a woman is Rh negative and her husband is positive, then all her pregnancies must be kept under careful obstetrical surveillance.

When your mother had children, the problem of Rh incompatibility was indeed an ominous one. But thanks to several medical advances, worry is now unwarranted.

First of all, if this is your first pregnancy, there is very little threat to the baby. Trouble doesn't start brewing until the Rh factor enters the mother's circulatory system during a delivery (or abortion or miscarriage) of a child who has inherited the Rh factor from his or her father. The mother, in a protective immune reaction to the "foreign" substance, develops antibodies. The antibodies themselves are harmless, until she becomes pregnant again. If the next baby is Rh positive, the mother's antibodies can cross the placenta into the fetal system, where they attack the fetal red blood cells. This can cause very mild to very serious anemia in the fetus, depending on the antibody levels in the mother. Rarely, antibodies can form in first pregnancies, when fetal blood leaks through the placenta into the mother's circulatory system.

Today, prevention of the development of Rh antibodies is the key to protecting the fetus when there is Rh incompatibility. Most doctors use a two-pronged attack. At 28 weeks, an expectant Rh-negative woman who shows no antibodies in her blood is given a dose of Rh-immune globulin. Another dose is administered within 72 hours of delivery or miscarriage. If the pregnancy ends in elective abortion, this vaccine is also administered.

If tests determine that a woman has developed Rh antibodies previously, amniocentesis (see page 47) can be used to check the blood type of the fetus. If it is Rh positive, and thus incompatible with the mother's, a close watch is kept on the condition of the fetus and on the mother's antibody levels. If problems seem imminent, an exchange of blood, replacing the fetus's Rh positive with Rh negative, *may* be necessary. When the incompatibility is severe, which is rare, the fetal transfusion can take place while the fetus is still in the uterus. More often, it can wait until immediately after delivery. In mild cases, when antibody levels are low, a transfusion may not be needed. But doctors will be ready to do one at delivery if necessary.

The use of Rh vaccines has reduced the need for transfusions in Rh incompatible pregnancies to less than 1%, and in the next few years may make this lifesaving procedure a modern medical miracle of the past.

HERPES

"I was anxious for a positive pregnancy test; but now that I am definitely pregnant, I'm terrified because I have genital herpes."

Herpes has generated more frightening headlines in the past few years than almost any other disease. And it's no wonder. With an estimated 5 to 20 million victims in the United States alone, this presently incurable infection may soon surpass gonorrhea and chlamydia as the most common sexually transmitted disease. Herpes in adults can be extremely painful, but it is relatively benign. It can, however, be deadly in a newborn infant, who has contracted the disease en route through the birth canal of an infected mother. Fortunately, such infection of infants, though on the increase, is still relatively rare (about 1 in 1,000) and, with proper medical care, avoidable. Today a woman with herpes need not pass on anything but her brown hair or her green eyes.

The twin keys to protecting the baby—whether it's the mother or her partner who is affected—are strict medical supervision and good personal hygiene:

❖ See an obstetrician regularly, starting before you conceive, or as early in pregnancy as possible.

❖ Refrain from sexual intercourse if you or your partner have an active infection.

❖ Wash your hands thoroughly with mild soap and water after using the toilet or having sexual relations; bathe or shower daily.

❖ Keep any lesions clean and dry, dusted with cornstarch.

❖ Wear cotton underpants; avoid garments that are constricting in the crotch area.

❖ Have a weekly viral culture (a smear of vaginal secretions is taken and tested) from the 34th or 36th week on, so that the presence or absence of an active infection can be determined before delivery.

The odds are good that you won't have an active infection at delivery, in which case there should be no problem. If, however, it turns out that your infection flares up when you're ready to deliver (your physician can determine this through examination or by recent positive cultures), you will almost certainly be delivered by cesarean section. This will assure that your baby won't become infected.

OTHER STDs (SEXUALLY TRANSMITTED DISEASES)

"I've heard that herpes can be dangerous to the fetus. Is this also true of other sexually transmitted diseases?"

The bad news: Yes, there are other STDs that present a hazard to the fetus. The good news: They are easily tested for and treated. Gonorrhea has long been known to cause conjunctivitis, blindness, and serious generalized infection in the fetus allowed to deliver through an infected birth canal. For this reason, pregnant women are routinely tested for the disease at their first prenatal visit (see page 92). If disease is found, it is treated immediately with antibiotics. As an added precaution, drops of silver nitrate are squeezed into every newborn's eyes at birth.

The bone and tooth deformities, the progressive nervous system damage, the stillbirths, and the delayed brain damage caused by syphilis have long been recognized, too. And testing for this disease is also routine at the first prenatal visit. Antibiotic treatment before the fifth month, when the infection usually begins to cross the placental barrier, will prevent damage to the fetus.

More recently recognized as potential dangers to the fetus are chlamydia and AIDS (Acquired Immune Deficiency Syndrome). Chlamydia is now reported more frequently than gonorrhea, and like gonorrhea can cause infertility if untreated; there is also the risk of pneumonia or eye infection in the baby born to an infected mother. Though both chlamydia and gonorrhea are treatable in the newborn, they can be prevented with prenatal antibiotic therapy. AIDS, too, can be transmitted from mother to child.

An expectant mother who believes she may have been infected with any STD should ask to be tested for the disease.

AN IUD STILL IN PLACE

"I've been wearing an IUD for two years and just discovered that I'm pregnant. We want to be able to keep the baby; is it possible?"

Getting pregnant while using birth control is always a little unsettling, but it does happen. The odds of it happening with an IUD are 1 to 5 in 100, depending on the type of device used and whether or not it has been properly inserted. A woman who conceives with an IUD in place and doesn't want to terminate her pregnancy has two choices—which she should discuss as soon as possible with her doctor: leaving the IUD in place or having the IUD removed. According to the research, her chances of delivering a full-term baby are better with the second choice, particularly when the IUD is removed as soon as possible after pregnancy is confirmed. When the IUD, with its removal-string protruding from the cervix, is left in for the term of the pregnancy, there is a significant chance that the fetus will spontaneously miscarry;[1] when it's removed, the risk is only 20%. If that doesn't sound reassur-

ing, keep in mind that the rate of miscarriage in all known pregnancies is estimated to be about 15% to 20%.

If you do continue your pregnancy with your IUD left in, you should, during the first trimester, be especially alert for such signs as bleeding, cramps, or fever, because the IUD puts you at higher risk for early pregnancy complications. (See Ectopic Pregnancy, page 99, and Miscarriage, page 100.) Notify your doctor of such symptoms promptly.

BIRTH CONTROL PILLS IN PREGNANCY

"I got pregnant while using birth control pills. I kept taking them for over a month because I had no idea I was pregnant. Now I'm worried about the effect this may have on my baby."

Ideally, you should stop using oral contraceptives three months, or for at least two normally occurring menstrual cycles, before you want to become pregnant. But conception doesn't always wait for ideal conditions, and occasionally a woman becomes pregnant while taking the Pill. In spite of what you might have read on drug insert warnings, there's no reason for alarm. Statistically, there is a very slightly increased risk of certain types of fetal malformation when the mother has conceived while on oral contracep-

---

1. If, however, the removal-string is not protruding from the cervix, the risk of miscarriage is reduced, and it may be safer to leave the IUD in place.

tives, but certainly not enough to warrant eight months of worry. A discussion of the subject with your practitioner should relieve your concern.

SPERMICIDES

"I conceived while using a spermicide with my diaphragm, and used it several times again before I knew I was pregnant. Could the chemicals have damaged the sperm before conception, or the embryo after it?"

It is estimated that between 300,000 and 600,000 women who become pregnant each year used spermicides around the time of conception and/or in the early weeks of pregnancy before finding out that they'd conceived. So the question of what effects spermicides may have during conception and pregnancy is of great significance to a great many expectant couples—and to those choosing a method of birth control.

Fortunately, the answers so far have been reassuring. No more than a tentative link has ever been suggested between the use of spermicides and the incidence of certain birth defects, specifically Down's syndrome and limb deformities. And the most recent and most convincing studies indicate that spermicides are probably *not* teratogenic, or damaging, to the unborn child. So according to the best information available, you and the other 299,999 to 599,999 mothers-to-be can relax—there appears to be nothing to worry about.

You may, however, be more comfortable with a different, and perhaps more reliable, method of birth control in the future. And because any chemical exposure of embryo or fetus is suspect, if you do continue to use a spermicide, you should plan on terminating its use before you decide to become pregnant again.

PROVERA

"Last month my doctor gave me Provera to bring on a late period. It turns out that I was pregnant. The package insert warns that pregnant women should never take this drug. Could my baby be malformed? Should I consider an abortion?"

Having taken the progesterone drug Provera during pregnancy, though it isn't recommended, is no reason to consider an abortion—as your obstetrician will probably tell you. It's not even a reason to worry. The drug company's warnings are not only for your protection, but for theirs: to protect themselves in case of a lawsuit. It's true that some studies show a 1 in 1,000 risk of certain birth defects when an embryo or fetus has been exposed to Provera, but that is only minimally higher than the same defects occurring in any pregnancy.

Whether Provera actually does cause birth defects or not isn't even certain. Some physicians who use Provera to prevent miscarriage believe that it only *seems* to cause defects—by occasionally helping a woman to sustain a blighted pregnancy that would have otherwise miscarried. It will probably take years more study on hundreds of thousands of pregnant women to determine definitely the effects—if any—of progesterone drugs on the fetus. But from what is presently known, it is believed that if Provera is actually a teratogen, it is a very weak one (see Playing Baby Roulette, page 72). Cross this one off your worry list.

DES

"My mother took DES when she was pregnant with me. Can this affect my pregnancy or my baby in any way?"

Before the dangers of using the synthetic estrogen drug diethylstilbestrol (DES) to prevent miscarriage were known, more than a million pregnant women took it. Now that their daughters, many of whom were born with structural abnormalities of the reproductive tract (the majority so slight that they are of no gynecological or obstetrical significance), are of childbearing age, they are concerned about the effects DES exposure will have on their own pregnancies. Happily, these effects appear to be minimal—it is estimated that at least 80% of DES-exposed women have been able to have children. However, when the abnormalities are serious, there appears to be an increased risk of ectopic pregnancy, miscarriage (particularly midtrimester), and premature delivery. Ectopic pregnancy is uncommon, even among DES-exposed women. But because it could be life threatening, it is impor-

tant to be aware of the symptoms and to get emergency medical attention immediately if they occur.

Though nothing can be done to save an ectopic pregnancy, it is possible to head off a late miscarriage or premature birth. These complications are generally related to an incompetent, or weakened, cervix. (See page 31 for treatment). Threatened premature labor can also often be successfully postponed with bed rest and the use of labor-halting drugs. To be sure that your cervix will be carefully monitored throughout your pregnancy (weekly or biweekly pelvic examinations may be necessary), let your obstetrician[2] know of your DES exposure at your first visit.

GENETIC PROBLEMS

"I keep worrying that I might have a genetic problem and not know it. Should I get genetic counseling?"

Probably all of us carry one or more deleterious genes for mild or serious genetic disorders. But fortunately, because most disorders (for example, Tay-Sachs or cystic fibrosis) require a matching one-from-mom, one-from-dad pair of genes—an unlikely possibility—they rarely manifest themselves in our children. One or both parents can be tested for some of these disorders before or during pregnancy. But testing only makes sense if there is a better-than-

2. Because of the slightly increased risk of complications, DES-exposed women are probably better off with an obstetrician overseeing their pregnancy care.

average possibility that both parents are carriers of a particular disorder. The clue is often ethnic or geographic origin. Jewish couples, for example, whose families came originally from eastern Europe should be tested for Tay Sachs. (In most cases, a practitioner will recommend a test for one parent; the second test is necessary only if the first is positive.) Black couples can be tested for the sickle cell anemia trait.

The diseases that can be passed on by one carrier parent (hemophilia), or by one affected parent (Huntington's chorea), have usually turned up in the family before and should be common knowledge. That's why it's important to keep records of family health histories.

Most expectant parents, happily, are at low risk for having genetic problems and need never see a genetic counselor. In many cases, an obstetrician will talk to a couple about the most common issues, referring to a genetic counselor those with a need for more expertise:

❖ Couples whose blood tests show them both to be carriers of a genetic disorder.

❖ Parents who have already borne one or more children with genetic birth defects.

❖ Couples who know of hereditary defects on any branch of either of their family trees.

❖ Closely related couples, because the risk of inherited disease in offspring is greatest when parents are related (for example, 1 in 8 for first cousins).

❖ Women over 35.

A genetic counselor is a sort of heredity bookmaker, trained to give such couples the odds of bearing a healthy child and to guide them in deciding whether or not to have children. If they are already pregnant, the counselor can suggest appropriate prenatal testing.

Genetic counseling has saved hundreds of thousands of high-risk couples from the heartbreak of bearing children with genetic or other serious problems. The best time to see a genetic counselor is before getting pregnant, or in the case of close relatives, before getting married. But it's not too late after pregnancy is confirmed.

If testing uncovers a serious defect in a fetus, the expectant parents are faced with the decision of whether or not to continue with the pregnancy. Though the decision is theirs, a genetic counselor can provide important input.

WHAT IT'S IMPORTANT TO KNOW:
ABOUT PRENATAL DIAGNOSIS

Is it a boy—or a girl? Will it have blond hair like grandma, green eyes like grandpa? Daddy's voice and mommy's flair for figures or— heaven forbid!—the other way around? The questions of pregnancy far outnumber the answers, providing lively material for nine months of dinner table debate, neighborhood speculation, and office pools.

But there's one question that isn't a topic for casual wagering. It's one most parents hesitate to talk about at all: "Is my baby okay?"

Until recently, that question, like that of the color of a baby's hair and eyes, could be answered only at birth. Today some (no doubt in the future it will be all) such questions are being answered as early as six weeks after conception, through prenatal diagnosis.

Because of inherent risks, small as they are, prenatal diagnosis isn't for everyone. Most parents will continue to play the waiting game, with the happy assurance that the odds are overwhelming that their babies are indeed "okay." But for those whose concerns represent more than normal prenatal jitters—whose age, health status, or family history makes their chances of having a baby who isn't okay greater than average—the benefits of prenatal diagnosis can far outweigh its risks.

In more than 95% of cases, prenatal diagnosis turns up no apparent abnormalities. In the remainder, the expectant couple's discovery that something is wrong with their baby isn't comforting. But, teamed with expert genetic counseling, the information can be used to make vital decisions about this and future pregnancies. Options include:

A Therapeutic Abortion. If testing suggests a defect that is fatal or very disabling, and interpretation and/or retesting by a genetic counselor confirms the diagnosis, many parents opt for terminating the pregnancy.

Most, after consulting with genetic counselors, try again, with hopes that test results—and thus pregnancy outcome—will turn out favorable the next time around.

Continuing the Pregnancy. For some parents, an abortion just isn't an option—no matter how seriously handicapped their baby may be. Assuming the third option (see below) isn't available in their case, prenatal diagnosis gives them the advantage of being able to prepare themselves emotionally and practically for the birth of a child with special needs.

Prenatal Treatment of the Fetus. This option is available in only a few instances, though in the future it can be expected to become more and more common. Treatment may consist of blood transfusion (as in Rh disease), surgery (to drain an obstructed bladder, for instance), or administration of enzymes or medication (such as steroids to accelerate lung development in the fetus who must be delivered).

The most commonly used methods of prenatal diagnosis follow.

AMNIOCENTESIS

The cells shed by the growing fetus into the amniotic fluid make this solution a reliable indicator of the fetal condition in the uterus. Thus, being able to extract some of the fluid through amniocentesis so that fetal cells can be cultured (grown) and examined for genetic defects is one of the most important advances in prenatal diagnosis. It is recommended when:

❖ The mother is over age 35. Between 80% and 90% of all amniocentesis is performed solely on the basis of advanced maternal age, primarily to determine if the fetus has Down's syndrome, which is most prevalent among children of older mothers.

❖ The couple has already had a child with a chromosomal abnormality, such as Down's syndrome, or with a metabolic disorder, such as Hunter's syndrome.

❖ The couple has already had a child or has a relative with a neural tube defect. (A test to determine alpha-fetoprotein, or AFP, levels in the mother's blood will probably be performed first.)

❖ The mother is a carrier of an x-linked genetic disorder, such as hemophilia, which she has a 50-50 chance of passing on to any son she bears. Amniocentesis can identify the sex of the fetus, although not whether the baby is affected. Fetoscopy (see page 50) can, however, detect some of these disorders.

❖ Both parents are carriers of autosomal recessive inherited disorders, such as Tay-Sachs disease or sickle cell anemia, and thus have a 1 in 4 chance of bearing an affected child.

❖ It is necessary to assess the maturity of the fetal lungs (among the last organs ready to function on their own) when an early delivery is contemplated to protect the well-being of mother or child.

When Is It Done? Diagnostic second-trimester amniocentesis is usually performed between the 16th and 18th weeks of pregnancy, though occasionally as early as the 14th or as late as the 20th week. Earlier than this there would be insufficient amniotic fluid; later might prove too late for an abortion should a defect be detected. Most tests, because cells must be cultured in the laboratory, take from 24 to 35 days to be completed, though a few, such as for Tay-Sachs disease, Hunter's syndrome, and neural tube defects, can be performed immediately.

Amniocentesis can also be performed in the last trimester to assess the maturity of fetal lungs.

How Is It Done? After changing into a hospital gown and emptying her bladder, the expectant mother is positioned on the examining table on her back, her body draped so that only her abdomen is exposed. The fetus and placenta are then located via ultrasound, so that the doctor will be able to steer clear of them during the procedure. The abdomen is shaved, swabbed with antiseptic solution, and numbed with an injection (the only painful part of the procedure) of a local anesthetic, similar to the novocaine used by dentists. Then a long, hollow needle (the only scary part of the procedure) is inserted through the abdominal wall into the uterus, and a small amount of amniotic fluid is withdrawn. The mother's vital signs and the fetal heart tones are checked before and after the procedure, which, from start to finish, shouldn't take more than an hour.

Unless it is a necessary part of the diagnosis, parents have the option not to be told their baby's sex when the report comes back, but to find out the old-fashioned way, in the delivery room. (Keep in mind that mixups, though rare, do happen.)

How Safe Is It? Most women experience no more than a few hours of cramping after the procedure; rarely there is slight vaginal bleeding or amniotic fluid leak. Although fewer than 1 in 200 women experience infection or other complications that lead to miscarriage, amniocentesis, like most other prenatal diagnostic tests, should be performed only when the benefits outweigh the risks.

ULTRASOUND

The advent of ultrasonography has made obstetrics a much more precise science and pregnancy much less worrisome for many expectant parents. Through the use of sound waves which bounce off internal structures, it allows visualization of the fetus without the hazards of x-ray. If the apparatus used has a TV-like viewing screen, it provides a unique opportunity to "see" your baby—and maybe even get a photo to show to friends and family—though it may take an expert to make heads or buttocks out of the blurry image.

Ultrasound may be recommended when the mother has a poor obstetrical history; for example, when she's had an ectopic (tubal) pregnancy, a hydatidiform mole (the placenta developed into a grape-like bunch of cysts which couldn't support an embryo), delivered a baby with birth defects or genetic disease, or had a cesarean section. It may also be used to:

❖ Rule out pregnancy by the seventh week if there's been a suspected false-positive.

❖ Determine causes for bleeding or spotting in early pregnancy, such as a tubal pregnancy or a blighted ovum (an embryo that has stopped developing and is no longer viable).

❖ Locate an IUD that was in place at the time of conception.

❖ Verify a due date by checking to see if it correlates with the baby's size.

❖ Locate the fetus prior to amniocentesis and during chorionic villi biopsy (see page 53).

❖ Determine the baby's condition if no heartbeat has been detected by the 14th week with a Doppler device, or no fetal movement by the 22nd week.

❖ Diagnose the existence of multiple fetuses, especially when the mother has taken fertility drugs and/or the uterus is larger than expected.

❖ Determine if rapid uterine growth is due to an excess of amniotic fluid.

❖ Determine the condition of the placenta. A deteriorating placenta, which does not nourish the fetus adequately, might be responsible for retarded fetal growth or fetal distress. Early delivery may be necessary.

❖ Determine if bleeding late in pregnancy is due to placenta previa, in which the placenta implants near or over the cervix.

❖ Evaluate the maturity of a fetus when early delivery, either induced or by cesarean, is being contemplated; or to evaluate the condition of a fetus that is believed to be postmature.

❖ Verify breech presentation or other uncommon fetal position prior to delivery.

When Is It Done? Depending on the indication, ultrasound is performed any time from the fifth week of gestation until delivery.

How Is It Done? The procedure itself is painless (except for the discomfort of a full bladder), and quick (5 to 10 minutes).

During the exam, the expectant mother lies on her back and her bare abdomen is spread with a film of oil or gel that improves conduction of sound. A transducer is then moved slowly over the abdomen, recording echoes as the sound waves bounce off parts of the baby. It may be possible, with the doctor's help, to see the beating of the heart, the curve of the spine, the head and arms and legs—depending on the position of the fetus. Sometimes even the genital organs are visible and the sex can be surmised. (If you don't want to know your baby's sex yet, inform the doctor in advance.)

How Safe Is It? In 25 years of clinical use and study, no known risks and a great many benefits have been associated with the use of ultrasound photography. Still, because risks may yet show up in the future, it is the position of a panel of experts who examined the use of ultrasound in pregnancy for the National Institutes of Health that the procedure should be used only when valid indications exist.

FETOSCOPY

Fetoscopy is science fiction turning fast into medical fact. In a voyage as fantastic as any penned by Isaac Asimov, a miniaturized, telescope-like instrument, complete with lights and lenses, is inserted through a tiny incision in the abdomen into the amniotic sac, where it can view and photograph the fetus. At the same time, fetoscopy allows the diagnosis, through tissue and blood sampling, of several diseases which amniocentesis can't detect. Still a relatively new procedure, its usefulness in certain high-risk pregnancies is speeding its acceptance in the obstetrical community. It is most commonly recommended when there is a family history of a blood disease, particularly when one or both parents are carriers, or of certain skin disorders.

When Is It Done? Usually after the 16th week.

How Is It Done? After the abdomen is swabbed with antiseptic and numbed with a local anesthetic, a tiny incision is made in the abdomen. With ultrasound monitoring to guide the instrument, a fiber-optic endoscope is passed through the incision into the uterus. With this miniature periscope, the fetus, placenta, and amniotic fluid can be observed, blood samples can be taken from the junction of the umbilical cord and the placenta, and/or a tiny bit of fetal or placental tissue removed for examination (a biopsy).

How Safe Is It? Fetoscopy is, at this point, still a relatively risky procedure, carrying between a 3% and 5% chance of fetal loss. Though this risk is greater than with other diagnostic tests, it is outweighed for the occasional woman who needs it by the benefit of discovering, and possibly treating, a defect in her fetus.

ALPHA-FETOPROTEIN SCREENING

Elevated levels in the mother's blood of alpha-fetoprotein (AFP), a substance produced by the fetus, can indicate a neural tube defect, such as spina bifida (a deformity of the spinal column) or anencephaly (an absence of all or part of the brain). But since AFP levels may also be abnormally high because of a multiple pregnancy or a miscalculation of due date (levels increase later in pregnancy), the test yields many false-positives. Abnormally low levels may indicate an increased risk of Down's syndrome.

The availability of test kits to the medical community has made routine AFP testing possible and increasingly popular. But because of the high number of false-positive readings these tests can produce, and because of the emotional and financial strain such readings can needlessly entail (a complete battery of follow-up tests can be costly), routine AFP screening is not recommended by either the American College of Obstetricians and Gynecologists or the American Academy of Pediatrics. Such testing, they suggest, should be reserved only for those at high risk—those who've already had a child with a neural tube defect or who have a family history of such defects.

When Is It Done? Between the 16th and 18th weeks.

How Is It Done? The first screening step is a simple maternal blood test. If AFP levels are found to be high, a second test is run. If levels are still high, then a series of follow-up procedures—including amniocentesis to obtain AFP levels in the amniotic fluid, and a sonogram to view the fetus—are performed to determine whether or not a neural tube defect actually exists. Out of 50 women with high readings on the initial blood test, only 1 or 2 will eventually be shown to have an affected fetus. In the other 48, the tests will show that there is more than one fetus, or that the pregnancy is further along than at first believed, or that the original readings were inaccurate.

How Safe Is It? The initial screening test poses no more risk to mother or baby than any other blood test. The major risk of the test is that a false-positive result may lead to follow-up procedures that do present some risk—and in some cases, to thera-

peutic abortions of perfectly normal fetuses. To be sure that the diagnosis is accurate, all tests should be performed only by trained personnel

---

Reducing Risk in Any Pregnancy

Good Medical Care. Even a low-risk pregnancy is put at high risk if prenatal care is absent or poor. Seeing a qualified practitioner regularly, beginning as soon as pregnancy is suspected, is vital for all expectant mothers. Choose an obstetrician experienced with your particular condition if you are in a high-risk category. But just as important as having a good doctor is being a good patient. Be an active participant in your medical care—ask questions, report symptoms—but don't try to be your own doctor. (See Choosing Your Practitioner, page 23.)

Good Diet. The Best-Odds Diet (see page 75) gives every pregnant woman the best odds of having a successful pregnancy and a healthy baby. It may also help to prevent gestational diabetes, hypertension, and preeclampsia.

Fitness. It's best to begin pregnancy with a well-toned, exercised body, but it's never too late to start deriving the benefits of fitness. Regular exercise prevents constipation and improves respiration, circulation, muscle tone, and skin elasticity, all of which contribute to a more comfortable pregnancy and an easier, safer delivery. (See page 161.)

Sensible Weight Gain. A gradual, steady, and moderate weight gain may help prevent a variety of complications, including diabetes, hypertension, varicose veins, hemorrhoids, low birth weight, or difficult delivery due to an overly large fetus. (See page 127.)

No Smoking. Quitting as early in pregnancy as possible reduces the many risks to mother and baby, includ-

ing prematurity and low birth weight. (See page 56)

Abstinence From Alcohol. Drinking very rarely or not at all will reduce the risk of birth defects, particularly of fetal alcohol syndrome, the result of high alcohol intake. (See page 54.)

Avoidance of Drugs. So little is known about the effects of drugs on fetal development that it is best to avoid taking any during pregnancy that are not absolutely essential and prescribed by your doctor.

Prevention of and Prompt Treatment for Infection. All infections—from common flu to urinary tract and vaginal infections to the increasingly common venereal diseases—should be prevented whenever possible. When contracted, however, infection should be treated promptly by a physician who knows you are pregnant.

Being Wary of the Superwoman Syndrome. Often well established in their careers and highly motivated in everything they do, today's mothers tend to be overachievers and over-doers. Getting enough rest during pregnancy is far more important than getting everything done, especially in high-risk pregnancies. Don't wait until your body starts pleading for relief before you slow down. If your doctor recommends that you begin your maternity leave earlier than you'd planned, take the advice. Some studies have suggested a higher incidence of premature delivery among women who work up until term, particularly if their job entails physical labor or long periods of standing.

using sophisticated equipment, and results should be evaluated by an experienced physician or competent genetic counselor.

CHORIONIC VILLI SAMPLING

Unlike amniocentesis, chorionic villi sampling (CVS) can detect fetal defects very early in pregnancy, when abortion is a less complicated and traumatic procedure. In certain cases (in the future, possibly in most), defects can be treated in utero, and healthy, normal babies delivered at term. Some experts believe CVS will become a routine screening procedure and will replace amniocentesis before the end of the decade.

Eventually, chorionic villi sampling will be able to detect virtually all of the 3,800 or so disorders for which a defective gene is responsible. At present, it is useful only in conditions where the detection technology exists. The indications for use are the same as those for amniocentesis, though CVS is not used to assess fetal lung maturity.

When Is It Done? Usually between the 8th and 12th week, sometimes as early as the 5th.

How Is It Done? This painless procedure may one day be performed routinely in a physician's office. At the moment it is done in major medical centers only. With the expectant mother on an examining table, a long thin catheter (tube) is inserted into her uterus through the vagina. Guided by a picture of the procedure on an ultrasound monitor, the doctor positions the catheter between the uterine lining and the chorion, the fetal membrane which will eventually form the fetal part of the placenta. A sampling of the chorionic villi (finger-like projections from this membrane) is then snipped or suctioned off for diagnostic study.

Since the villi, like the chorion, are of fetal origin, examining them can give a complete picture of the genetic makeup of the developing fetus. Because more cells are collected and because they multiply more rapidly, CVS results are available sooner than in amniocentesis— theoretically within days, more generally within a week.

How Safe Is It? This procedure is relatively new, but early studies conclude it is "acceptably safe and reliable." The chorionic villi, from which the cells are taken for the test, disappear as the fetus matures, so there is believed to be no danger in removing them. The risk of complications leading to miscarriage appears to be about 3 in 200 (about three times that of amniocentesis—a risk many are willing to take in return for earlier information on the fetus. Occasionally an abnormality called mosaicism may be detected in the villi but may not exist in the fetus; then amniocentesis is used for verification.

3
Throughout Your Pregnancy

What You May Be Concerned About

Pregnant women have always worried. What about, however, has changed considerably over the generations, as obstetrical medicine—and expectant parents—find out more and more about what does and does not affect the health and well-being of our unborn. Our grandmothers, vulnerable to a variety of old wives' tales, feared that seeing a monkey while pregnant would result in monkey-like offspring, or that slapping their bellies in fright would leave their babies with hand-shaped birthmarks. We, vulnerable instead to a daily deluge of modern media tales (usually as frightening, sometimes as unfounded), have other fears: Am I breathing in too much polluted air or drinking unsafe water? Is my job, or my husband's smoking, or that cup of coffee I had this morning hazardous to my baby's health?

What about that x-ray I had at the dentist's? As a basis for worry, these concerns can make pregnancy unnecessarily nervewracking. As a basis for action, they can give you a better sense of control and greatly improve the odds of your having a healthy baby.

ALCOHOL

"I had a few drinks on several occasions before I knew I was pregnant. I'm afraid that alcohol may have harmed my baby."

"Behold, thou shalt conceive, and bear a son; now beware, drink no wine or strong drink," an angel tells Samson's mother in the Book of Judges. Lucky lady. She was able to start ordering Perrier when her son was just a gleam in his father's eye. But not many of us receive such advance notice of our pregnancies. And because we're often unaware that we're pregnant until we are into our second month, we're apt to have done things we wouldn't have done if only we had known. Like having a few, a few times too often. Which is why this concern is one of the most common brought to the first prenatal visit.

Fortunately, it's also one of the concerns that can most easily be put aside. There's no evidence that a few drinks on a couple of occasions early in pregnancy will prove harmful to your baby. And one recent study showed that women who had had two or three such drinking binges early in pregnancy weren't any more likely to have babies with structural defects or growth retardation than teetotalers.

Heavy daily doses of alcohol throughout pregnancy, such as those consumed by heavy drinkers or alcoholics, however, *are* connected with a wide variety of problems, including fetal alcohol syndrome (FAS)—a condition in which infants are born undersized, usually mentally deficient, with multiple deformities (particularly of the head and face, the limbs, and the central nervous system), and a high neonatal mortality rate. What "heavy drinker" means varies from study to study, but it's generally considered to be a person who consumes five or six drinks—beer, wine, or distilled spirits—a day. The risks are certainly dose related: The more you drink, the more potential danger to your baby. And they are compounded by other drug use.

But even at lower daily intakes throughout pregnancy, alcohol appears to cause a variety of very serious problems, including increased risk of miscarriage, prematurity, complications during labor and delivery, and possible developmental lags in later infancy and childhood. Though many women manage to drink lightly during pregnancy— one glass of wine nightly, for instance—and still deliver healthy babies, there is no assurance that this is a wise practice. The safe daily alcohol dose in pregnancy, if any, is not known.

That's partly because each fetus, like each mother, has a different genetic makeup and responds differently to drugs like alcohol. And since alcohol enters the fetal bloodstream in approximately the same concentrations present in the mother's blood, each drink a pregnant woman takes is shared with her baby. This leads us to suggest that although you shouldn't worry about what you've already had to drink, it would be prudent to stop drinking for the rest of your pregnancy— except perhaps for a celebratory glass of wine on a birthday or anniversary. (Always taken *with* a meal, since food reduces the absorption of alcohol.)

That's as easily done as said for some women—those who develop a distaste for alcohol in early pregnancy which may linger through delivery. For others, particularly those who habitually "unwind" with cocktails or take wine with dinner, abstinence may require a concerted effort, possibly including a change in lifestyle. If you drink to relax, for example, try substituting other methods of relaxation: music, warm baths, massage, exercise, reading. If drinking is part of a daily ritual that you don't want to give up, try a Virgin Mary (a Bloody Mary minus the vodka) at brunch, sparkling cider or non-alcoholic malt beverages at dinner, a grapefruit or orange juice spritzer (half juice, half seltzer, with a twist) or a Mock Strawberry Daiquiri or Virgin Sangria (see page 89) at cocktail hour—served at the accustomed time, in the accustomed glasses, with the accustomed ceremony. If your husband joins you on the wagon (at least while in your company), the ride will be considerably smoother.

The sooner a heavy drinker stops drinking during pregnancy, the less risk to her baby. The heavy drinker who refuses to abstain or to seek help from Alcoholics Anonymous or an alcoholism clinic is often advised to consider terminating her pregnancy.

CIGARETTE SMOKING

"I've been smoking for 10 years. Will this hurt my baby?"

Happily, there's no clear evidence that smoking prior to pregnancy—even 10 or 20 years of it—will harm a developing fetus. But it's well documented that continuing to smoke during pregnancy—particularly beyond the fourth month—can cause a wide variety of prenatal complications, everything from miscarriage and bleeding early in the first trimester

to premature separation of the placenta and premature rupture of the membranes in the last. There is also strong evidence that the expectant mother's smoking directly affects her baby's development in utero for the worse.

The most widespread risk is low birth weight, with all its concomitant dangers—especially perinatal death (just before, during, or after birth). But babies of three-pack-a-day smokers also have a quadrupled risk of low Apgar scores (the standard scale used to evaluate infants at birth), which means they just aren't as healthy as other babies. And there's evidence that, on the average, they may never catch up to the children of non-smokers, that they may have long-term physical and intellectual deficits, and may also be hyperactive. At age 14, one study showed, children of smokers tended to be more prone to respiratory disease, to be shorter than children of non-smokers, and to be less successful in school.

It was once believed that the reason for the difficulties these children display was poor prenatal nutrition: The mothers smoked rather than ate. But recent studies show this isn't the case; smoking mothers who eat as much and gain as much weight as non-smoking mothers still give birth to smaller babies. The cause seems to be carbon monoxide poisoning and a reduction of oxygen to the fetus through the placenta. Gaining a huge amount of weight—40 pounds or more—may somewhat reduce the risk of a smoking mother having an undersized baby, but this excess weight poses other risks to the mother and child.

In effect, when you smoke, your baby is living in a smoke-filled womb. His heartbeat speeds, he coughs and sputters, and, worst of all, he can't grow and thrive as he should. Cutting down on the number of cigarettes you smoke may help just a bit: The more cigarettes you smoke, the greater the risk to your baby. But in most cases, cutting down is illusory because the smoker just compensates by taking more frequent and deeper puffs and smoking more of each cigarette, as she also does when she tries to reduce risk by using low-tar or low-nicotine cigarettes.

The news, however, isn't all bad. Some studies show that women who quit smoking early in pregnancy—no later than the fourth month—can reduce the risk of damage to the fetus to the level of the non-smoker. Sooner is better, but quitting even in the last month can help preserve oxygen flow to the baby during delivery. For some smoking women, quitting will never be easier than in early pregnancy, when they develop a sudden distaste for cigarettes—probably the warning of an intuitive body. If you're not lucky enough to have such a natural aversion, try quitting with the help of Smoke Enders or other smoking cessation groups.

You may experience withdrawal symptoms when you quit smoking; the exact symptoms vary from person to person. Some of the most common are a craving for tobacco, irritability, anxiety, restlessness, dullness, and sleep and gastrointestinal disturbances. Some people also find that concentration, judgment, and both physical and mental performance are impaired. In most cases, the symptoms won't last more than a few days, though occasionally some effects of withdrawal linger longer. The benefits, however, will last a lifetime—for you and your baby. (For more tips on habit breaking, see page 58.)

WHEN OTHER PEOPLE SMOKE

"I quit smoking, but my husband still goes through two packs a day. I keep worrying that somehow this may hurt our baby."

Smoking, it has become more and more apparent, doesn't just affect the person with the cigarette in his mouth—it affects everyone around him. Including a developing fetus whose mother happens to be nearby. So if your husband (or anyone else who lives in your home or works at the next desk) smokes, your baby's body is going to pick up nearly as much contamination from tobacco smoke by-products as if *you* were lighting up.

If your husband says he can't quit smoking, ask him to at least do all his smoking out of the house or in a different room, away from you. Quitting, of course, would be better, not just for his own health, but for the baby's long-term well-being. Studies show that parental smoking—mother's or father's—can cause respiratory problems in the infant and child after birth and impaired lung development into adult-

Breaking the Smoking Habit

Identify Your Motivation for Smoking. For example, do you smoke for pleasure, stimulation, or relaxation? To reduce tension or frustration, to have something in your hand or mouth, to satisfy a craving? Perhaps you smoke out of habit, lighting up without thinking about it. Once you understand your motivations, you should be able to substitute other satisfactions.

Identify Your Motivation for Quitting. When you're pregnant, there's a clear one.

Choose Your Method of Withdrawal. Do you want to go cold turkey—or taper off? Either way, pick a "last day" that isn't too far off. Plan a full day of activities for that date—things you don't associate with smoking.

Try to Sublimate Your Urge to Smoke. Use any and all of the following that you think will help:

❖ If you smoke mainly to keep your hands busy, try playing with a pencil, beads, a straw; knit, polish silver, create a new nutritious recipe, write a letter, play the piano, learn to paint, make rag dolls, do jigsaw or crossword puzzles, challenge someone to a game of chess or Scrabble—anything that will make you forget to reach for a cigarette.

❖ If you smoke for oral gratification, try a substitute: raw vegetables, popcorn, a whole-wheat breadstick, gum made with sorbitol, a toothpick, an empty cigarette holder. Do avoid empty-calorie nibbles.

❖ If you smoke for stimulation, try to get your lift from a brisk walk, an absorbing book, good conversation. Be sure your diet contains all essential nutrients and that you eat frequently, to avoid feeling draggy because of low blood sugar.

❖ If you smoke to reduce tension and relax, try exercise instead. Or relaxation techniques. Or listening to soothing music while knitting. Or a long walk. Or a massage. Or making love.

❖ If you smoke for pleasure, seek pleasure in other pursuits, preferably in no-smoke situations. Go to a movie, visit baby boutiques, tour a favorite museum, attend a concert or a play, have dinner with a friend who is allergic to smoke. Or try something more active, like tennis doubles.

❖ If you smoke out of habit, avoid the settings in which you habitually smoke; frequent places with no-smoking rules instead. Stay away from heavy smokers.

❖ If you connect smoking with a particular beverage, food, or meal, avoid the food or beverage, eat the meal in a different locale. (Say you smoke two cigarettes with breakfast but you never smoke in bed. Have breakfast in bed for a few days.)

❖ When you feel the urge to smoke, take several deep breaths with a pause between each. Hold the last breath while you strike a match. Exhale slowly, blowing out the match. Pretend it was a cigarette and crush it out.

If You Do Slip Up and Have a Cigarette, Don't Despair. Just get right back on your program, knowing that every cigarette you *don't* smoke is going to help your baby.

Look at Smoking as a Non-Negotiable Issue. When you were a smoker, you couldn't smoke in a theater, or a subway, or a department store, even in some restaurants. That was that. Now you have to tell yourself that you can't smoke, period. That is that.

hood. (If you choose to nurse and smoke, tobacco poisons will contaminate the milk your baby drinks.)

You probably won't be able to get your co-workers to kick their habits, but you might be able to persuade them to take their cigarettes elsewhere when you're around. (In some communities and at some companies, you'll get official support in your efforts to create non-smoking spaces.)

MARIJUANA AND OTHER DRUG USE

"I've been a social smoker of marijuana—indulging only at parties—for about 10 years. Could this have altered my chromosomes enough to damage the baby I'm now carrying? And is smoking pot during pregnancy dangerous?"

As with cigarette smoking over 20 years ago, all the evidence on the effects of marijuana use is not yet in. Consequently, those who choose to smoke it today are guinea pigs testing a substance whose dangers may not be fully documented for some time to come. And since marijuana crosses the placenta, mothers who smoke it during pregnancy make guinea pigs out of their unborn children as well.

It is usually recommended that couples trying to conceive abstain from marijuana use, since it can interfere with conception. But if you are already pregnant, you needn't worry about your past smoking—there is no present evidence that it will harm your fetus.

Smoking *during* pregnancy, however, is a story that appears to have a less happy ending. Studies show that women who use marijuana at least once a month during pregnancy are: more than twice as likely to show meconium staining of the amniotic fluid during labor (a complication which can indicate fetal distress); more likely to suffer hyperemesis (severe and chronic vomiting, which can interfere seriously with prenatal nutrition), to gain inadequate weight, and to be anemic; more likely to have dangerously rapid labor, prolonged or arrested labor, or to require a cesarean section; slightly more likely to have low-birth-weight babies; twice as likely to have babies needing resuscitation after delivery. Though it may not have a direct toxic effect on a developing fetus, marijuana *does* affect placental function and the fetal endocrine system, and can interfere with the successful completion of pregnancy. Based on the available evidence, the United States surgeon general has warned that marijuana use during pregnancy may be hazardous to a baby's health.

So treat marijuana as you would any other drug during pregnancy: Don't take it unless it is medically required and prescribed. If you have already smoked early in your pregnancy, don't worry. Since placental function becomes more important as pregnancy progresses, it's very unlikely any harm was done. Any pregnant woman who can't seem to break her marijuana habit should seek professional help as soon as the pregnancy is confirmed.

Pregnant women who use other

"recreational" drugs are also putting their babies in jeopardy. Not enough is known about their risks, and their benefits are hardly worth such potential danger. Using street drugs, the exact compositions of which are always unknown to the purchaser, presents added hazards. And addictive drugs, such as heroin, can "hook" not only mother but fetus as well, with devastating results at birth.

CAFFEINE

"I find it difficult to get through my day without my two cups of coffee. I've read, though, that caffeine can cause birth defects and low-birth-weight babies. Is this true?"

According to the most recent scientific studies, probably not. Caffeine (found in coffee, tea, colas, and other soft drinks, and in a related form in chocolate) does cross the placenta and enter the fetal circulation. But, though early animal studies showed numerous harmful effects from caffeine on developing animal fetuses, human studies to date have shown no harm from moderate use—up to three cups of coffee or the equivalent in each 24-hour period—during pregnancy.

Still, there are some valid reasons to give up caffeinated coffee (and tea and colas) during pregnancy, or at least to cut down consumption. First of all, caffeine has a diuretic effect, drawing fluid and calcium—both vital to maternal and fetal health—from the body. If you're having a problem with frequent urination anyway, caffeine intake will compound it. Second, coffee and tea, especially when taken with cream and sugar, are filling without being nutritious and can spoil your appetite for good food. Colas are not only filling but loaded with a wide range of questionable chemicals and either diet sweeteners, which may or may not be safe to consume when you're expecting, or empty sugar calories. (Saccharin use is definitely not recommended during pregnancy. Aspartame [Equal, Nutrasweet] does not seem to be harmful to the fetuses of women who have no difficulty handling phenylalanine. Still it would be prudent to avoid frequent use until more studies confirm the safety.) Third, caffeine could exacerbate your normal pregnancy mood swings and also interfere with adequate rest. Finally, the fact that many women lose their taste for coffee early in pregnancy suggests that mother nature considers the substance to be unsuitable for pregnant women.

How Do You Break the Caffeine Habit? The first step, finding your motivation, is easy in pregnancy: giving your baby the healthiest possible start in life. Next you need to determine why you indulge. If it's just a matter of taste or the comfort of a hot drink that turns you on to coffee or tea, then you can switch to a naturally decaffeinated beverage (but no more than two cups a day, unsweetened, or you won't have room for the good stuff). If you drink cola for taste we can't recommend substituting caffeine-free soft drinks, because no soft drink has a place in pregnancy; if it's refreshment you're thirsting for, you'll find that juices and plain or carbonated water are better thirst quenchers than colas, anyway. If it's the caffeine lift you crave, you'll get a more natural, longer-lasting boost from exercise and good food, especially protein, or from doing something that exhilarates you: dancing, jogging, making love. Though you'll doubtless sag for a few days after giving up caffeine, you'll soon feel better than ever. (Of course, you will still experience the normal fatigue of early pregnancy.)

If you drink coffee, tea, or cola for something to do, do something else—something good for your baby. Knit him or her a sweater, go for a walk or shop for a crib, scrub a bunch of vegetables for dinner. If you drink your caffeinated beverage as part of a daily ritual (the coffee break, reading the paper, watching TV), change the time and place of that ritual, and change the beverage that accompanies it.

Minimizing Caffeine Withdrawal Systems. But as any coffee, tea, or cola addict is well aware, it is one thing to want to give up caffeine and another thing to do it. If you're a heavy imbiber and quit cold turkey, you can expect to experience withdrawal symptoms, including headache, fatigue, and lethargy. But these uncomfortable side effects can be minimized:

❖ Keep your blood sugar, and thus your energy level, up. Eat frequently, especially when headache strikes, and concentrate on high protein and complex-carbohydrate foods. Vitamin supplements may help, too.

❖ Get some outdoor exercise every day. It will also, believe it or not, raise your energy level.

❖ Be sure to get enough sleep—which will probably be easier without caffeine.

❖ If you drink large quantities of coffee or other caffeine-containing beverages, cutting down over a period of a few days may be the best way to reduce the severity of withdrawal symptoms.

MICROWAVE EXPOSURE

"I've read that exposure to microwave ovens is dangerous to a developing fetus. Should I unplug ours until after the baby's born?"

A microwave oven can be a working mother-to-be's best friend, helping to make nutritious eating-on-the-run possible. But like so many of our modern miracles, there's talk it may also be a modern menace. Whether or not we can be zapped by exposure to microwaves is still very controversial. Much more research needs to be done before the answer is known. It is believed, however, that two types of human tissue—the developing fetus and the eye—are particularly vulnerable to the effects of microwaves because they have a poor capacity to dissipate the heat the waves generate. So rather than unplugging your microwave oven, you should take some precautions. First of all, be sure your oven doesn't leak. (Meters are available for checking leaks;

some cities provide this service.) Second, don't stand near the oven when it is in operation. Finally, follow the manufacturer's directions very carefully.

TOXOPLASMOSIS

"My test for toxoplasmosis came back positive. The doctor said I may have to have an abortion and I'm heartsick."

Having a positive titer for toxoplasmosis is not very unusual. But actually having the infection during pregnancy is. The parasitic organism that causes the disease, Toxoplasma gondii, is transmitted to humans via both cat feces and raw meat. The condition in adults is so mild that its symptoms (a slight rash, some achiness, swollen glands, a low-grade fever) often go unnoticed. But while a woman infected during pregnancy is at no risk, her fetus may suffer serious illness, lasting damage, or might even die.

But before you consider terminating your pregnancy, your doctor will certainly want to do some more testing to confirm an active infection. Experts recommend taking a second blood sample and running it through the test for toxoplasmosis and, at the same time, rerunning the original sample. If the titer shows a rise between the first and second samples and if IGM antibodies are also high, there is probably an active infection. But 95% of the time, the retests prove negative.

On the rare occasions when infection in the mother is confirmed, an expectant couple needs to look at the facts and discuss them with their doctor, and possibly a genetic counselor.

The risk of a fetus becoming infected in the first trimester is relatively small, probably less than 25%, but the risk of serious damage from the infection is high. In the second trimester the likelihood of infection is a little higher, but the risk of damage a little less. In the last trimester, the baby is most likely to be infected, but the risk of serious damage is smallest. Unfortunately, there is no way to test for fetal infection, though occasionally an ultrasound can pick up damage to the brain that's already been done.

At least 1 in 3 women are already immune when they conceive (the rate is higher for women who eat raw or very rare meat or who have cats at home) and have no chance of passing the infection along to their offspring. Those who are not immune can prevent infection in these ways:

❖ Avoid other people's cats and strays. Have any cats at home tested for active infection. Board in a kennel or ask a friend to care for any infected cat for at least six weeks— the period of infection. Keep others infection-free by not feeding raw meat or allowing them to roam out of doors, hunt mice or birds, or fraternize with other cats. Have someone else handle the litter box.

❖ Don't garden in soil or let your children play in sand where cats may have deposited feces. Wash home-grown produce with detergent (rinsing thoroughly) and/or peel or cook it.

❖ Don't eat meat that is raw or that hasn't been cooked to at least 140 degrees (rare). In restaurants, order meat well-done.

X-RAYS

"I had an x-ray series at the dentist before I found out I was pregnant. Could this have hurt my baby?"

Don't worry. First of all, dental x-rays are directed far away from your uterus. Second, a lead apron shields your uterus and your baby effectively from any radiation.

The safety of other types of x-rays during pregnancy, however, is more controversial. No one knows exactly what a safe dose of radiation is, or what all the potential dangers are. There is believed to be some risk to the fetus from direct radiation, at least during the first trimester. Fortunately, the risk is being reduced as x-ray equipment is improved and refined, delivering lower doses of radiation and becoming more precise in focusing directly on the desired area.

Of course, it still isn't wise to take unnecessary risks, no matter how small. But necessary risks are another matter. The Committee on Radiology of the American Academy of Pediatrics says that because the possibility of birth defects resulting from x-ray exposure to pregnant women is extremely low, even abdominal x-ray examination need not be postponed if it is genuinely needed during pregnancy. If you need an x-ray:

❖ Always inform the doctor ordering the x-ray and the technician performing it that you are pregnant.

❖ Never have an x-ray, even a dental x-ray, during pregnancy when the benefit does not outweigh the risk. Your doctor or dentist can help you determine that. (Read Weighing Risk vs. Benefit, page 73.)

❖ Do not have an x-ray if any safer diagnostic procedure can be used instead.

❖ If an x-ray is necessary, be certain that it is taken in a licensed or regularly inspected facility. Equipment should be up-to-date, in good condition, and operated by well-trained, conscientious technicians under the supervision of a full-time radiologist. The x-ray beams should, when possible, be adjusted so that only the minimum area necessary is exposed to radiation; other areas, especially the uterus, should be shielded with a lead apron.

❖ Follow the technician's directions precisely, being especially careful not to move during the shot, so that retakes won't be needed.

❖ Most important, if you've had an x-ray, or need an x-ray, don't waste your time worrying about the possible consequences. Your baby is in more danger every time you forget to buckle your seat belt.

GETTING SICK

"I'm afraid that if I get sick my baby will suffer. And if I get a fever, there's nothing I can safely take."

Pregnancy is one of those times when an ounce of prevention is worth a pound of cure—and is a lot safer, too. You won't have to worry about what to take for a cold if you avoid catching one, and the best ways to do that are:

❖ Keep your resistance up. Eat the best diet possible (see the Best-Odds Diet, page 75), get enough sleep, and don't wear yourself down by running yourself ragged.

❖ Avoid sick people like the plague. Stay away from those you know are sick (sit far from coughers and sneezers on the bus), and never shake hands with them (this exchanges not only greetings but germs).

❖ If your children are down with a cold or flu, you can't avoid them entirely. But you can avoid handling their linens and soiled tissues, finishing up their lunches or drinking from their cups, and kissing them on the face. See that they wash their hands frequently and cover their mouths when they cough or sneeze. Use disinfectant on telephones and other commonly used surfaces. Ask your husband, mother, or a non-pregnant friend to play nurse-maid as much as possible. If a child comes down with a rash of any kind—unless you know you've already had, or been vaccinated for, German measles (rubella)[1] and chickenpox—stay away from them completely and contact your doctor at once.

---

1. Your doctor will have done a rubella titer as part of your first prenatal exam. Be sure to ask whether or not you are immune.

If, despite all your efforts, you come down with a cold or the flu (most pregnant women do at some point in the nine months), you can feel reassured that mild illness, though uncomfortable for you, is very unlikely to be harmful to your baby.

It's the traditional medical treatments—antihistamines, aspirin, and antibiotics—that can cause problems. Don't take any of these, or any other medication, without your doctor's advice; he or she will know which are safe in pregnancy and which will be effective in your case. Aspirin use is not a good idea, particularly late in pregnancy when it could lead to childbirth complications and bleeding. If you've already taken aspirin, though, don't panic. There is no evidence that a couple of them will be harmful, unless they are taken just prior to delivery. Less is known about the effects of acetaminophen (non-aspirin products like Tylenol or Datril), and many physicians okay them for very occasional use during pregnancy. Others do not. Ibuprofen also may be recommended by some physicians during the first six months of your pregnancy, but it shouldn't be used at all in the third trimester. (These pain relievers, incidentally, will not cure colds and will not relieve most cold symptoms. Over-the-counter cold medications and cough syrups may relieve symptoms, but they are generally not recommended—particularly early in pregnancy, before the fetus is well developed.)

Fortunately for you and your baby, some of the best cold and flu remedies are the safest ones, too:

❖ Nip your cold in the bud, before it blossoms into a nasty case of bronchitis or another secondary infection. With the very first sneeze, go to bed or at least plan on getting a little extra rest.

❖ When you're lying down or sleeping, keep your head slightly elevated to facilitate breathing.

❖ Don't starve your cold, fever—or baby. Stay on the Best-Odds Diet whether you have an appetite or not, forcing yourself to eat if need be. Be sure to have some citrus fruit or juice every day, but don't take extra vitamin C supplements without medical advice.

❖ Flood yourself with fluids. Your body will be losing fluids you and your baby urgently need through fever, sneezes, and runny nose. Keep a thermos of hot grapefruit or orangeade (½ cup unsweetened frozen juice concentrate to 1 quart of boiling water) next to your bed, and drink at least one cupful an hour. Also try the Jewish penicillin: chicken soup. Medical researchers have proven that it really does help.

❖ Keep your nasal passages moist with a humidifier, and by spraying the inside of your nose with an atomizer filled with salt water.

❖ If your throat is sore or scratchy, or you're coughing, gargle with salt water (1 teaspoon of salt to 8 ounces of water) at the temperature of hot tea.

❖ Bring down a fever naturally. Take cool showers or baths, or sponge with tepid water; drink cool beverages, and wear light bedclothes. If your fever reaches 102 degrees or more, call your doctor immediately. (High body temperature for extended periods isn't good for the baby.)

❖ If your cold or flu is really bad and interferes with eating or sleeping, or if you're coughing up greenish or yellowish sputum, call your doctor. He or she may want to prescribe a topical medication that won't cross the placenta, or if there is a risk of complications, an antibiotic or antihistamine that is safe during pregnancy.

Remember that you and your doctor must weigh risk against benefit when it comes to using medications. Don't put off calling the doctor, or refuse to take a prescribed medication you are assured is safe, because you've heard all drugs are harmful during pregnancy. They aren't.

DIARRHEA

"I've got an intestinal virus and my midwife took me off dairy products until the diarrhea stops. Is that safe?"

A couple of days off your diet won't hurt your baby, but prolonged diarrhea might. So take your practitioner's advice. Do take your vitamin-mineral supplements if you can, get plenty of fluids (diluted juices, water, decaffeinated teas) and as many calories as possible through dry toast, baked potato (no skins), boiled or steamed white rice, banana, and other permitted foods.

Bedrest will also hasten your recovery. If your diarrhea hasn't cleared up in 24 to 48 hours, medication may be prescribed.

TAKING MEDICATIONS

"How do I know which medicines, if any, are safe to take during pregnancy, and which aren't?"

No drug, prescription or over-the-counter, is 100% safe for 100% of the people 100% of the time. When you're pregnant, every time you take a drug there are two individuals at risk, one very small and vulnerable. On the other hand, even during pregnancy there are many situations in which medications are absolutely essential to life and/or health. Whether you will take a particular medication at a particular time during pregnancy will be something you and your physician will have to decide by weighing the risk a drug might pose against the benefit it offers (see page 73). You should take *no* medication without medical consultation, and only take medication that is absolutely necessary.

Which drug you take in a particular situation will depend on the latest information available on drug safety in pregnancy. The many lists of safe, possibly safe, possibly unsafe, and definitely unsafe drugs may provide some assistance, but most are outdated and unreliable by the time they're published. Package inserts and labels are of little use, since most warn not to use the product during pregnancy without a physician's orders, even when the product is believed safe. Your best sources of information will be:

❖ A well-informed physician (not all are familiar with drug safety in pregnancy).

❖ The Food and Drug Administration—your regional office, or the Public Health Service, FDA, Parklawn Building, 5600 Fisher's Lane, Rockville, MD 20857.

❖ The March of Dimes—try your local office first, or contact the National Foundation/March of Dimes, 1275 Mamaroneck Avenue, White Plains, NY 10605.

HOUSEHOLD HAZARDS

"The more I read, the more I'm convinced that the only way to protect my baby in this day and age is to spend the next nine months locked up in a sterile room. Even my home isn't safe."

The threats you and your baby face from the increasing number of environmental hazards, including those in your own backyard, quickly pale when compared to those faced by your great-grandmothers, when modern obstetrical medicine was in its infancy. All of today's environmental perils combined (alcohol, tobacco, and other drugs excepted) are far less menacing to you and your baby than one untrained midwife with unwashed hands was to your ancestresses. So in spite of all the trumpeting about the perils around us, we repeat: Pregnancy and childbirth have never been so safe.

But while you won't need to give up your home and move to that sterile room, a little caution is certainly warranted when dealing with household hazards:

Household Cleaning Products.

Since many cleaning products have been in common use for the better part of the century and no correlation has ever been noted between clean homes and birth defects, it's unlikely that disinfecting your toilet bowl or polishing your dining-room table will in anyway compromise the well-being of your baby. In fact, much the opposite is probably true: The elimination of germ-carrying bacteria by chlorine, ammonia, and other cleaning agents can protect your baby by preventing infection.

No studies have proven that the occasional incidental inhalation of ordinary household cleansers has any detrimental effect on the developing fetus; on the other hand, no studies have proven frequent inhalation completely safe. If you've already been "exposed" to cleansers, there's no reason for concern. But for the rest of your pregnancy, clean with prudence. Let your nose, and the following tips, be your guide in screening out potentially hazardous chemicals:

❖ If the product has a strong odor or fumes, don't breathe it in directly. Use it in an area with plenty of ventilation, or don't use it at all.

❖ Use pump sprays instead of aerosols.

❖ Never (even when you're not pregnant) mix ammonia with chlorine-based products; the combination produces very hazardous fumes.

❖ Try to avoid using products such as oven cleaners and dry-cleaning fluids whose labels are plastered with warnings about toxicity.

❖ Wear gloves when you're cleaning. Not only will they spare your hands a lot of wear and tear, they'll prevent the absorption through the skin of potentially toxic chemicals.

Tap Water. Water ranks second only to oxygen on the list of things essential to life. Though starvation certainly isn't medically recommended, humans can survive for at least a week without food, but only a few days without water. In other words, you've got more to worry about if you *don't* drink the water than if you do.

It's true that water once posed a serious threat to the lives it sustained, carrying deadly typhoid and other diseases. But modern treatment has eliminated such threats, at least in developed areas of the world. Though there are some who suspect that a new threat to the unborn now exists in the very chemicals that are used to purify water, there is no conclusive evidence that this is true. Any possible hazard is eliminated in cities that use filters instead of chemicals in the water purification process.

Most drinking water in the United States is safe and drinkable. But in a few areas, chemical seepage from factories, dumping areas, and farms has led to potentially hazardous contamination. If this is the case in your home town, you're probably well aware of it. If so, or even if you're only suspicious, here's how to make sure you're drinking to your—and your baby's—health:

❖ Check with your local Environmental Protection Agency (EPA) or health department about the purity and safety of community drinking water. If there is a possibility that the quality of your water (because of pipe deterioration, because your home borders on a waste disposal area, or because of odd taste or color) might differ from the rest of the community's, arrange for one or the other of these agencies to test it.

❖ If your tap water looks suspicious or has an "off" taste, invest in a carbon filter for your kitchen sink. (It will last longer if it is used only for cooking and drinking water and not for the dishwasher and other purposes.) Or use bottled water for drinking and cooking.

Insecticides. Though some insects, such as gypsy moths, pose a considerable threat to trees and plants, and others, such as roaches and ants, to your esthetic sensibilities, they rarely pose a health risk to human beings—even pregnant ones. And it's generally safer to live with them than to eliminate them through the use of chemical insecticides, some of which have been linked to birth defects.

Of course, your neighbors and/or your super (if they don't happen to be pregnant or have small children) may not agree. If neighborhood spraying is currently being done, avoid being outdoors as much as possible until the chemical odors have dissipated, about two to three days. When indoors, keep the windows closed. If your super is spraying apartments for roaches or other insects, ask him to skip yours. If he's already sprayed, stay out of the apartment for a day or two if that's possible, and ventilate with open windows for as long as is feasible. The chemicals are only potentially dangerous as long as the fumes linger. Have someone scrub all of the food preparation surfaces in or near the sprayed area.

On your own property or in your apartment, try to take the natural approach to pest control. Pull weeds instead of spraying them. Have someone remove gypsy moth larvae or other insect pests manually from trees and plants, or, as one doctor did in his neighborhood, try to convince those responsible for spraying to use a soap-and-water mixture, which kills bugs by clogging up their breathing passages, instead of chemicals. The soap-and-water technique may take two sprayings, but it will work. Kill cockroaches and ants with boric acid (sprinkled in heavy-bug-traffic areas), which is harmless (unless ingested) to humans and human fetuses and is probably more effective than the insecticides most frequently used. Bug "motels" are also safe to use.

If you have been accidentally exposed to insecticides or herbicides, don't be alarmed. Brief, indirect exposure isn't likely to have done any harm to your baby. What does increase the risk is frequent, long-term exposure, the kind which working daily around such chemicals (as in a factory) would entail.

Paint Fumes. In the entire animal kingdom, the period before birth (or egg laying) is passed in hectic preparation for the arrival of the new offspring. Birds feather their nests, squirrels line their tree-trunk homes with leaves and twigs, and human mothers and fathers sift madly through volumes of wallpaper and fabric samples.

And almost invariably (if a safe "asexual" color can be decided on) painting of the baby's room is involved. Which, in the days of arsenic- or lead-based paints, might have posed some threat to the health of the unborn. But modern latex paints are much safer. They dry quickly, give off fewer fumes, and rarely contain lead. Still, painting isn't the best avocation for an expectant mother—even for one who's trying desperately to keep busy in those last weeks of waiting. Balancing on ladder tops is precarious, to say the least, and paint odors can bring on an attack of nausea. Try, instead, to get the expectant father, or someone else, to handle this aspect of preparations.

While the painting is being done, try to be out of the house. Whether you're there or not, be sure to keep windows open for ventilation. Avoid entirely exposure to paint removers, which are highly toxic, and steer clear of removing paint (whether chemicals or sanders are used).

AIR POLLUTION

"It seems it isn't even safe to breathe when you're pregnant. Will air pollution hurt my baby?"

Living in a bus terminal or sleeping nightly in a toll booth on a congested highway might, of course, expose your fetus to excessive pollutants while depriving it of essential oxygen. Ordinary breathing in the big city, however, isn't as risky as you might think, particularly when you consider the alternative. Millions of women live and breathe in major cities across the nation and give birth to millions of healthy babies. Even in the 1960s, when pollution was at its worst levels in such smoggy places as Los Angeles and New York, there was no documented damage to the unborn.

Day-to-day breathing, then, will have no detrimental effect on your baby. Even enough carbon monoxide to cause illness in the mother appears not to have deleterious effects on the fetus early in pregnancy (although carbon monoxide poisoning later in pregnancy might). It's common sense, however, to avoid extraordinarily high doses of most pollutants. Here's how:

❖ Avoid smoke-filled rooms for extended, repeated periods. Keep in mind that cigars and pipes, because they aren't inhaled, release even more smoke into the air than cigarettes do. Ask family, guests in your home, and co-workers not to smoke in your presence.

❖ Have the exhaust system on your car checked to be sure there is no leakage of noxious fumes and that the exhaust pipe isn't rusting away. Never start your car in the garage with the door closed; keep the tailgate on a station wagon closed when the engine is running; avoid waiting in gas lines with other cars spewing out carbon monoxide; keep your car's air vent closed when driving in heavy traffic.

❖ If a pollution alert is called in your city, stay indoors as much as you can, with the windows closed and the air conditioner, if you have one, running. Follow any other instructions given by the city for residents who are at particular risk.

❖ Don't run, walk, or bicycle along congested highways, or exercise out of doors when there's a pollution alert, since you breathe in more air—and pollution—when you're active.

OCCUPATIONAL HAZARDS

"You hear a lot about dangers on the job, but how do you know if your workplace is safe?"

The hazards of the workplace, and the threats they may pose to the reproductive capabilities of both male and female workers and to the well-being of their unborn children, have only just begun to be explored and identified. Conclusive answers have been elusive, as they are whenever cause-and-effect connections between environmental factors and poor pregnancy out-

comes are sought. First of all, it's hard to separate out all the various possible contributing risk factors in a woman's life, or to prove that an unfavorable outcome wasn't caused by a genetic accident. Second, though animal studies often yield interesting results, there's no way to ascertain whether the results apply to humans, since experiments on humans aren't, of course, feasible.

Therefore, effects on humans can be determined only through epidemiological studies. These studies can be done in two ways: Large groups of women who are exposed to certain substances can be looked at to see if they show an increase in one or more types of poor pregnancy outcome (miscarriages, birth defects, etc.). Or small groups of women who have poor outcomes can be studied to see if there is a common risk factor shared by all of them. Either way, such studies give us clues but not definitive answers.

From what we presently know, it is clear that some workplaces do present hazards for the pregnant woman (e.g., chemical factories, operating rooms, x-ray departments). Other workplace hazards so far have fallen into gray areas because not enough research has been done to establish their safety—or lack of it. What some of the research has already indicated, and will probably continue to indicate, is that there is a great deal of unwarranted concern about potential risks on the job.

The use of a video display terminal, such as that on a word processor or other computer, is one of the most common occupational preoccupations of pregnant women. Because display terminals emit radiation, pregnant women who worked with them daily and suffered miscarriages, or whose infants were stillborn or born with defects, have charged that the machines were responsible. Studies so far seem to indicate these problems were random and not related to the display terminals; the levels of radiation emitted, experts say, were far too low (less even than that of sunshine) to be causative factors. It's been suggested, rather, that the stress under which many workers operate a VDT may be the real culprit in these tragedies. The issue is still, however, controversial, and the National Institute of Occupational Safety and Health (NIOSH) has undertaken a two-year study to try to clarify it. In the meantime, responsible manufacturers are striving, through technological refinement, to reduce any potential risks their machines may pose.

Of course, there are many occupational risks that are real and proven, and a pregnant woman should be alerted to them. The Occupational Safety and Health Administration (OSHA) lists a number of substances which pregnant women should avoid, among them: alkylating agents, anesthetic gases, arsenic, benzene, carbon monoxide, chlorinated hydrocarbons, diethylstilbesterol, dimethyl sulfoxide, dioxin, ionizing radiation, organic mercury compounds, organophosphate pesticides, polychlorinated biphenyls.

Some workers, such as doctors and nurses who work in operating rooms, x-ray technicians, and certain lab or pharmacy workers, are probably aware of the substances they're exposed to on the job. Others may not be. By law, you have the right to know, and your employer is under obligation to tell you. (Information on workplace hazards can also be obtained by contacting the National Institute of Occupational Safety and Health, Clearing House for Occupational Safety and Health Information, 4676 Columbia Parkway, Cincinnati, OH 45226; or the Occupational Safety and Health Administration, 200 Constitution Avenue NW, Washington, DC 20210; information about the safety of machinery or other equipment that you operate on the job can often be secured by writing directly to the manufacturer's corporate medical director.) If your job does expose you to hazards, either ask to be transferred temporarily to a safer post or, finances permitting, begin your maternity leave early.

Though chemicals pose the most direct occupational threats, they don't pose the only ones. Teachers and social workers who deal with young children are likely to come into contact with potentially dangerous infections, such as rubella. Laundry workers and those in the health care field may be exposed to a variety of infections; animal handlers, meat cutters and inspectors to toxoplasmosis. Fortunately, unlike exposure to chemicals, exposure to infection can usually be avoided, either through immunization or the use of gloves and masks or other precautions. (See the individual infections, such as Toxoplasmosis, page 62.)

WHAT IT'S IMPORTANT TO KNOW:
PLAYING BABY ROULETTE

When a gambler playing roulette puts down a bet on his lucky number, the odds are very high against the wheel coming to a stop there. It's the same when a pregnant woman plays baby roulette (intentionally or inadvertently), exposing her baby to teratogens, substances potentially harmful to the fetus. Almost all of the time the baby roulette wheel will pass innocuously by, and the baby won't be affected.

Although the gambler will call it luck, where the roulette wheel stops depends on the weight of the wheel, the friction it encounters, the force with which it is spun. And though baby roulette may also appear to be a game of chance, it, too, is dependent on a variety of factors:

How Strong Is the Teratogen?
Whereas thalidomide, a drug used in the early 1960s, caused very severe deformities in all fetuses who were exposed in utero at a particular time in their development, some sex hormones, also considered teratogens, cause defects in only about 1 in 1,000 fetuses. Fortunately, drugs as potent as thalidomide are extremely rare. In fact, a study of the effects of common drugs on 50,000 pregnancies found no drug similar to it in teratogenic effect. Other teratogens (such as x-ray, chemicals, and so on) also vary in the strength of their effect.

Is the Fetus Genetically Susceptible to the Teratogen?
Just as not everybody exposed to cold or flu germs succumbs, not every fetus who is exposed to a teratogen is susceptible to its effects.

When Was the Fetus Exposed to the Teratogen?
Thalidomide, despite its horrifying potential, caused no damage when taken after the 52nd day of pregnancy. Malformations caused were specific to the part of the body that was developing at the time of ingestion and depended on the susceptibility of that part. Likewise, rubella virus causes congenital damage in more than a third of fetuses exposed during the first month, but risk after the third month is probably under 1%.

How Much Exposure Was There?
Most teratogenic effects are dose related. One brief diagnostic x-ray will be unlikely to cause a problem. A series of heavy-dose radiation treatments could. Smoking lightly for the first few months will not be likely to harm a fetus; heavy smoking for the entire pregnancy increases certain risks very significantly.

What Is the Mother's General Nutritional Status?
Some animal experiments show defects apparently caused by a drug are actually caused by poor nutrition; the drug only reduced appetite, and thus water and food intake. Just as you will resist a

cold virus more effectively if you are well nourished and not rundown, so will your fetus resist teratogens better if he or she is well nourished—through you, of course.

Are Several Factors Combining to Increase Risk? The trio of poor diet, smoking, and alcohol abuse, the duet of smoking and tranquilizers, and other "losing combinations" can greatly increase risk.

Is Some Unknown Protective Factor in Play? Even when all factors appear identical, not all fetuses are affected in the same way. In experiments with fetal mice of identical genetic strains who were exposed to the same teratogens at identical stages in development and at identical dosages, only 1 in 9 were born malformed. No one knows exactly why, though perhaps someday medical science will come up with the solution to this mystery.

WEIGHING RISK VS. BENEFIT

Should today's pregnant woman fear for her baby's life and well-being because he or she is developing in a world filled with environmental threats? Absolutely not—and for several reasons. First of all, drugs and other environmental factors account for less than 1% of all birth defects. The general risk is extremely slight, even if you have already been exposed to a specific teratogen. Second, if you haven't, knowing what the risks are can help you to avoid them, improving your

baby's odds still more. Third, in spite of the dire warnings making headlines and highlighting news programs daily, never have the chances of having a healthy, normal baby been better.

Of course, nothing in life is totally without risk. But in dealing with risks, we learn to weigh them against benefits. This is never more important than during pregnancy, when each decision potentially affects the safety and well-being of not one but two lives. When you're faced with the decision of whether or not to smoke, to have a before-dinner cocktail, to nibble on a chocolate bar instead of an apple while watching TV, you are going to be weighing risk against benefit. Are the benefits, if any, you are going to derive from smoking, drinking, or junk-food snacking worth the risks to your baby?

Well, most of the time, your answer will probably be no. But once in a while you may decide that a little risk will be worth it. One glass of wine, for example, to toast your anniversary. The risk to your baby is practically nil. And the benefit (a more festive anniversary) is really important. Or a big chunk of cake for your birthday—a lot of empty calories, true. But just this once they won't really deprive baby of necessary nutrients, and after all, it *is* your birthday.

Some risk vs. benefit decisions are easy. For instance, regular heavy alcohol consumption throughout pregnancy can handicap your child for life (see page 54). Giving up the pleasure you derive from drinking may take considerable effort, but your choice is clear: Give it up, or don't have the baby.

Or say you have an infection and are running a fever that's high enough to pose a threat to your baby. Your doctor won't hesitate to use medication—the safest possible drug at the lowest effective dose—to wipe out the infection and bring down the fever. In this case, the benefit of drug use far outweighs its possible harm. A mild fever, on the other hand, won't hurt your baby and will help your body fight an infection. So before resorting to medication, your doctor will probably give your body a chance to cure itself, on the grounds that the possible risk of taking the drug outweighs its potential benefits.

Other decisions are not so clear cut. What if you have a terrible cold with sinus headaches which have been keeping you up at night? Should you take a cold tablet to help you get some rest? Or should you suffer through sleepless nights which won't do you or the baby any good? The best way to approach such decisions is:

❖ Determine if there are alternative no-risk ways of obtaining the benefits you seek—perhaps through non-drug approaches (see page 65). Try them. If they don't work, continue to evaluate your original option, in this case, cold tablets.

❖ Ask your physician about risks and benefits. It's important to remember that not all drugs are known to cause birth defects, and that many have been used safely in pregnancy. New studies are turning up more information on drug safety, or lack of it, daily. Your practitioner has access to this information.

❖ Do some research on your own. For the latest information on the safety of a particular drug during pregnancy, check with the Federal Drug Administration or the March of Dimes. (See page 66.)

❖ Determine if there are ways of increasing the benefits or decreasing the risks (taking the safest, most effective pain reliever in the smallest effective doses for the shortest possible time), and try to ensure that if you do take the risk, you will receive the benefit (take your cold tablet before you go to bed, when you are most likely to get that needed rest).

❖ In consultation with your practitioner, review all the information you've gathered—weighing risks against benefits—and make your decision.

During pregnancy you will be challenged to make intelligent decisions in dozens of situations, weighing risk against benefit. Each decision you make will impact on your chance of having a healthy baby. But an occasional wrong decision isn't likely to be catastrophic— it will change the odds only very slightly. If you've already made a few not-so-terrific choices and there's no way to undo them, forget them. Just try to make better decisions for the rest of your pregnancy. And remember, the odds are very much in your baby's favor!

4
The Best-Odds Diet

There's a tiny new being developing inside you. The odds are already fairly good that he or she will be born healthy. But you have the chance to improve those odds significantly, to come as close as possible to guaranteeing your baby not just good health, but excellent health—with every bite of food you put in your mouth.

That's not just idle theory. A study done at the Harvard School of Public Health is a dramatic illustration of how closely the state of a baby's health at birth is tied to its mother's diet during pregnancy. Of the women in the study who had good-to-excellent diets, fully 95% had babies in excellent or good health. Only 5% of their babies were in fair or poor health. On the other hand, only 8% of women on really awful diets (composed largely of junk foods) had babies in excellent or good health, and 65% of their infants were in the poorest health condition—stillborn, premature, functionally immature, or with congenital defects.

Of course, most of the women in the study (like most pregnant women) were on neither excellent diets nor extremely poor ones. Their diets were average, and so was the health of their children. Eighty-eight percent had babies in good or fair health. But only 6% had infants in really excellent health—which is, after all, what most of us want for our children.

If your eating habits aren't the most disciplined or virtuous to begin with, following the Best-Odds Diet will probably present you and your willpower with quite a challenge. But when you consider the result of your extra efforts—better odds for your baby's health—we think you'll agree it's a challenge worth taking. (And because the Best-Odds Diet nourishes your baby without putting excess weight on you, the odds of your quickly regaining your figure will also be improved.)

NINE BASIC PRINCIPLES FOR NINE MONTHS OF HEALTHY EATING

Make Every Bite Count. You've got only nine months of meals and snacks with which to give your baby the best possible start in life. Make every one of them count. Before you close your mouth on a forkful of food, consider, "Is this the best I can give my baby?" If it will benefit your baby, chew away. If it'll benefit only your sweet tooth or appease your appetite, put your fork down.

All Calories Are Not Created Equal.

For example, 150 empty candy-bar calories are not equal to the 150 calories in ⅓ of a cup of mineral- and vitamin-packed raisins. Nor are the 100 calories in 10 high-fat potato chips equal to the 100 in a baked potato. So choose your calories with care, selecting quality over quantity. (Your baby will benefit a lot more from 2,000 nutrient-rich calories daily than 4,000 mostly empty ones.)

Starve Yourself, Starve Your Baby.

Just as you wouldn't consider starving your baby after it's born, you shouldn't consider starving it in utero. The fetus can't live well off your flesh, no matter how ample. It needs regular nourishment at regular intervals. Never, never skip a meal.[1] Even if you're not hungry, the baby is. If persistent heartburn or a constant bloated feeling is spoiling your appetite, spread your daily requirements out over six small meals a day instead of three large ones.

---

1. That means never fasting during pregnancy, either. An Israeli study showed a jump in deliveries just after Yom Kippur, the Day of Atonement, indicating that fasting late in pregnancy could trigger an early delivery.

Become an Efficiency Expert.

Fill your daily nutritional requirements in the most efficient way possible within your caloric needs. Eating six tablespoons of peanut butter (if you can get it down) at 600 calories, or about 25% of your daily allotment, is a considerably less efficient way of getting 25 grams of protein than eating 3½ ounces of water-packed tuna at 125 calories. And eating a cup and a half of ice cream (about 450 calories) is a far less efficient way of getting 300 milligrams of calcium than drinking a glass of skim milk (90 calories). Fat, because it has more than twice as many calories per gram as either proteins or carbohydrates, is a particularly inefficient food selection. Choose lean meats over fatty ones, low-fat milk and dairy products over full fat, broiled foods over fried; spread butter lightly; sauté in a teaspoon of fat rather than a quarter cup.

Carbohydrates Are a Complex Issue.

Some women concerned about gaining too much weight during pregnancy mistakenly drop carbohydrates from their diets like so many hot potatoes. True, simple carbohydrates (like white bread, white rice, refined cereals, cakes, cookies, pretzels, sugars, syrups) are nutritionally weak—supplying little but calories. But complex carbohydrates (whole-grain breads and cereals, brown rice, vegetables, dried beans and peas, and, of course, hot potatoes—especially in their skins) and fresh fruit supply essential B vitamins, trace minerals, protein, and important fiber. Good not only for your baby, but for you. They'll help keep nausea and constipation in check, and because they are filling but not fattening, they'll help keep your weight down, too.

Sweet Nothings: Nothing But Trouble.
No calorie is as empty, and therefore as wasted, as a calorie of sugar. In addition, researchers are finding that sugar may be not only void of value, but harmful—possibly implicated in diabetes, heart disease, depression, hyperactivity. That's why the Best-Odds Diet recommends eating no refined sugars (brown, white, turbinado, honey, maple syrup, corn syrup) at all during pregnancy. Every calorie they supply could better come from foods which yield a higher return nutritionally for your baby.

Eat Foods That Can Remember Where They Came From.
If your green beans haven't seen their native fields for months (having been boiled, processed, preserved, and canned since harvesting), they probably don't have much of their natural goodness left to offer your baby. Choose fresh vegetables first, or if they're not in season, the quick-frozen variety. To cook, steam or stir fry lightly, so they'll retain their vitamins and minerals. Fruits, too, should be eaten fresh and unsweetened. Avoid prepared foods that are full of chemicals, sugar, salt, and low in nutritive value. Choose a fresh chicken breast over chicken roll, fresh (preferably whole-wheat) noodles and cheese over a dehydrated casserole mix, an unsweetened baked apple in place of a slice of apple pie.

Make Good Eating a Family Affair.
If there are subversive elements at home, urging you to bake chocolate chip cookies or to add potato chips to your shopping list, it's a sure bet that the Best-Odds Diet won't stand a chance. To avoid sabotage, put the whole household on the diet with you. Bake naturally sweet Fruity Oatmeal Cookies (page 88) instead of chocolate chip; bring home whole-wheat pretzels or toasted sunflower seeds instead of potato chips. In addition to a healthier baby and a relatively slimmer you, there will be the postpartum bonus of a fitter, trimmer husband and older children (if you have them) with better eating habits. Continue the Best-Odds Diet for the whole family after delivery and you will be giving each member the best odds for a longer and healthier life.

Don't Sabotage Your Diet.
The best prenatal diet strategy in the world is easily undermined when the expectant mother ignores three potential dangers to her developing offspring: alcohol, cigarettes, and caffeine. Read about these under individual listings in this book, and reinforce your good dietary habits accordingly.

THE BEST-ODDS DAILY DOZEN

Calories. The old adage that a pregnant woman is eating for two is true. But it's important to remember that one of the two is a tiny developing fetus whose caloric needs are significantly lower than yours—a mere

300 a day. That means that if you eat enough calories to sustain your pre-pregnancy weight, you only have to consume 300 to 500[2] additional calories daily during your pregnancy.[3] In spite of the numerous pregnancy diets you may see that seem to recommend you eat enough food to feed a family of four, ingesting more calories than this is not only unnecessary but unwise.

There are four exceptions to this basic formula. In each of these cases the expectant mother should discuss her calorie needs with her practitioner: the overweight woman, who, with proper nutritional guidance, can possibly do with fewer calories; the seriously underweight woman, who certainly needs more; the adolescent, who is still growing herself and has special nutritional needs; and the woman carrying multiple fetuses, who will have to add 300 calories for each of them.

Having to eat 500 extra calories a day sounds like a food lover's dream, but sad to say, it isn't. By the time you've guzzled your four glasses of milk (total of 380 calories) and taken your required extra grams of protein, you've probably come close to exceeding your allowance.

Protein. The amino acids that compose proteins are the building blocks of human cells, and they are particularly important when you're building a new baby. Lack of protein seems to have as much to do with babies being small for their gestational ages as does lack of calories. So at minimum, the pregnant woman should have 75 grams of protein every day. We think 100 grams, the amount usually recommended for high-risk pregnancies, is safer since the larger quantity may help prevent your pregnancy from becoming high risk. The Best-Odds Diet Food Selection Groups shows you how easily and deliciously you can get your 100 grams—without exceeding your calorie limit. If you come up short on any particular day, simply eat a couple of hard-boiled egg whites (most of an egg's protein is found in the white), each of which will provide 3 grams of high-quality protein for a mere 15 calories.

Vitamin C Foods. You and baby both need vitamin C daily for growth, tissue repair, wound healing, development of strong bones and teeth, and various other metabolic processes. In addition to the small amount the prenatal supplement you take every day contains, eat at least one vitamin C–rich food daily. Vitamin C content is most available in foods that are fresh and uncooked, as exposure to heat, light, and air destroys it over time. (See Vitamin C Foods, page 82, for good food choices that are high in vitamin C.)

2. Because metabolism speeds up in pregnancy, you may need the higher quantity, particularly in mid and late pregnancy. The only way you can tell if you are getting the right number of calories is to see if you are gaining the right amount of weight (see page 127). Adjust your intake according to your weekly gain—but be sure you never cut out necessary nutrients along with the calories.

3. To find out how many calories it takes to sustain your prepregnancy weight, multiply your prepregnancy weight by 12 if you're sedentary, 15 if you're moderately active, and up to 22 if you're very active.

Calcium. Back in elementary school you probably learned that growing children need plenty of calcium for strong bones and teeth. Well, so do growing fetuses on their way to becoming growing children. Calcium is also vital for muscle, heart, and nerve development, blood clotting, and enzyme activity. Be diligent about your four-glasses-of-milk-a-day, or the equivalent in high-calcium foods. One of the great things about milk is that it can be hidden in so many foods: soups, casseroles, breads, cereals, desserts—particularly by using non-fat dry milk, ⅓ of a cup of which equals a glass of fluid milk. (One terrific way to sneak 2 cups of milk into one: Double-the-Milk Shake, page 87.) For those who can't tolerate milk, the Food Selection Groups provide a variety of adequate equivalents.

Green Leafy and Yellow Vegetables and Fruits. These rabbit-favorites supply the Vitamin A that's important for healthy cell growth (your baby's cells are multiplying at a fantastic rate), for healthy skin, bones, and much more. They also provide vital doses of vitamin E, riboflavin, folic acid, B$_6$, numerous minerals, and constipation-fighting fiber. Even if you're not a vegetable lover, you're sure to find some of those that you can stomach in the Food Selection Groups. (If all vegetables are completely offensive early in pregnancy, short-term substitution of vegetable juice is acceptable.) Have two to three servings a day.

Other Fruits and Vegetables. In addition to the deep green and yellow and vitamin C produce, you should have at least one other fruit or vegetable daily—for added fiber, vitamins, and minerals. A variety are suggested in the Food Selection Groups.

Cereals and Grains. Whole-grain foods (made from wheat, oats, rye, barley, corn, rice, millet, triticale, soy, and so on) are packed with vitamins, particularly the B vitamins that are needed for just about every part of your developing baby's body. They are also rich in trace minerals like zinc and selenium, which have been getting so much publicity lately, and in the equally well-publicized constipation-combating fiber. Starchy grain foods may also help reduce early-pregnancy morning sickness. The different types of grains are pretty much interchangeable, but the more variety the better. Be adventurous. Bread your chicken with a mixture of whole-wheat flour or breadcrumbs and wheat germ; add triticale to your rice pilaf. Just one caveat: use only *whole* grains. Refined flours, even when they are enriched, are lacking in trace minerals and fiber.

The Iron-Rich Foods. Since large amounts of iron are essential for the developing blood supply of the fetus, you'll need more during these nine months than at any other time in your life. Get as much as you can from natural sources (see Food Selection Groups). But because it's often difficult to fill your iron requirement through diet alone, make sure your vitamin supplement contains iron, too.

High-Fat Foods. This requirement is definitely easier to exceed than to fill exactly, since fat is so concentrated. A tablespoon of oil in your salad dressing and one of butter on your bread will do it for the day. Be aware that fat used in cooking counts, too. So if you've fried your eggs in a tablespoon of margarine, you must subtract that from your day's allotment. See the Food Selection Groups for the recommended quantities.

Salty Foods. At one time the medical establishment prescribed limiting salt (sodium chloride) during pregnancy, because it contributed to water retention and bloating. Now it is believed that some increase in body fluids is necessary and normal, and that a moderate amount of sodium is needed to maintain adequate fluid levels. Still, very large quantities of salt and very salty foods (such as pickles, soy sauce, and potato chips) aren't good for anyone, pregnant or not. High sodium intake is closely linked to high blood pressure, a condition which can cause a variety of potentially dangerous complications in pregnancy, labor, and delivery. To be sure that you are getting your quota of iodine, use iodized salt. As a general rule, salt your food only to taste.

Fluids. You're not only eating for two, you're drinking for two. If you've always been a non-drinker— one of those people who goes through the day with barely a sip of anything—now's the time to change your habits. As body fluids increase during pregnancy, so does your need for fluid intake. Your baby, too, needs fluids. Most of his body, like yours, is composed of water. Extra fluids also help keep your skin soft, lessen the likelihood of constipation, rid your body of toxins and waste products, and reduce the risk of urinary tract infection. Be sure to get at least eight glasses a day— more, if possible. Of course, they don't all have to come straight from the tap. You can count milk, fruit or vegetable juices, small quantities of naturally decaffeinated coffee (from which caffeine has been removed without the use of chemicals) or tea, soups, or plain soda water (seltzer, not club soda—which usually has added salt).

Supplements. Think of your vitamin supplement as extra health insurance. Even if you eat the very best diet when you're pregnant, you can't be sure of getting all the nutrients you and your baby need from your daily food intake. First of all, especially early in pregnancy, nausea, heartburn and indigestion, or food aversions may interfere with your eating the right foods. Second, storage, cooking, and exposure to air can rob food of vitamins. And third, the requirements for some nutrients in pregnancy are so high that it is virtually impossible to get enough from your diet alone.

A good supplement formulation should contain, in addition to the usual vitamins and minerals found in multivitamin pills: calcium, iron, vitamin B_{12} (particularly important for vegetarians), folic acid, and such trace minerals as zinc and selenium.

Remember, however, the emphasis here is on *supplement:* No pill, no matter how power packed, can replace a good diet. It's very important that most of your vitamins and minerals come from foods, because that is the way nutrients can be most effectively utilized. Fresh foods (not processed) contain not only the nutrients that we know about and that can be synthesized in a pill, but a great many others that are as yet undiscovered. Thirty years ago, a pregnancy pill didn't contain zinc and the other trace minerals we now know to be necessary to good health. But whole-wheat bread has always contained it. Likewise, food supplies fiber and water (fruits and vegetables are loaded with both) and important calories and protein—none of which come packaged in a pill. (Incidentally, beware of those pills claiming to be equivalent to daily vegetable requirements—those claims are totally fraudulent.)

And don't think that because a little is good, a lot is better. Any vitamin supplementation beyond the RDA (the recommended daily allowance) should be considered medication and should be used only under medical supervision, when benefit outweighs risk.

THE BEST-ODDS DIET FOOD SELECTION GROUPS[4]

PROTEIN FOODS

Every day have four of the following, or a combination of these foods equivalent to four servings. Servings contain between 18 and 25 grams of protein, and you should consume 75 to 100 grams a day.

3 8-ounce glasses of skim or low-fat milk or buttermilk
¾ cup low-fat cottage cheese
2 ½ ounces Parmesan or Edam cheese
3 ounces Swiss or cheddar cheese
2 ½ ounces low-fat cheese
4 large egg whites
2 large whole eggs, plus 1 egg white
3 ½ ounces tuna
2 ½ ounces chicken or turkey, without skin
3 ½ ounces fish or shrimp
5 ounces clams, crabs, lobster
3 ounces lean beef or pork
3 ounces veal
4 ounces fatty beef
3 ½ ounces lean lamb or liver
5 or 6 ounces tofu (bean curd)
Texturized vegetable protein[5]
1 serving of a complete protein combination (box, page 83)

HIGH-PROTEIN SNACKS

Nuts and seeds
Whole-grain baked goods
Soy baked goods

---

4. Many foods fill more than one nutritional requirement, so Food Selection Groups may overlap. The same 3 glasses of milk, for example, will give you 3 calcium servings and 1 protein portion.

5. Recipes vary; some have a high protein/calorie ratio, others low, so read nutrition labels, remembering you need 20 to 25 grams of protein per serving.

Yogurt
Hard cheese
Hard-boiled eggs
Wheat germ

VITAMIN C FOODS

Have at least one of the following, or a combination equal to one, every day. Your body can't store this vitamin, so be careful not to skip a day.

½ large grapefruit
1 small grapefruit
1 cup grapefruit juice
1 large fresh orange
6 ounces orange juice
3 tablespoons orange juice concentrate
¾ cup lemon juice
1 medium mango
⅔ cup cubed papaya
½ small cantaloupe
⅔ cup strawberries
1½ large tomatoes
1¼ cups tomato juice
1 cup vegetable juice
1½ cups shredded raw cabbage (or cole slaw)
1 small red or green pepper
⅔ cup broccoli
¾ cup raw or 1 cup cooked cauliflower
¾ cup cooked fresh kale
½ cup collard greens, cooked in minimal water
1 cup cooked kohlrabi
4 ounces raw spinach

CALCIUM-RICH FOODS

Take four servings of these foods daily or any combination that is equivalent to four servings. Vegetarians who don't drink milk should also take a calcium supplement, because the calcium in some vegetarian products is not easily absorbed by the body. You need 1,280 to 1,300 milligrams daily.

8 ounces skim or low-fat milk or buttermilk
½ cup evaporated skim or low-fat milk
1¾ cups low-fat cottage cheese
1½ ounces cheddar or American cheese
1¼ ounces Swiss cheese
1 cup yogurt
⅓ cup non-fat dry milk
4 ounces canned salmon with bones
3 ounces canned sardines with bones
3½ ounces canned Pacific mackerel with bones
2 to 3 tablespoons ground sesame seeds
Soy milk and soy protein[6]
⅔ cup collard greens
1½ cups cooked fresh kale
1⅓ cups cooked fresh mustard or turnip greens
2 cups broccoli
2½ tablespoons blackstrap molasses

CALCIUM-RICH SNACKS

Almonds
Apricots
Dried figs
Baked goods made with sesame seeds or soy flour

---

6. Soy formulas vary; check the nutrition label to determine calcium equivalence, remembering you need 1,280 to 1,300 milligrams daily.

For Vegetarians

The following are good for all pregnant women; however, non-vegetarians should count only one serving a day in their protein allowance.

VEGETARIAN COMPLETE PROTEIN COMBINATIONS

Choose 1 serving (10 to 13 grams protein) from the legumes list plus 1 serving (10 to 13 grams protein) from the grains list for a complete protein combination.

LEGUMES

1 cup cooked beans: broad, cow (black eyed)
¾ cup soybeans or soy grits
¾ cup mung beans
1 cup chick peas
1 cup lentils

GRAINS

1 ½ cups grains:[7] brown rice, groats, barley, millet, bulgur
1 ⅓ cups wild rice
2 ounces (before cooking) soy pasta
2 to 4 ounces (before cooking) whole-wheat pasta (depending on protein content)
2 ounces (before cooking) Superoni or soy pasta
⅔ cup (before cooking) oats
¾ cup seeds: sesame, sunflower, pumpkin
1 ounce pine nuts
½ cup Brazil nuts or peanuts
2 ounces cashews, walnuts, or pistachios

DAIRY COMPLETE PROTEIN COMBINATIONS

Choose 1 serving (about 10 grams protein) from the legumes and grains list and 1 serving (about 12 grams protein) from the dairy food list for a complete protein.

LEGUMES AND GRAINS

1 portion beans, peas, lentils, grains, pasta, noodles (see above)
2 slices whole-grain bread
⅔ cup oatmeal
1 ½ ounces ready-to-eat cereal

DAIRY FOODS

2 ounces cheddar, American, Swiss, low-fat cheese
½ cup cottage cheese
¼ cup Parmesan cheese
⅓ cup non-fat dry milk plus 2 tablespoons wheat germ
2 ½ tablespoons peanut butter
1 cup yogurt plus 2 tablespoons wheat germ
2 eggs plus 1 egg white

---

7. These grains are low in protein; enrich with 2 tablespoons of wheat germ per serving.

GREEN LEAFY AND YELLOW VEGETABLES AND FRUITS

You need two or three a day, one of which should be raw. Try to eat one yellow and one green daily:

2 or 3 fresh or dried apricots
½ medium mango
1 cup cubed papaya
⅔ cup dried yellow peaches
1 medium persimmon
½ cup canned pumpkin
½ cup beet greens
⅔ cup broccoli or turnip greens
1 raw carrot, or ⅓ cup cooked
½ cup collard greens
3 ½ ounces endive or escarole
½ cup kale or mustard greens
8 large leaves dark green leafy lettuce
3 ½ ounces fresh spinach, ½ cup cooked
⅔ cup winter squash
1 small sweet potato or yam
⅔ cup Swiss chard

OTHER FRUITS AND VEGETABLES

Have at least one of the following daily; two would be better:

1 apple or ½ cup unsweetened applesauce
6 to 7 asparagus spears
1 small banana
1 cup bean sprouts
¾ cup green beans
⅔ cup blueberries, blackberries, raspberries, lingonberries
⅔ cup Brussels sprouts
⅔ cup pitted fresh cherries
⅔ cup grapes
1 wedge honeydew melon (⅛ melon)
1 cup fresh mushrooms
1 medium nectarine or peach
9 pods okra
½ cup parsley
1 medium pear
1 medium slice fresh or canned unsweetened pineapple
1 medium potato
⅔ cup zucchini

WHOLE GRAINS AND OTHER COMPLEX CARBOHYDRATES

Have four or five of the following every day:

1 slice whole-wheat, whole-rye, other whole-grain or soy bread
½ cup cooked brown rice
½ cup cooked wild rice
½ cup cooked whole-grain cereal (oatmeal, Wheatena, Ralston)
1 ounce unsweetened whole-grain ready-to-eat cereal (Shredded Wheat, Nutri-Grain, Grape Nuts, etc.)
¼ cup wheat germ
½ cup cooked millet, bulgur, triticale, kasha (buckwheat groats)
½ cup cooked whole-grain, soy, or high-protein-type pasta
2 × 2 × 1-inch corn bread (made with non-degerminated meal)
½ cup beans or peas

IRON-RICH FOODS

Small amounts of iron are found in most of the fruits, vegetables, grains, and meats you will eat every day. But try to have some of the following higher-iron-content foods daily, along with your supplement:

Dried fruit (raisins, apricots, prunes, peaches, currants)
Liver and other organ meats (use infrequently)
Beef
Sardines
Blackstrap molasses
Soy baked goods
Spinach

HIGH-FAT FOODS

Have 2 tablespoons a day unless you are gaining weight too quickly, in which case limit your fat intake to 1 tablespoon, selected from the following:

Polyunsaturated vegetable oils
Margarine high in polyunsaturates (limit 1 tablespoon per day)
Butter (limit 1 tablespoon per day)
Mayonnaise (limit 1 tablespoon per day)

One of the following can be substituted for a tablespoon of fat:
½ small avocado
3 tablespoons light cream
2 tablespoons heavy (whipping) cream
2 tablespoons cream cheese
4 tablespoons sour cream
20 almonds
3 tablespoons peanuts, pecans, or walnuts

BEST-ODDS RECIPES

These recipes are designed not only to pacify your sweet and snacking tooth, but also to give you party "cocktail" suggestions and a few breakfast ideas.

CREAM OF TOMATO SOUP

Makes 3 servings

In a saucepan, melt over low heat:
   1 tablespoon margarine or butter
Add and blend over very low heat for 2 minutes:
   2 tablespoons whole-wheat flour
Gradually blend in over low heat:
   1¾ cups evaporated skim milk
Continue cooking over low heat, stirring occasionally, until thickened. Stir in until smooth:
   3 cups tomato or vegetable juice
   4 tablespoons tomato paste
   Salt and pepper to taste
   Fresh or dried oregano and basil to taste (optional)
Continue cooking over low heat for 5 minutes, stirring frequently. Serve soup warm, topped with, if desired:
   A scoop of low-fat cottage cheese
   A sprinkling of Parmesan cheese or wheat germ

1 serving = 1 calcium-rich food serving plus 1 vitamin C food (plus 1 green leafy, if vegetable juice is used)

POWER-PACKED OATMEAL

Makes 1 serving

Bring to a boil in a small saucepan:
> **1 ¼ cups water**

Add, stirring to mix thoroughly:
> **½ cup rolled oats**
> **2 tablespoons wheat germ (if constipation is a problem, substitute unprocessed bran for all or part of wheat germ)**
> **Salt to taste**

Lower the heat and cook 5 minutes or longer, according to desired texture, adding additional water if necessary. Remove the pan from the heat and stir in:
> **⅓ cup instant non-fat dry milk**

Serve immediately.

SWEET VARIATION: Add 2 tablespoons raisins and 1 tablespoon frozen apple juice concentrate (optional) when you add the oats; ground cinnamon (optional) to taste when you add the milk.

SAVORY VARIATION: Add pepper, grated Parmesan or cheddar cheese (remember to count the cheddar as part of your milk requirement) to taste when you add the milk.

1 serving = 1 grain serving plus 1 calcium-rich food serving plus 1 protein serving plus high fiber

BRAN MUFFINS

Makes 12 to 16 muffins

In a small saucepan, simmer 5 minutes over low heat, stirring:
> **⅔ cup raisins**
> **¼ cup frozen apple juice concentrate, thawed, undiluted**
> **4 tablespoons frozen orange juice concentrate, thawed, undiluted**

Combine in mixing bowl and blend:
> **1 ½ cups whole-wheat flour**
> **½ cup wheat germ**
> **1 ½ cups unprocessed bran**
> **1 ¼ teaspoons baking soda**
> **½ cup chopped nuts**
> **1 teaspoon ground cinnamon (optional)**

Beat together in a separate bowl:
> **1 ½ cups low-fat buttermilk**
> **¾ cup frozen apple juice concentrate, thawed, undiluted**
> **2 egg whites, slightly beaten**
> **⅓ cup instant non-fat dry milk**
> **2 tablespoons melted margarine or butter, cooled**

Combine the dry and liquid ingredients, blending thoroughly in a few strokes. Fold in the raisins with their cooking juice. Fill non-stick muffin tins, or paper muffin cups placed in regular tins, to ⅔ full. Bake in a preheated 350°F oven for about 20 minutes, or until a toothpick inserted in the center of a muffin comes out clean.

1 large muffin = 1 grain serving plus high fiber

WHOLE-WHEAT BUTTERMILK PANCAKES

Makes approximately 12 pancakes (3 servings)

Note: Allow 1 hour preparation time for batter to settle.

Purée in a blender:
1 cup low-fat buttermilk
1 teaspoon frozen apple juice concentrate, thawed, undiluted
¾ cup whole-wheat flour
5 tablespoons wheat germ
⅓ cup non-fat dry milk
Dash of salt to taste
Ground cinnamon to taste (optional)
Stir in:
2 teaspoons baking powder
In a mixing bowl, beat until stiff:
2 large egg whites
Quickly beat the buttermilk-flour mixture into the egg whites. Let the batter stand for 1 hour, then heat a non-stick skillet. When it is hot, brush on:
Margarine or butter
Stir the batter and spoon it onto the skillet to make pancakes of the desired size. When the surface of the pancakes begins to bubble and the undersides are nicely browned, turn and brown the other side. Continue making the pancakes until the batter is used up (you will need between 2 and 3 teaspoons more butter or margarine). Serve them with:
Unsweetened applesauce
Unsweetened preserves (fruit only) or apple butter
Plain low-fat yogurt

VARIATION: Add ¼ cup raisins to the batter.

1 serving = 1 grain serving plus 1 protein serving plus ½ calcium-rich food serving plus high fiber

DOUBLE-THE-MILK SHAKE

Makes 1 serving

Note: Freeze the banana, peeled and wrapped in a plastic bag, 12 to 24 hours ahead of time.

Purée in a blender:
1 cup skim or low-fat milk
⅓ cup non-fat dry milk
1 frozen, overripe banana, cut into chunks
1 teaspoon vanilla extract
Dash of ground cinnamon, or to taste (optional)

BERRY VARIATION: Add ½ cup berries, fresh or unsweetened frozen (thawed), and 1 tablespoon frozen apple juice concentrate (thawed, undiluted) before blending; omit the cinnamon.

"CREAMSICLE" VARIATION: Add 2 tablespoons frozen orange juice concentrate (thawed, undiluted); omit the cinnamon.

One banana shake = 2 calcium-rich food servings plus ⅔ protein serving plus 1 fruit serving

One berry variation = 2 calcium-rich food servings plus ⅔ protein serving plus 2 fruit servings

FIG BARS

Makes about 36 cookie bars

Cream together in a bowl:
>**1 tablespoon fructose**
>**4 tablespoons (½ stick) margarine or butter**

Add, and continue to cream:
>**½ cup plus 2 tablespoons frozen apple juice concentrate that has been heated until warm**

Add, and mix to form a dough:
>**1½ cups whole-wheat flour**
>**1 cup wheat germ**
>**1½ teaspoons vanilla extract**

Divide dough in two, forming each half into a rectangular bar. Wrap them, separately, in wax paper and chill for 1 hour.

Combine in a saucepan, and cook together over low heat until soft:
>**1 pound dried figs, chopped**
>**½ cup frozen apple juice concentrate, thawed, undiluted**

Remove from the heat and add, stirring until smooth:
>**2 tablespoons ground almonds or other nuts**

On a large non-stick cookie sheet that has been lightly greased with oil or non-stick spray, roll out one rectangular bar of dough until it is very thin, evening out the edges as much as possible. Over this evenly spread the fig mixture. Roll out the second rectangle of dough between two sheets of wax paper to the same size as the first rectangle. Remove one sheet of wax paper, and flip the dough as neatly as possible over the fig mixture. Press down lightly, and even out the ends with a sharp knife.

Bake in a preheated 350°F oven for 15 to 30 minutes or until lightly browned. Cut into squares or diamond shapes while still hot.

2 or 3 cookies = 1 nutritious snack plus high fiber

FRUITY OATMEAL COOKIES

Makes 24 2-inch cookies

Place in a saucepan and simmer together until the fruit softens:
>**10 dates, pitted**
>**6 tablespoons frozen apple juice concentrate, undiluted**

Purée mixture in a blender or a food processor, then pour it into a bowl, and add:
>**2 tablespoons vegetable oil**
>**1½ cups rolled oats (or a mixture of oats and raw wheat flakes)**
>**1 cup raisins**
>**¼ to ½ cup chopped nuts**
>**Ground cinnamon to taste**

Beat lightly in a separate bowl:
>**1 egg white**

Fold gently into the cookie mixture. Drop the batter in tablespoonsful onto a greased cookie sheet. Bake in a preheated 350°F oven for 10 to 12 minutes.

2 or 3 cookies = 1 nutritious snack plus high fiber

FRUITED YOGURT

Makes about 1 cup

Purée in a blender:
> **¾ cup plain low-fat yogurt**
> **½ teaspoon fresh grated orange peel**
> **½ cup fresh or frozen (thawed) unsweetened strawberries**
> **1 tablespoon frozen orange juice concentrate, thawed, undiluted**
> **5 teaspoons frozen apple juice concentrate, thawed, undiluted**
> **½ teaspoon ground cinnamon, or to taste (optional)**

1 cup = 1 fruit serving plus ¾ calcium-rich food serving

MOCK STRAWBERRY DAIQUIRI

Makes 4 servings

Purée in blender:
> **2 cups washed, hulled fresh or frozen (unsweetened) strawberries (or substitute 2 very ripe bananas, cut into small pieces)**
> **1 cup ice cubes, cracked (decrease to ½ cup if using frozen berries)**
> **¼ cup frozen apple juice concentrate, undiluted, or to taste**
> **1 tablespoon lime juice**
> **1 teaspoon rum extract**

Serve cold in tall glasses.

1 serving = 1 fruit serving

VIRGIN SANGRIA

Makes 5 to 6 servings

Combine in a large pitcher:
> **3 cups unsweetened grape juice**
> **¾ cup frozen apple juice concentrate, thawed, undiluted**
> **1 tablespoon lime juice**
> **1 tablespoon lemon juice**

Stir to blend, and add:
> **1 small unpeeled lemon, sliced and seeded**
> **1 small unpeeled orange, sliced and seeded**
> **1 small unpeeled McIntosh apple, cored, cut into eighths**

Stir well, and chill. Add just before serving:
> **¾ cup seltzer (unsalted club soda)**

Serve in wine glasses over ice.

1 serving = 1 fruit serving

FARINA-BANANA PUDDING

Makes 2 servings

In a small saucepan, bring to a boil:

1 cup water

½ cup frozen apple juice concentrate, thawed, undiluted

½ cup apple juice

Stir in, lower heat, and cook until thickened:

½ cup farina (iron-enriched)

2 tablespoons wheat germ

Cool. Stir in:

⅔ cup instant non-fat dry milk

1 teaspoon vanilla extract

½ teaspoon ground cinnamon (optional)

Set inside. In a mixing bowl, beat until stiff:

2 egg whites

Beat into the egg whites:

2 very ripe bananas, mashed and sprinkled with lemon juice

Gently fold egg whites into farina mixture. Mound in individual sherbet glasses and chill. If desired, serve with:

Chopped nuts

1 portion = 1 protein serving plus 1 grain serving plus 1 fruit serving plus 1 calcium serving

CAROB BROWNIES

Makes 1 8 x 8-inch square, 32 1 x 2-inch brownies

Cook in a small saucepan over low heat for 10 minutes:

3 tablespoons butter or margarine

½ cup plus 1 tablespoon frozen apple juice concentrate, thawed, undiluted

½ cup raisins

Remove from heat and add:

1 teaspoon vanilla extract

In a medium-size bowl, mix together:

⅔ cup whole-wheat flour

1 teaspoon baking powder

¼ cup unsweetened carob powder

½ cup chopped walnuts

Combine the apple juice mixture with the carob mixture, blending quickly. Pour into a non-stick 8 x 8-inch brownie tin. Bake in a preheated 350°F oven for 10 minutes. Check with a toothpick for doneness. Let cool in the pan, then cut the brownies into squares.

2 squares = 1 higher-fiber, high-protein, high-iron snack

Part 2

NINE MONTHS AND COUNTING:

From Conception to Delivery

5
The First Month

WHAT YOU CAN EXPECT AT YOUR FIRST PRENATAL VISIT

The first is the most comprehensive of all the prenatal visits.[1] A complete medical history will be taken, and certain tests and procedures will be performed only at this exam. Each practitioner's routine will be slightly different. In general, the examination will include:

Validation of Your Pregnancy. Your practitioner will want to check the following: the pregnancy symptoms you are experiencing; the date of your last normal menstrual period, to determine your estimated date of confinement (EDC) or due date (see page 22); your cervix and uterus, for signs and approximate duration of the pregnancy. If there's any question, a pregnancy test may be ordered, if you haven't already had one.

A Complete History. Come prepared by checking home records and refreshing your memory of the following: your personal medical history (chronic illness, previous major illness or surgery, medications you are presently taking or have taken since conception, known allergies, including drug allergies); your family medical history (genetic disorders and chronic diseases); your social history (age, occupation, habits, such as: smoking, drinking, exercise, diet); your gynecological and obstetrical history (age at first menstrual period, usual length of menstrual cycle, duration and regularity of menstrual periods; past abortions, miscarriages, and live births; course of past pregnancies, labors, and deliveries).

A Complete Physical Examination. This may include: assessment of your general health through examination of heart, lungs, breasts, abdo-

---

1. See appendix for an explanation of the procedures and tests performed.

WHAT YOU MAY LOOK LIKE

By the end of the first month, your baby is a tiny, tadpole-like embryo, smaller than a grain of rice. In the next two weeks, the neural tube (which becomes the brain and spinal cord), heart, digestive tract, sensory organs, and arm and leg buds will begin to form.

and weight, usual and present; inspection of extremities for varicose veins and edema (swelling from excess fluid in tissues), to serve as a baseline for comparison at subsequent visits; inspection and palpation of external genitalia; examination of your vagina and cervix with a speculum inserted internally; examination of your pelvic organs bimanually (with one hand in the vagina and one on the abdomen) and also through the rectum and vagina; assessment of the size and shape of your bony pelvis.

A Battery of Tests. This may include: a Pap smear for cancer detection; gonorrhea culture; blood tests to determine blood type, Rh type, hematocrit or hemoglobin (to check for anemia), and rubella titer; a VDRL (for syphilis); urinalysis to check for glucose (sugar), albumin (protein), white blood cells, blood, and bacteria; tuberculin skin test; sickle cell or Tay-Sachs screening, if indicated.

An Opportunity for Discussion. Bring a list of questions, problems, and symptoms. This is also a good time to talk about fears, philosophy of childbirth, and so on.

men; measurement of your blood pressure to serve as a baseline reading for comparison at subsequent visits; measurement of your height

WHAT YOU MAY BE FEELING

You may feel all of these symptoms at one time or another, or only one or two.

PHYSICALLY:

❖ Absence of menstruation (though you may stain slightly when your

period is expected or when the fertilized egg implants in the uterus[2]

2. It is rare, but a woman may still menstruate in the first two or three months. *Any* bleeding, of course, should be reported to your practitioner.

❖ Fatigue and sleepiness

❖ A need to urinate frequently

❖ Nausea, with or without vomiting, and/or excessive salivation (ptyalism)

❖ Heartburn and indigestion, flatulence, and bloating

❖ Food aversions and cravings

❖ Breast changes (most pronounced in women who have breast changes prior to menstruation): fullness, heaviness, tenderness, tingling; darkening of the areola (the pigmented area around the nipple); sweat glands in the areola become prominent (Montgomery's tubercles), like large goose bumps; a network of bluish lines appear under the skin as blood supply to the breasts increases (though these lines may not appear until later)

EMOTIONALLY:

❖ Instability comparable to premenstrual syndrome, which may include irritability, mood swings, irrationality, weepiness

❖ Misgivings, fear, joy, elation—any or all of these

WHAT YOU MAY BE CONCERNED ABOUT

FATIGUE

"I'm tired all the time. I'm worried that I won't be able to continue working."

It would be surprising if you weren't tired. In some ways, your pregnant body is working harder even when you're resting than a nonpregnant body is when mountain-climbing; you just can't see its efforts. For one thing, it's manufacturing your baby's life support system, the placenta, which won't be completed until the end of the first trimester. For another, it's adjusting to the many other physical and emotional demands of pregnancy, which are considerable. Once your body is adjusted and the placenta is complete (around the fourth month), you should have more energy. Until then, you may need to work fewer hours or take a few days off if you're really dragging. But if your pregnancy continues normally, there is absolutely no reason why you shouldn't stay at your job. Most pregnant women are happier if they keep busy.

Since your fatigue is legitimate, don't fight it. Consider it a signal from your body that you need more rest. That, of course, is more easily suggested than done. But it is worth a try.

Baby Yourself. And your baby—as much as possible, and don't feel guilty about it. Don't try to be Super-Mom-to-Be. Getting enough rest is more important than having your house pass the white-glove test. Keep evenings free of unessential activities. Spend them off your feet when you can, reading, watching TV, scouring baby-name books. If you have older children, play quiet games with them. If you can afford the luxury of an afternoon nap, by all means indulge. If you can't sleep, lie down with a good book. A nap at the office isn't a reasonable goal, of course, but putting your feet up at your desk or in the ladies' lounge during lunch hour is.

Let Others Baby You. Accept your mother-in-law's offer to vacuum and dust the house when she's visiting. Let your dad take the older kids to the zoo on Sunday. Enlist your husband for chores like laundry and marketing.

Get an Hour or Two More Sleep Each Night. Skip the 11 o'clock news and turn in earlier; ask your husband to fix breakfast so you can turn out later.

Be Sure That Your Diet Isn't Deficient. First-trimester fatigue is often aggravated by a deficiency in iron, protein, or just plain calories. Double check the Best-Odds Diet (page 75) to make certain you're filling all of your requirements. And no matter how tired you're feeling, don't be tempted to rev your body up with caffeine, candy bars, and cake. It won't be fooled for long, and after the temporary lift, your blood sugar will plummet, leaving you more fatigued than ever.

When fatigue is severe, especially when it is accompanied by fainting, pallor, breathlessness, and/or palpitations, the possibility of anemia should be considered. (See page 133.)

Though fatigue will probably ease up by month four, you can expect it to return in the last trimester—probably as nature's way of preparing you for those long sleepless nights once the baby has arrived.

MORNING SICKNESS

"I haven't had any morning sickness. Can I still be pregnant?"

Morning sickness, like a craving for pickles and ice cream, is one of those truisms about pregnancy that ain't necessarily so. Only one third to one half of expectant women ever experience the nausea and/or vomiting of morning sickness. If you're among those who never suffer from it, you can consider yourself not only pregnant, but lucky, too.

"My morning sickness lasts all day. I'm afraid I'm not able to keep down enough good food to nourish my baby."

Fortunately, morning sickness (a misnamed malady, because it can strike morning, noon, or night— or even all day long) rarely interferes with proper nutrition enough to harm the developing fetus. And for most women, it doesn't last past the third month—though an occasional expectant mother won't experience it until well into the second trimester and a few, particularly those expecting twins, may enjoy its dubious pleasures for a full nine months.

What causes morning sickness? No one knows for sure, but there's no shortage of theories. It is known that the command post for nausea and vomiting is in a special area in the brain stem. A myriad of physical reasons why this area may be over-stimulated during pregnancy have been suggested, including the high level of the pregnancy hormone HCG in the blood in the first trimester and the rapid stretching of the uterine muscles. The problem is compounded by the relative relaxation of the muscle tissue in the digestive tract, which makes digestion less efficient, and excess acid in the stomach caused by not eating or eating the wrong foods.

But these physical triggers alone can't explain morning sickness, since most are common to all pregnancies and yet not all pregnant women experience nausea and vomiting. Several illuminating facts seem to support the theory that emotional factors augment the physical. For one thing, morning sickness is unknown in some more primitive societies where lifestyles are simpler, more relaxed, and less demanding (although it did exist in ancient Western civilization). For another, many women suffering from hyper-emesis, or excessive vomiting, recover without treatment as soon as they are placed in the relatively tranquil environment of a hospital, away from their families and the problems of day-to-day living. And studies also show that many of these women are highly hypnotizable, which means they are very susceptible to the power of suggestion—and our society surely suggests that morning sickness is an expected part of pregnancy. Also quite revealing is that some women suffer debilitating nausea and vomiting with unwanted, unplanned pregnancies, yet experi-ence no morning sickness at all in pregnancies they are happy about. Physical or mental fatigue also seems to increase the possibility of nausea striking. As does carrying multiple fetuses—probably because of a multiplication of both physical and emotional stresses.

Unfortunately, medical experts are even less certain of the cure for morning sickness than they are of its cause. They do, however, agree that there are many ways of alleviating its symptoms and minimizing its effects. See which work best for you:

❖ Eat a diet high in protein and complex carbohydrates (see the Best-Odds Diet, page 75)—both of which fight nausea. So does good nutrition, so eat as well as you can under the circumstances.

❖ Take plenty of fluids—especially if you're losing them through vomiting. If they are easier to get down than solids when your stomach is upset, use them for getting your nutrients. Concentrate on any of the following you can handle: Double-the-Milk Shakes (see page 87); fruit or vegetable juices; soups, broths, and bouillons. If you find fluids make you queasier, eat solids with high water contents, such as fresh fruits and vegetables—particularly lettuce, melons, and citrus fruits.

❖ Take a prenatal vitamin supplement (see page 98) to compensate for nutrients you may not be getting. But take it when you are least likely to chuck it back up. Your doctor may recommend an additional ration of 50 milligrams of B$_6$, which seems to help relieve nausea in some women. *Do not take any medication for morning sickness.* Benedictin, the only product approved by the FDA for the treatment of morning sickness, was withdrawn from the market in 1983 because of questions about its safety.

❖ Avoid the sight, smell, and taste of foods that make you feel queasy. Don't be a martyr and prepare a sausage and onion hero for your husband if it makes you rush to the bathroom.

❖ Eat often—before you feel hungry. When your stomach is empty, its acids don't have anything to eat but its own lining. This can trigger nausea. So can the low blood sugar caused by long stretches between meals. Six small meals are better than three large. Carry nutritious snacks (dried fruit, whole-grain crackers) with you for convenient snacking.

❖ Eat before nausea strikes. Food will be easier to get down and, by filling your stomach, may prevent an attack.

❖ Eat in bed—for the same reasons you eat often: to keep your stomach full and your blood sugar at an even keel. Before you go to sleep at night, have a snack that is high in protein and complex carbohydrates: a glass of milk and a bran muffin, for example. Twenty minutes before you plan to get out of bed in the morning, have a high-carbohydrate snack: a few whole-wheat crackers, or rice cakes, or a handful of raisins. Keep them next to your bed so you don't have to get up for them, and in case you wake up hungry in the middle of the night.[3]

❖ Get some extra sleep and relaxation. Both emotional and physical fatigue increase morning sickness.

❖ Greet the morning in slow motion—rushing tends to aggravate nausea. Don't jump out of bed and rush out the door. Stay in bed digesting your crackers for 20 minutes, then rise slowly to a leisurely breakfast. This may seem impossible if you have other children, but try to wake up before they do to give yourself a little quiet time, or let your husband handle their early morning needs.

FREQUENT URINATION

"I'm in the bathroom every half hour. Is it normal to be urinating this often?"

Most—though by no means all—pregnant women do make frequent detours to the toilet both in the first and last trimesters. One of the reasons for an initial increase in urinary frequency is the higher volume of body fluids and the improved efficiency of the kidneys, which helps rid the body more quickly of waste products. Another is the pressure of the growing uterus, which is still in the pelvis next to the bladder. The pressure is

---

3. If you start to associate a particular carbohydrate snack (crackers, for instance) with your nausea, switch to a different snack.

often relieved once the uterus rises into the abdominal cavity, around the fourth month. It probably won't return until the baby "drops" in the ninth month and again presses on the bladder. But because the arrangement of internal organs varies slightly from woman to woman, the degree of frequency may also vary.

"How come I'm not urinating frequently?"

No noticeable increase in the frequency of urination may be perfectly normal for you, especially if you ordinarily urinate often. You should, however, be certain you're getting enough fluids (at least eight glasses a day). Not only can insufficient fluid intake be the cause of infrequent urination, it could also lead to urinary tract infection.

BREAST CHANGES

"I hardly recognize my breasts anymore—they're so swollen and tender. Will they stay that way, and will they sag after I give birth?"

Get used to the chesty look. Although it may not be fashionable, it's one of the hallmarks of pregnancy. Your breasts are enlarging (even more than they do premenstrually) because of the increased amounts of estrogen and progesterone your body is now producing. This, and the other changes that occur in the breasts during pregnancy, are all aimed at preparing you to feed your baby when it arrives. The areola (the pigmented area around the nipple) darkens, spreads, and may be spotted with even darker areas. This darkening may fade but not disappear entirely after birth. The little bumps you may notice on the areola are sebaceous (sweat) glands, which become more prominent during pregnancy and return to normal afterwards. The complex road map of blue veins that traverses the breasts—often quite vivid on a fair-skinned woman—represents a mother-to-baby delivery system for nutrients and fluids. After delivery or nursing, they will disappear.

What you won't have to get used to, fortunately, is the sometimes agonizing sensitivity of your breasts. Though they will continue to grow throughout your pregnancy—possibly increasing as much as three cup sizes—they are not likely to remain tender-to-the-touch past the third or fourth month. As for whether or not they will sag after the baby is born, that is at least partly up to you. Stretching and sagging of the breast tissue result from a lack of support during pregnancy—not from pregnancy itself—though the tendency to sag may be genetic. No matter how firm your breasts are now, protect them for the future by wearing a good support bra daily. If your breasts are particularly large or have a tendency to sag, it's a good idea to wear a bra even at night.

VITAMIN SUPPLEMENTS

"Should I be taking vitamins?"

Virtually no one gets a nutritionally perfect diet every day, especially early in pregnancy when morning sickness is a common appetite suppressant. A daily vitamin supplement is your dietary insurance: a guarantee that your baby won't get cheated if you make an occasional slip-up. In addition, some studies have shown that women who take vitamin supplements prior to pregnancy and during the first month can significantly reduce the risk of neural tube problems (such as spina bifida) in their babies. Good supplements, formulated especially for expectant mothers, are available over-the-counter. (See page 80 for what the supplement should contain.) But never use vitamin pills to replace a good diet, only to supplement it. Any vitamins that supply more than the recommended daily allowance for pregnant women should be considered drugs and be taken only under medical supervision, when benefit outweighs risk.

ECTOPIC PREGNANCY

"I've been having occasional cramping. Could I have an ectopic pregnancy without knowing it?"

The fear of ectopic, or tubal, pregnancy lurks somewhere in the mind of nearly every newly pregnant woman who has heard of this abnormal type of implantation. Fortunately, for the vast majority it's an unfounded fear. A fear that can be dismissed completely by the eighth week of pregnancy, by which time most tubal pregnancies have been diagnosed and terminated.

Only about 10 in 1,000 pregnan-

cies are ectopic—that is, take place outside the uterus, usually in the fallopian tubes. A good many of these are diagnosed before a woman even realizes she is pregnant. So chances are that if your doctor has confirmed your pregnancy through a blood test and a physical exam and you've had no signs of ectopic pregnancy, then you can cross this worry off your list.

There are several factors that can make women more susceptible to ectopic pregnancies. They include:

❖ A previous ectopic pregnancy.

❖ Previous pelvic inflammatory disease.

❖ Previous abdominal or tubal surgery with postoperative scarring.

❖ Unsuccessful tubal ligation (sterilization surgery), or tubal ligation reversal.

❖ An IUD in place when conception occurs (an IUD is more likely to prevent conception in the uterus than outside it—thus the increase in the relative incidence of ectopics in IUD users).[4]

❖ Possibly, multiple induced abortions (the evidence isn't clear).

❖ Possibly, exposure to diethylstilbestrol (DES) in the womb, especially if it resulted in significant structural abnormalities of the reproductive tract.

Rare as ectopic pregnancies are, every pregnant woman—particularly those at high risk—should

---

4. But having worn an IUD previously does not appear to increase risk.

be familiar with the symptoms. Occasional cramping, probably the result of ligaments stretching as the uterus grows, is not one of them. But any or all of the following might be, and do require the immediate evaluation of a physician. If you can't reach your physician, go at once to the emergency room at the hospital his or her office or service recommends.

❖ Colicky, crampy pain with tenderness, usually in the lower abdomen—on one side initially, though the pain can radiate throughout the abdomen. Pain may worsen on straining of bowels, coughing, or moving. If tubal rupture occurs, pain becomes very sharp and steady for a short time before diffusing throughout the pelvic region.

❖ Brown vaginal spotting or light bleeding (intermittent or persistent), which may precede pain by several days or weeks. There may be no bleeding without rupture of the tube; with rupture, heavy bleeding may begin.

❖ Nausea and vomiting in about 25% to 50% of women—though this may be difficult to distinguish from morning sickness.

❖ Dizziness or weakness, in some women. If the tube ruptures, fast weak pulse, clammy skin, and fainting are common.

❖ Shoulder pain, in some women.

❖ Feeling of rectal pressure, in some women.

Should these symptoms prove to indicate ectopic pregnancy, quick medical attention can often save the patient's fallopian tube and fertility.

THE CONDITION OF YOUR BABY

"I'm very nervous because I can't really feel my baby. Could it die without my knowing it?"

A t this stage, with no noticeable enlargement of the abdomen or obvious fetal activity, it's hard to imagine that there's really a living, growing baby inside you. But the death of a fetus or embryo that isn't expelled from the uterus in a miscarriage is very rare. When it does happen, the woman loses all signs of pregnancy, including breast tenderness and enlargement, and may develop a brownish discharge, though no frank bleeding. Upon examination, the physician will find that the uterus, rather than growing, has diminished in size.

If at any time all of your pregnancy symptoms should disappear, call your doctor for an appointment. That's a more positive approach than sitting at home worrying.

MISCARRIAGE

"Between what I read and what my mother tells me, I'm afraid everything I've done, am doing, and will do might cause a miscarriage."

F or many expectant women, the fear of miscarriage keeps their joy guarded in the first trimester.

Some even refrain from spreading their happy news until the fourth month, when they begin to feel secure that the pregnancy will indeed continue. And for most of them—probably 90%—it will.

Though it is hard for parents to believe it at the time, when a miscarriage *does* occur it is usually a blessing. Early miscarriage is generally a natural selection process in which a defective embryo or fetus (defective because of environmental factors, such as radiation or drugs; because of poor implantation in the uterus; because of genetic abnormality, maternal infection, random accident, or unknown reasons) is discarded before it has a chance to develop.

Happily, most women who have one miscarriage do not become habitual aborters. In fact, having a miscarriage is so common that many doctors believe that virtually every woman will have at least one sometime during her reproductive life. Many of these miscarriages go unnoticed, occurring even before a woman knows she is pregnant and passing for an unusually heavy and crampy menstrual period.

There is still much to be learned about the reasons for early miscarriage, but several factors are believed *not* to cause the problem. They include:

❖ Previous trouble with an IUD. Scarring of the endometrium (the lining of the uterus) because of IUD-triggered infection could prevent a pregnancy from implanting in the uterus, but should not cause miscarriage once implantation is well established. Nor should previous difficulty holding an IUD in position affect a pregnancy.

❖ History of multiple abortions.[5] Scarring of the endometrium from multiple abortions, as from IUD-caused infections, could prevent implantation but should not otherwise be responsible for early miscarriage.

❖ Usual and accustomed physical activity, such as hanging curtains, moving light furniture, tennis, and so on.[6]

❖ Emotional upset—resulting from an argument, stress at work, or family problems.

❖ A fall or other minor accidental injury to the mother. But serious injury could hurt the fetus, so safety precautions—such as wearing a seat belt and not climbing on rickety chairs—should always be observed.

There are several factors, however, that *are* believed to increase the risk of spontaneous abortion. Some are one-time events and should not affect future pregnancies (for example: a severe infection such as pneumonia; a high fever; rubella, x-rays, or drugs that harm the fetus; an IUD in place when conception

5. Though not a cause of early miscarriage, repeated dilatations from abortions or other procedures may result in a weakened or incompetent cervix—often a cause of late miscarriage. (See page 152.)

6. In a high-risk pregnancy, the physician may limit these activities or even prescribe strict bed rest. But you should limit activity only on direction of your doctor.

Possible Signs of Miscarriage

When to Call Your Doctor Immediately, Just in Case

❖ When you experience bleeding with cramps or pain in the center of your lower abdomen. (Pain on one side in early pregnancy could be triggered by an ectopic pregnancy, and also warrants a call to the doctor.)

❖ When pain is severe or continues unabated for more than one day, even if it isn't accompanied by staining or bleeding.

❖ When bleeding is as heavy as a menstrual period, or staining continues lightly for more than three days.

When to Get Emergency Medical Attention

❖ When you have a history of miscarriage, and experience either bleeding or cramping or both.

❖ When bleeding is so heavy you soak several pads in an hour, or when pain is so severe you can't bear it.

❖ When you pass clots or grayish material along with the blood—which may mean a miscarriage has already begun. If you can't reach your doctor, go to the nearest emergency room or the one recommended by his or her office or source. The doctor may want you to save the material you pass (in a jar, plastic bag, or other clean container) so he or she can try to determine whether or not the miscarriage is simply threatening, is complete, or is partial and requires a D and C (dilatation and curettage) to complete it.

occurs). Other risk factors, when they are detected, can be controlled in future pregnancies (poor nutrition; smoking; Rh incompatibility; hormonal insufficiency; and certain maternal medical problems). A few miscarriage risk factors are still not easily overcome (such as a malformed uterus, though some can be surgically corrected, and certain chronic maternal illnesses).

When Not to Worry. It's important to recognize that each cramp, ache, or bit of spotting isn't necessarily warning of an impending miscarriage. Just about every normal pregnancy will include at least one of these usually innocuous symptoms at one time or another:[7]

❖ Mild cramps or achiness on one or both sides of the abdomen. This is probably due to the stretching of ligaments that support the uterus. Unless cramping is severe, constant, or accompanied by bleeding, there's no need to worry.

❖ Staining a bit around the time you might have expected your period or about 7 to 10 days after conception, when the little ball of cells that is going to develop into your baby attaches itself to the uterine wall. Slight bleeding at these times is common and doesn't necessarily indicate a problem with your pregnancy— as long as it isn't accompanied by lower abdominal pain.

---

7. You should routinely tell your practitioner about *any* pains, cramping, or bleeding. In most cases his or her response will put your worries to rest.

If You Suspect Miscarriage. If you experience any of the symptoms listed in the box on page 102, put a call in to your practitioner. If your symptoms are listed under "get emergency medical attention" and your practitioner is not available, leave a message for him or her, and either call the emergency medical squad or go straight to the nearest emergency room.

While waiting for help, lie down if you can, or rest in a chair with your feet up. This may not prevent a miscarriage if it's about to happen, but it will help you to relax. It should also help you to relax to know that most women who have episodes of bleeding in early pregnancy carry to term and have normal, healthy babies.

If, on examination, the doctor finds the cervix dilated, it will be assumed that a miscarriage has occurred or is in progress. In such a case nothing can be done to prevent the loss of the fetus. In many cases the fetus will already have died prior to the onset of miscarriage—triggering the spontaneous abortion.

On the other hand, if the fetus is shown to be alive either through ultrasound or a Doppler device and there is no dilatation, the chances are very good that the threatened miscarriage will not occur. Some physicians will suggest no particular treatment on the theory that a doomed pregnancy will abort, therapy or no, and a healthy pregnancy will hang in there (also with or without therapy). Others—particularly when a woman has a history of miscarriage, or when it is believed that implantation is imperfect—will impose bed rest and restrictions on activities, including sexual intercourse. Female hormones, once given routinely for early bleeding, are no longer used because there is doubt about their efficacy and concern that they can harm the fetus if the pregnancy continues.

Sometimes, when a miscarriage does occur, it isn't complete—only parts of the placenta, sac, and embryo are expelled. If you've had, or believe you've had, a miscarriage, and bleeding and/or pain continue, phone your doctor immediately. A D and C will probably be required to stop the bleeding. It's a simple but important procedure in which the doctor dilates the cervix and scrapes or suctions out any remaining fetal or placental tissue. Your physician will probably also want to evaluate material passed or scraped out for clues to the cause of the miscarriage.

Losing a baby, even this early, is traumatic. But don't let guilt compound your misery—*a miscarriage is not your fault.* Do allow yourself to grieve. Sharing your feelings with your spouse, your practitioner, a friend, will help. In some communities, there are support groups for couples who have experienced pregnancy loss. Ask your practitioner if there is one in your area.

Probably the best therapy is getting pregnant again soon. Before you do, discuss the possible causes of the miscarriage with your doctor and, if feasible, take steps to correct them before you conceive again.

Whatever the cause of your miscarriage, many doctors suggest waiting three to six months before starting a new pregnancy—though sexual relations can often be resumed after six weeks. Think of this waiting period positively. Take advantage of it by improving your diet and health habits. The odds are excellent that next time around you'll have a normal pregnancy and a healthy baby.

"I don't really feel pregnant. Could I have miscarried without knowing it?"

Worry that you might miscarry without realizing it, though common, is unwarranted. Once a pregnancy is established, the signs that it is aborting are not something which can be inadvertently overlooked. Simply not "feeling pregnant" is not a reason for concern. Share your concerns with your practitioner at your next visit, which will undoubtedly be reassuring.

WHAT IT'S IMPORTANT TO KNOW:
GETTING REGULAR MEDICAL CARE

In the past decade, the self-care health movement has instructed Americans in everything from taking their own blood pressure and pulse to home-treating muscle strains and evaluating a scratchy throat or an aching ear. The impact it has had on the effectiveness of our health care has been unquestionably positive—cutting down on the number of trips we make to our doctors and making us better patients when we do go. Best of all, it's made us aware of the responsibility we each have for our own health, and it has the potential of making us a lot healthier in the years to come.

Even in pregnancy, as you can see throughout this book, there are countless steps you can take to make your own nine months safer and more comfortable, your labor and delivery easier, and your expected end product healthier. But to try to go it alone, even for a few months, is to abuse the concept of self-care—which is built on the foundation of a cooperative partnership between you and your health professional.

Regular professional input in pregnancy is crucial. One major study found that women who had many prenatal visits (an average of 12.7) had bigger babies with better survival rates than those who had few prenatal visits (an average of 1.4).

A SCHEDULE OF PRENATAL VISITS

Ideally, your first visit to a physician or nurse-midwife should take place while that baby is still a gleam in daddy's (and your) eye. That's an ideal many of us, especially those whose pregnancies are unplanned, can't always manage. Second best, and still very good, is a visit as soon as you suspect you have conceived. An internal exam will help confirm your pregnancy, and a physical will uncover any potential problems that may need monitoring. After that, the schedule of visits will vary depending on the practitioner you are seeing and whether or not yours is a high-risk pregnancy. In an unevent-

When to Call the Practitioner

It's best to set up an emergency protocol with your practitioner before an emergency strikes. If you haven't, and you are experiencing a symptom that requires immediate medical attention, try the following. First call the practitioner's office. If he or she isn't available and doesn't call back within a few minutes, call the office again and leave a message saying what your problem is and where you are headed. Then go directly to the nearest emergency room or call the emergency medical squad.

When you report any of the following to your practitioner, be sure to mention any other symptoms you may be experiencing, no matter how remote they may seem from the immediate problem. Also be sure to be specific, mentioning how long the symptom has existed, how frequently it recurs, what seems to relieve or exacerbate it, and how severe it is.

❖ Severe lower abdominal pain, on one or both sides, that doesn't subside: notify your practitioner the same day; if it is accompanied by bleeding, or nausea and vomiting, call immediately.

❖ Slight vaginal spotting: notify your practitioner the same day.

❖ Heavy bleeding (especially when combined with abdominal or back pain): call immediately.

❖ A gush of fluid from the vagina, which indicates the rupture of the amniotic sac: call immediately.

❖ A sudden increase in thirst, accompanied by a paucity of urination, or no urination at all for an entire day: call immediately.

❖ Swelling or puffiness of hands, face, eyes: call the same day. If very sudden and severe, or accompanied by headache or vision difficulties: call immediately.

❖ Severe headache that persists for more than two or three hours: call the same day. If accompanied by vision disturbances or sudden puffiness of eyes, face, hands: call immediately.

❖ Painful or burning urination: call the same day. If accompanied by chills and fever over 102 degrees, and/or backache: call immediately.

❖ Absence of noticeable fetal movement for more than five days through the fifth month: call the same day. From the sixth month on, absence of noticeable movement for 24 hours: call immediately.

❖ Vision disturbances (blurring, dimming, double vision) that persist for two or three hours: call immediately.

❖ Fainting or dizziness: notify the doctor the same day.

❖ Chills and fever over 100 degrees (with no cold or flu symptoms): call the same day. Fever over 102 degrees: call immediately.

❖ Severe nausea and vomiting, vomiting more often than two or three times a day in the first trimester, vomiting later in pregnancy when you haven't before: notify the doctor the same day. If vomiting is accompanied by pain and/or fever: call immediately.

❖ Sudden weight gain of more than two pounds that does not seem related to excessive eating: notify the doctor the same day. If accompanied by edema of the hands and face and/or headache or visual disturbances: call immediately.

ful low-risk pregnancy you can probably expect to see your practitioner monthly up until the end of the 32nd week. After that you may begin going every two weeks until the last month, when weekly visits are usual.

For what you can expect to happen at each prenatal visit, see the monthly chapters.

TAKING CARE OF THE REST OF YOU

You're understandably preoccupied with obstetrical matters during pregnancy. But though your health care should begin with your belly, it shouldn't end there. And don't just wait for problems to occur. Do pay a visit to your dentist; most dental work, particularly the preventive kind, can be done safely during pregnancy (see page 63). See your allergist, if necessary. You probably won't begin a new course of injections now, but if your allergies are severe, he or she will want to monitor your condition. Your family doctor or a specialist should also be monitoring any chronic illnesses or other medical problems that don't fall under the purview of the obstetrician; if you're seeing a nurse-midwife for pregnancy, you should see your family physician for *all* medical problems.

If new problems come up while you're pregnant, don't ignore them. Even if you've noticed symptoms which seem relatively innocuous, it's more important than ever to consult with your physician promptly. Your baby needs a *wholly* healthy mother.

6
The Second Month

WHAT YOU CAN EXPECT AT THIS MONTH'S CHECKUP

If this is your first prenatal visit, see What You Can Expect at Your First Prenatal Visit (page 92). If this is your second exam, you can expect your practitioner to check the following, though there may be variations depending upon your particular needs and your practitioner's style of practice:[1]

❖ Weight and blood pressure

❖ Urine, for sugar and protein

❖ Hands and feet for edema (swelling), and legs for varicose veins

❖ Symptoms you have been experiencing, especially unusual ones

❖ Questions or problems you want to discuss—have a list ready

---

WHAT YOU MAY BE FEELING

You may feel all of these symptoms at one time or another, or only one or two. Some may have continued from last month, others may be new. Don't be surprised, no matter what your symptoms, if you don't feel pregnant yet.

PHYSICALLY:

❖ Fatigue and sleepiness

❖ A need to urinate frequently

❖ Nausea, with or without vomiting, and/or excessive salivation (ptyalism)

❖ Constipation

❖ Heartburn and indigestion, flatulence and bloating

---

1. See appendix for an explanation of the procedures and tests performed.

❖ Food aversions and cravings

❖ Breast changes: fullness, heaviness, tenderness, tingling; darkening of areola (the pigmented area around the nipple); sweat glands in the areola become prominent (Montgomery's tubercles), like large goose bumps; a network of bluish lines appear under the skin as blood supply to the breasts increases

❖ Occasional headaches, possibly due to a reaction to hormones (similar to headaches in women taking birth control pills)

❖ Occasional faintness or dizziness

❖ Clothes may begin to feel tight around waist and bust, abdomen may appear enlarged, probably due to bowel distention rather than uterine growth

EMOTIONALLY:

❖ Instability comparable to premenstrual syndrome, which may include irritability, mood swings, irrationality, weepiness

❖ Misgivings, fear, joy, elation—any or all of these

WHAT YOU MAY LOOK LIKE

By the end of the second month, the embryo is more human-looking, about 1¼ inches long from head to buttocks (one-third of it is the head), and weighs about ⅓ ounce. It has a beating heart, and arms and legs with the beginnings of fingers and toes. Bone starts to replace cartilage.

WHAT YOU MAY BE CONCERNED ABOUT

VENOUS CHANGES

"I have unsightly blue lines under the skin, on my breasts and abdomen. Is that normal?"

Very normal. They are part of the network of veins that expand to carry the increased blood flow that comes with pregnancy. Not only are the veins nothing to worry about, they are a sign that your body is doing what it should. They show up earliest in very slim women. In other women the venous network may be less visible, not noticeable at all, or may not become obvious until later in pregnancy.

"Since I became pregnant I've got awful-looking spidery purplish-red lines on my thighs. Are they varicose veins?"

They aren't pretty, but they aren't varicose veins. They are spider nevi, or telangiectases, which can result from the hormone changes of pregnancy. They will fade and disappear after delivery.

"My mother and grandmother both had varicose veins during pregnancy and had trouble with them ever after. Is there anything I can do to prevent the problem in my own pregnancy?"

Because varicosities often run in families, you're wise to think about prevention now. Especially since varicose veins tend to worsen with subsequent pregnancies.

Normal, healthy veins carry blood from the extremities back to the heart. Because they are working against gravity, they are designed with a series of valves that prevent back flow. In some people these valves are missing or faulty, causing blood to pool in the veins and resulting in the bulging of varicosities. Veins that are easily distended, or distensible, can further contribute to the condition. The problem is more common in people who are obese, and occurs four times more often in women than in men. In women who are susceptible, the condition often surfaces for the first time during pregnancy. There are several reasons for this: increased pressure from the uterus on the pelvic veins; increasing pressure on leg veins; augmented blood volume; and pregnancy hormones which relax the muscle tissue in the veins, causing them to open wider.

The symptoms of varicose veins aren't difficult to recognize, but they vary a great deal in severity. The swollen veins may cause severe pain, mild achiness, a sensation of heaviness, or may even be entirely asymptomatic. A slight outline of bluish veins may be visible, or serpentine veins may bulge from ankle to upper thigh or vulva. In severe cases the skin covering the veins becomes swollen, dry, and irritated. Occasionally, thrombophlebitis (an inflammation of a vein associated with a blood clot) may develop at the site of a varicosity.

Fortunately, varicose veins during pregnancy can often be prevented, or the symptoms minimized:

❖ Avoid excessive weight gain.

❖ Avoid long periods of standing or sitting; when sitting or lying down, elevate legs above the level of the heart when possible.

❖ Wear support pantyhose or elastic stockings, putting them on before getting out of bed in the morning and removing them at night before going to sleep.

❖ Do not wear a tight girdle—especially a panty-leg girdle—or stockings or socks with elastic tops that cut off circulation.

❖ Get plenty of exercise—a brisk 20-to-30-minute walk every day.

❖ Be sure to get enough vitamin C, which some physicians believe helps to keep veins healthy and elastic.

Surgical removal of varicose veins isn't recommended during pregnancy, although it can certainly be considered afterward. Most cases, however, will clear up or improve spontaneously after delivery, usually by the time prepregnancy weight is reached.

COMPLEXION PROBLEMS

"My skin is breaking out the way it did when I was a teenager."

The glow of pregnancy that some women are lucky enough to exude is due not simply to happiness, but to an increased secretion of oils caused by hormonal changes. And so, alas, are the less-than-glowing breakouts of pregnancy that other women experience (particularly those whose skin ordinarily breaks out before their periods). Though such breakouts are hard to eliminate entirely, the following may help keep them to a minimum:

❖ Be faithful to the Best-Odds Diet—it's good for your skin as well as for your baby.

❖ Don't pass a tap without filling your glass—water is one of the most effective pore-purifiers around.

❖ Wash your face often with a gentle cleanser. Avoid skin-clogging greasy creams and makeups.

❖ If your practitioner approves, take a vitamin B$_6$ supplement (25 to 50 milligrams). This vitamin is sometimes useful in treating hormonally induced skin problems.

For some women, dry skin, often with itching, is a pregnancy problem. Moisturizers may be helpful. So may taking plenty of fluids and keeping rooms well humidified in the heating season. Too-frequent washing or bathing, particularly with soap, tends to increase dryness, so don't overdo it.

WAISTLINE EXPANSION

"Why does my waist seem to be expanding already? I thought I wouldn't 'show' until the third month at least."

Your expanding waistline may very well be a legitimate product of pregnancy, especially if you started out slender, with little excess flesh for your growing uterus to hide under. Or it may be the result of bowel distention, very common in early pregnancy. On the other hand, it's also quite possible that your "show" may be nothing but fat around your middle—an indication that you're gaining weight too quickly. If you've gained more than 3 pounds so far, analyze your diet—you are very likely taking in too many calories, possibly empty ones. Review the Best-Odds Diet, and read about weight gain on page 127.

LOSING YOUR FIGURE

"I'm afraid I'll lose my figure forever—and so is my husband."

This is a very understandable fear—particularly for someone who is conscious of her figure to begin with. But it is also one over which you can have complete control. Many women do look fat and flabby after childbirth because they gained too much, ate the wrong foods, or didn't get enough exercise during pregnancy—and *not* simply because they were carrying a child. The weight gain of pregnancy has just one legitimate purpose: to nurture the developing fetus. If only enough weight to serve that purpose is gained and a woman keeps physically fit, her figure should return to normal within a few months after the baby is born, especially if she is breastfeeding. See the Best-Odds Diet, and read about weight gain on page 127.

With the right prenatal care, you can look better than ever after pregnancy, because you will have learned how to take optimum care of your body. Your husband can look better after pregnancy, too, benefiting from your healthier lifestyle.

HEARTBURN AND INDIGESTION

"I have indigestion and heartburn all the time. Will this affect my baby?"

While you are painfully aware of your gastrointestinal discomfort, your baby is blissfully oblivious to it and unaffected by it— as long as it isn't interfering with your eating the right foods.

Though indigestion can have the same cause (usually overindulgence) during pregnancy as when you're not pregnant, there are additional reasons why it may be plaguing you now. Early in pregnancy, your body produces large amounts of progesterone and estrogen, which tend to relax smooth muscle tissue everywhere, including that in the gastrointestinal tract. As a result, food moves more slowly through your system, resulting in bloating. This is uncomfortable for you but good for the baby, because the slow-down allows better absorption of nutrients into your bloodstream and, subsequently, through the placenta into your baby's system.

Heartburn results when the sphincter that separates the esophagus from the stomach becomes lax, occasionally allowing food and harsh digestive juices to back up from stomach to esophagus. The stomach acids irritate the sensitive esophageal lining, causing a burning sensation right about where the heart is, thus: heartburn—which, of course, has nothing to do with your heart. During the last two trimesters the problem is compounded by your blossoming uterus, which presses up on your stomach, pushing it and its contents farther up toward the esophagus.

It's nearly impossible to have an indigestion-free nine months; it's just one of the less pleasant facts of pregnancy. There are, however, some pretty effective ways of avoiding heartburn and indigestion most of the time, and of minimizing the discomfort when it strikes:

❖ Avoid gaining too much weight: Excess weight puts excess pressure on the stomach.

❖ Don't wear clothing that is tight around your abdomen and waist.

❖ Eat slowly, taking small mouthfuls and chewing thoroughly.

❖ Eliminate from your diet any food that causes discomfort. Most common offenders are: hot and highly seasoned foods; fatty foods; processed meats (hot dogs, bologna, sausage, bacon); chocolate, coffee, alcohol, carbonated beverages; spearmint and peppermint (even in the form of gum).

❖ Don't smoke.

❖ Avoid bending over at the waist; bend instead with your knees.

❖ Sleep with the head of your bed elevated about six inches.

❖ Relax.

❖ If all else fails to relieve your symptoms, ask your doctor if you can take antacids and over-the-counter medications for heartburn which have no contraindications in pregnancy. Do not take preparations containing sodium or sodium bicarbonate.

FOOD AVERSIONS AND CRAVINGS

"Certain foods—particularly green vegetables—that I've always liked taste funny now. Instead, I have cravings for foods that are less nutritious."

The pregnancy cliché of a harried husband running out in the middle of the night, raincoat over his pajamas, for a pint of ice cream and a jar of pickles to satisfy his wife's cravings probably occurs more often in the heads of cartoonists than in real life. Not many pregnant women's cravings carry them—or their husbands—that far.

But most of us do find that our tastes in food change somewhat in early pregnancy. The long-favored theory that these changes are signals (that our bodies are craving something they need, or warning us off something they shouldn't have) sounds reasonable. And sometimes it works. As when the black coffee that used to be the mainstay of your workday becomes totally unappealing. Or the cocktail before dinner seems too strong even when it's weak. Or you suddenly can't get enough citrus fruit. On the other hand, when you can't stand the sight of fish, or broccoli suddenly tastes bitter, or you crave ice-cream sandwiches, you can't credit your body with sending accurate signals.

The fact is that body signals relating to food are notoriously unreliable, probably because we've departed so significantly from the food chain in nature that we can no longer interpret them correctly. Before ice-cream sandwiches were invented, when food came from nature, a craving for carbohydrates and calcium would have steered us toward fruits or berries and milk or cheese. With the wide variety of tempting (but often unwholesome) foods available today, it's no wonder our bodies are confused.

You can't totally ignore cravings and aversions. But you can deal with them without putting your baby's nutritional needs in jeopardy. If you crave something that's good for you and baby, by all means go ahead and eat it. If you crave something that you know isn't good, then look for a satisfactory substitute: raisins, dried apricots, or a glass of apple juice instead of a candy bar; unsalted or lightly salted whole-wheat pretzels instead of the usually oversalted, nutritionally vacant variety.

If you feel a sudden aversion to coffee or alcohol or chocolate ice cream, great. It will make giving them up for the duration all the easier. If it's fish or broccoli or milk you can't tolerate, you don't have to force-feed yourself, but you do have to find compensating sources of the nutrients they supply. (See the Best-Odds Diet for substitutes.)

Most cravings and aversions disappear or weaken by the fourth month. And those that don't may be mostly triggered by emotional needs—the need for a little extra attention, for example. If both you and your husband understand this need, it should be easy to deal with. You might, instead of requesting a middle-of-the-night pint of Rocky Road, settle for some quiet cuddling or a romantic bath-for-two (or, rather, three).

MILK AVERSION

"I can't tolerate milk, and drinking four cups a day would make me ill. Will my baby suffer if I don't drink milk?"

First of all, it's not the milk your baby needs, it's the calcium. Since milk is the most convenient source of calcium in the American diet, it's the one most often recommended for filling the greatly increased requirement during preg-

nancy. But there are many substitutes which fill the nutritional bill just as well. Many people who are lactose-intolerant (can't digest the milk sugar, lactose) can tolerate some kinds of dairy products, such as hard cheeses, fully processed yogurts, and the new LactAid milk, in which 70% of the lactose has been converted to a more easily digested form. If you can't tolerate these, you can still get all the calcium your baby requires by eating the nondairy foods listed under Calcium-Rich Foods, page 82.

If your problem with milk isn't physiological, but just a matter of distaste, there are plenty of ways to get the calcium you need without offending your taste buds. You'll find them all in the Calcium-Rich Foods list.

A MEATLESS DIET

"I eat chicken and fish but no red meat. Can I supply my baby with all the nutrients he needs without meat?"

Your baby can be just as happy and healthy as any beef-eating mother's offspring. Fish and poultry, in fact, nourish your baby in the most efficient way possible, giving you more protein and less fat for your calories than beef, pork, lamb, and organ meats. And all the important nutrients found in red meats are found in plentiful supply elsewhere in a balanced diet—especially in poultry and fish, whole grains (wheat germ, whole-wheat cereals and breads, brown rice), eggs, fresh green leafy and deep yellow vegetables, dried fruits, and milk products.

A VEGETARIAN DIET

"I'm a vegetarian and in perfect health. But everyone—including my doctor—says that I have to eat meat and fish, eggs and milk products to have a healthy baby. Is this true?"

V egetarians of every variety can have healthy babies without compromising their dietary principles. But they have to be even more careful in planning their diets than meat-eating mothers-to-be, particularly in being sure to get all of the following:

Adequate Protein. For the ovo-lacto vegetarian, who eats eggs and milk products, adequate protein intake can be assured by taking ample quantities of both. A vegan (a strict vegetarian who eats neither milk nor eggs) has to depend on combinations of vegetable proteins (see Vegetarian Complete Protein Combinations, page 83). Some meat analogues are good protein sources; others are low in protein and high in calories. Read the labels.

Adequate Calcium. This is no problem for the vegetarian who takes dairy products, but adroit maneuvering is needed for those who don't. Use the Calcium-Rich Foods list, page 82, to be sure of meeting your calcium needs. Soy products are useful because they are fairly high in calcium, but don't use soy milks loaded with sucrose (sugar, corn syrup, honey). Instead use a pure soybean extract. For added insurance, vegans should also take a prescribed calcium supplement.

Vitamin B$_{12}$. Vegetarians, particularly vegans, often don't get enough of this vitamin because it is found primarily in animal foods. So they should be certain to take a vitamin supplement that includes B$_{12}$ as well as folic acid and iron.

Vitamin D. This vitamin is not naturally found in foods except for fish liver oils. Most milk is fortified with vitamin D, but for those who don't drink milk, this vitamin should be included in their supplement. (Be careful, however, not to take vitamin D in doses beyond pregnancy requirements, which can be toxic.)

Enough of Everything Else. Vegetarians need to have heartier-than-average appetites, because in addition to all of the above, they'll have to find room for the rest of the foods recommended for all pregnant women in the Best-Odds Diet. This doesn't mean they have to gain more weight. Since vegetarian food is generally lower in fat (and thus in calories) than meat foods, eating more of it shouldn't be more fattening.

JUNK-FOOD JUNKIE

"I'm addicted to junk foods—doughnuts for breakfast; fast-food burgers, fries, and Cokes for lunch. I'm afraid that if I can't break these bad habits, my baby will be undernourished."

Y ou're right to worry. Before you became pregnant, your dietary indiscretions hurt only you; now they can hurt your baby as well. Make a daily diet of doughnuts, fast-food burgers, and Cokes, and you'll be denying your baby adequate nourishment during the most important nine months of his or her life. Eat the junk food on top of a balanced diet, and baby won't be the only one growing.

Happily, any addiction can be broken. Heroin. Tobacco. Even junk food. Here are several ways to make withdrawal almost as painless as it is worthwhile:

First of All, Change the Locale of Your Meals. If you munch a pastry at your desk, have breakfast at home before you go to work. If you can't resist a burger at lunch, go to a restaurant that doesn't serve burgers, or bring a sandwich from home.

Stop Thinking of Eating as a Catch-as-Catch-Can Proposition. Start thinking of every bite as a chance to help your baby grow and thrive. Don't grab what is easiest. Plan ahead and pick what is best.

Don't Give Temptation a Tumble. Don't bring boxes of cookies, candy, bags of chips, soft drinks, into the house (other family members will survive without it—will do better in fact). When the coffee wagon bell rings, don't answer it; keep wholesome snacks like raisins, nuts, whole-wheat breadsticks, fruit, juices, and hard-boiled eggs in your desk or purse instead. When you're about to pass your favorite ice-cream parlor, cross the street.

Don't Use Lack of Time as an Excuse for Sloppy Eating. It takes no more time to make a tuna sandwich to take to the office than to stand on line at Burger King. And in fact, it takes less time to cut a fresh peach into a container of yogurt than to bake a peach pie. If the prospect of preparing a real dinner every night seems overwhelming, cook enough for two or three dinners at once and give yourself alternate nights off. And keep it simple: fancy sauces aren't nutritious, only high in calories.

Don't Use a Tight Budget as an Excuse for Eating Junk Foods. A glass of orange juice or milk is cheaper than a can of Coke. A broiled chicken breast and baked potato cost a lot less than a Big Mac and fries.

Quit Cold Turkey. Don't tell yourself you can have just one cola today or just one doughnut. That almost never works when you're trying to break an addiction. Just make up your mind that junk food is out—at least until you deliver. You may be surprised to find, once the baby's born, that your new good eating habits will be as hard to break as your old bad ones.

Study the Best-Odds Diet. Make it part of your life.

EATING FAST FOOD

"I go out with friends for fast food after a movie about once a month. Do I have to skip this for the rest of my pregnancy?"

Treating yourself to an occasional dinner at a fast-food restaurant is acceptable during pregnancy—but only if you order with care and restraint. First of all, try to pick a place that offers a salad bar. That way you will be sure to get your quota of leafy green and yellow vegetables, and possibly a serving of cheese as well. Make a main course of a single burger, a fish or chicken sandwich, a taco, or perhaps a couple of slices of pizza—preferably with whole-wheat crust. Forego the fries (you can snitch a couple from a friend), sodas, pasty pies, and shakes (they often contain little or no milk and are loaded with sugar, artificial flavors and colors, and saturated fats). Drink juice, milk, or plain water, and bring along your own fruit to munch for dessert.

CHEMICALS IN FOODS

"With additives in packaged foods, insecticides on vegetables, PCBs in fish, DES in meat, and nitrates in hot dogs, is there anything I can safely eat during pregnancy?"

Reports of hazardous chemicals in just about every item in the American diet are enough to scare the appetite out of anyone— especially a pregnant woman afraid not only for her own well-being but for that of her unborn child. Thanks to the media, "chemical" has become synonymous with "danger," and "natural" with "safe." But neither generalization is true. Everything we eat is made up of chemicals. Some chemicals are harmless (even beneficial); some are not. And although "natural" is often better

than artificial or unnatural, it can also be deadly. A "natural" mushroom can be poisonous; "natural" eggs, butter, and animal fats are associated with heart disease, and "natural" sugar and honey cause cavities.

So forget about classifying foods into natural and chemical. Think instead about foods that are safe to eat during pregnancy and those that are not. When in doubt (and for many food ingredients, safety during pregnancy is unknown), leave it out. But don't be fanatic. There are no food ingredients which in small occasional doses are known to cause birth defects. And, of course, most American women eat a wide variety of foods during pregnancy—never reading a single label—and have perfectly normal babies.

Still, you will want to be as prudent as possible and avoid regularly eating foods that *might* be hazardous. Use the following as a guide in deciding what to drop into your shopping cart and what to pass up:

❖ Use the Best-Odds Diet as your basic food plan; it automatically steers you clear of most potential perils.

❖ Don't use foods sweetened with saccharine or aspartame (their effects on the fetus are not yet known).

❖ Whenever possible, cook from scratch; you'll not only avoid many questionable ingredients but you will get more nutrients from your foods.

❖ Contact your local Environmental Protection Agency (EPA) or

Health Department for a list of fish in your area that have not been contaminated with PCBs or other chemicals. As a general rule ocean fish, for example tuna, sea bass, sole, flounder, and snapper, are safer than river and lake varieties. Never eat raw fish or seafood, and avoid (even cooked) seafood which is sometimes contaminated, such as clams.

❖ Generally avoid foods preserved with nitrates and nitrites: frankfurters, salami, luncheon meats, smoked fish and meats.

❖ Whenever you have the choice between products with or without artificial colorings, flavorings, preservatives, and other additives, opt for the one that's additive-free.

❖ Don't use MSG or flavor enhancers that contain it.

❖ Eat lean cuts of meat and poultry, cutting off fat and skin—they store chemicals that are fed to livestock. Don't eat organ meats (liver, kidneys, etc.) very often, for the same reason.

❖ Give all your fruits and vegetables a detergent bath (in the same detergent you use to hand wash dishes) and rinse thoroughly before using them, to remove chemical residues; scrub skins when possible. It is not necessary to buy organically grown produce; studies show it often has as much chemical residue as supermarket fruits and vegetables, and it is much more costly.

READING LABELS

"I'm eager to feed my baby well, but I find that it's difficult to know what I'm getting when I go to the supermarket."

Labels aren't always designed to help you as much as to sell you. Be aware when buying and learn to read the small print, including the list of ingredients and the nutritional label.

The ingredients listing will tell you, in order of predominance, exactly what is in the product. You will know whether the first ingredient in a cereal is sugar (you'll want to pass that one by), or a whole grain (you may want that one). You will also have a rough idea of whether a product is high in salt, fats, or additives.

The nutritional label appears on more than half the products on your grocer's shelves, and it is particularly valuable for a pregnant woman counting her protein and calories, as it gives the grams of the former and the number of the latter in each serving. The listing of percentages of the government's recommended daily allowance, however, is less useful, because the RDA for pregnant women is different from the RDA used on package labels. Still, a food high in a wide variety of nutrients is a good product to purchase.

While it's important to read the small print, it's just as important to ignore the large print. When a box of English muffins trumpets loudly "made with whole wheat, bran, and honey," reading the small print may show that the major (first) ingredient is *white*, not whole-wheat, flour and that the muffins contain precious little honey or bran (these are near the bottom of the ingredient list).

"Enriched" and "fortified" are also banners to be wary of. Adding a few vitamins to a poor food doesn't make it a good food. That's true of cereals that are 50% sugar (the nutritional label also gives you information on the percentage of sugar in many products) but have a few pennies' worth of vitamins added. You're much better off with a bowl of oatmeal which has acquired its vitamins naturally.

WHAT IT'S IMPORTANT TO KNOW:
PLAYING IT SAFE

The home. The highway. The backyard. The most significant risks faced by pregnant women are not medical but accidental.

Accidents often seem "accidental," that is, to happen by chance. Yet most are the direct result of carelessness—often on the part of the victim herself—and many can be avoided with a little extra caution and common sense. There are a wide variety of steps you can take to prevent injuries and accidents:

❖ Recognize that you're not as agile as you were prepregnancy. As your abdomen grows, your center of gravity will shift, making it more difficult for you to keep your balance. You will also find it difficult to see your feet. These changes will contribute to your becoming more accident-prone.

❖ Always fasten your seat belt in autos and on airplanes.

❖ Never climb on a shaky chair or ladder, or better still, never climb.

❖ Don't wear high, spiky heels, sloppy slippers, or thongs that can snap, all of which encourage falls and twisted ankles. Don't walk on slippery floors in your stocking feet or in smooth-soled shoes.

❖ Be careful getting in and out of the tub; be sure your tub and shower are equipped with non-skid surfaces and sturdy grab bars.

❖ Check your house and backyard for hazards: rugs without skid-proof bottoms, especially at the top of stairs; toys or junk on stairways; poorly lit stairs and hallways; wires strung across the floor; overwaxed floors; icy sidewalks and steps.

❖ Observe the safety rules of whatever sport you play; follow all the tips for safe exercise and activity on pages 161–169.

❖ Don't overdo. Fatigue is a major contributor to accidents.

7
The Third Month

WHAT YOU CAN EXPECT AT THIS MONTH'S CHECKUP

This month you can expect your practitioner to check the following, though there may be variations depending upon your particular needs and your practitioner's style of practice:[1]

❖ Weight and blood pressure

❖ Urine, for sugar and protein

❖ Fetal heartbeat

❖ Size and shape of uterus, by ex-ternal palpation, to see how it correlates to due date or estimated date of confinement (EDC)

❖ Height of fundus (the top of the uterus)

❖ Hands and feet for edema (swelling), and legs for varicose veins

❖ Questions or problems you want to discuss—have a list ready

WHAT YOU MAY BE FEELING

You may feel all of these symptoms at one time or another, or only a few of them. Some may have continued from last month, others may be new. You may also have additional, less common symptoms.

PHYSICALLY:

❖ Fatigue and sleepiness

❖ A need to urinate frequently

❖ Nausea, with or without vomiting, and/or excessive salivation

❖ Constipation

---

1. See appendix for an explanation of the procedures and tests performed.

- Heartburn and indigestion, flatulence and bloating
- Food aversions and cravings
- Breast changes: fullness, heaviness, tenderness, tingling; darkening of the areola (the pigmented area around the nipple); sweat glands in the areola become prominent (Montgomery's tubercles), like large goose bumps; network of bluish lines under skin expands
- Additional veins visible as blood supply to abdomen and legs also increases
- Occasional headaches
- Occasional faintness or dizziness
- Clothes begin to feel tight around waist and bust, if they hadn't previously; abdomen may appear enlarged by end of month
- Increasing appetite

EMOTIONALLY:

- Instability comparable to premenstrual syndrome, which may include irritability, weepiness
- A new sense of calmness

WHAT YOU MAY LOOK LIKE

By the end of the third month, this tiny human, now a fetus, is 2½ to 3 inches long and weighs about ½ ounce. More organs are developing; circulatory and urinary systems are operating; the liver produces bile. Reproductive organs are developed, but the gender is difficult to distinguish externally.

- Misgivings, fear, joy, elation—any or all

WHAT YOU MAY BE CONCERNED ABOUT

CONSTIPATION

"All my pregnant friends seem to have problems with constipation. I don't; in fact, I've been more regular than ever. Is my system working right?"

Pregnant women are so programmed by mothers, friends, books, even doctors, to expect constipation that those who do become constipated accept it as normal and inevitable, and those who don't worry that there's something wrong.

There's a sound rationale for this programming, and for constipation being such a common complaint of pregnancy. For one thing, relaxation of the musculature of the bowel, due to the high levels of certain hormones circulating during pregnancy, makes elimination sluggish and less efficient. For another, the pressure from the growing uterus on the bowels inhibits their normal activity.

But there's no sound reason for believing constipation is inevitable with every pregnancy. Many women never experience it—probably because they are compensating for the sluggishness of their bowels with proper diet and exercise. Some of these women may also have more frequent bowel movements because of the additional food and the added fiber they are eating.[2] As long as the stools aren't loose, watery, bloody or mucusy, there's no cause for alarm.

Women who *do* suffer from constipation can overcome the problem and head off one of the common results of irregularity, hemorrhoids (see page 174). Here's how:

Enlist Fiber into Your Diet. Eat fresh fruits and vegetables (lightly cooked or raw, with skins left on when possible), whole grains (cereals and breads), and dried fruits (raisins, prunes, apricots). In general, follow the Best-Odds Diet—it also gives you the best odds against constipation. But if you usually eat little fiber, add high-fiber foods to your diet gradually or you may find your stomach upset.

Drown Your Opponent. Constipa-

tion doesn't stand a chance against an ample fluid intake. Most fluids—particularly water and fruit and vegetable juices—are effective in softening stool and keeping food moving along the digestive tract. Some people find cups of hot water flavored with lemon (but no sugar) especially useful. If constipation is severe, prune juice may do the trick.

Start an Exercise Campaign. Fit a brisk walk of at least half an hour into your daily routine; supplement it with as much as you like of any exercise you enjoy that is safe during pregnancy (see Exercise During Pregnancy, page 161).

FLATULENCE (GAS)

"I'm very bloated from gas and worry that the pressure, which is so uncomfortable for me, might also be hurting the baby."

Snug in a safe uterine cocoon, protected by impact-absorbing amniotic fluid, your baby is impervious to your intestinal distress. If anything, he or she probably is soothed by the bubbling and gurgling of your gastric Muzak.

The only possible threat to your baby's well-being is if bloating—which often worsens late in the day—is preventing you from eating regularly and properly. To avoid this risk (and to minimize your own discomfort), take the following measures:

Stay Regular. Constipation is a common cause of gas and bloating.

---

2. Iron supplements may contribute to diarrhea *or* to constipation. If your supplement seems to unsettle your system, ask your practitioner to suggest a different formula.

Don't Gorge. Large meals just add to the bloated feeling. They also overload your digestive system, which isn't at its most efficient to begin with during pregnancy. Instead of three large meals a day, eat six small ones.

Don't Gulp. When you rush through meals or eat on the run, you're bound to swallow as much air as food. This captured air forms painful pockets of gas in your gut.

Keep Calm. Particularly during meals: Tension and anxiety can make you swallow air.

Steer Clear of Gas-Producers. Your stomach knows what they are—possibly onions, cabbage and cabbage-family members such as Brussels sprouts and broccoli, fried foods and sugary sweets (which you shouldn't be having now anyway), and, of course, the notorious beans.

WEIGHT GAIN

"I only gained one pound in my first trimester. My friend, who's also pregnant, gained six. What's enough, and what's too much?"

Weight gain that is just enough for one woman may be too much or too little for another. The extremely underweight woman is probably doing her baby a favor by gaining 6 pounds (as long as they're gained by eating highly nutritious foods) in the first trimester, or doing him or her an injustice by gaining only 1. The obese mother-to-be, on the other hand, is doing no one a favor by gaining weight rapidly, and can probably afford to gain only 1 pound (or even none) in the first trimester (as long as she eats adequate amounts of nutritious foods) without jeopardizing her baby's health. For the woman who is average, however, 6 pounds is probably too much and 1 not enough. Two to 4 would be just right (see page 127).

STRETCH MARKS

"I'm afraid I'm going to get stretch marks. Can they be prevented?"

For many women—especially those who favor bikinis—stretch marks are more to be dreaded than flabby thighs. Nevertheless, 90% of all women will develop these pink or reddish, slightly indented streaks on their breasts, hips, and/or abdomen sometime during pregnancy.

As their name implies, stretch marks are caused by stretching of the skin, generally due to a large and/or rapid increase in weight. Expectant mothers who have good, elastic skin tone (because they either inherited it or earned it through years of excellent nutrition and exercise) may slip through several pregnancies without a single telltale striation. Others may be able to minimize, if not prevent, stretch marks by keeping weight gain steady, gradual, and moderate. Promoting elasticity in your skin by nourishing it well with the Best-Odds Diet (page 75) may help, but no expensive cream, lotion, or oil will prevent or alleviate stretch marks—although they may be fun for your husband to rub on your tummy, and will prevent your skin from drying.

If you do develop stretch marks during pregnancy, you can console yourself with the knowledge that they will gradually fade to a silvery sheen after delivery. It may also help to think of them less as a disfigurement than as a medal of motherhood.

ASPIRIN, NON-ASPIRIN, AND HEADACHES

"Last week I took two aspirins for a pounding headache. Now I read that aspirin can cause birth defects. Could I have hurt my baby?"

O f the millions of Americans who opened their medicine cabinet today and reached for a bottle of aspirin, few thought twice—or even once—about its safety. And for most people occasional aspirin use is very helpful and perfectly harmless. But during pregnancy, aspirin, like so many other ordinarily innocuous over-the-counter remedies, becomes a potential hazard.

If you've unwittingly taken one or two aspirins on one, or even a few, occasions in the first two trimesters, don't worry—they won't hurt your baby. For the rest of your pregnancy, however, be aware that like any drug, aspirin should be taken only when absolutely necessary, and then only with your physician's approval.

Research shows that there may be a link between frequent doses of aspirin taken at any time during ges-

tation and problems in fetal development. But during the third trimester, even one or two aspirins can be risky. Because it is an antiprostaglandin, and prostaglandins are involved in the mechanism of labor, aspirin can prolong both pregnancy and labor and lead to other complications during delivery. And since it interferes with blood-clotting, if taken during the two weeks before delivery, aspirin may lead to hemorrhage during labor and bleeding problems in the newborn.

Taking an aspirin-substitute in place of aspirin isn't the logical solution in pregnancy. Acetaminophen, sold under trade names like Tylenol, Datril, and Anacin III, has been used widely only since the 1970s, and all of its possible risks aren't yet known. It *is* known that it can cause liver damage in the user, and there is speculation that it might also damage the liver of a fetus whose mother takes it in large doses during pregnancy. So take acetaminophen only if absolutely necessary, and then *only* with the approval of your practitioner.

Both aspirin and acetaminophen are hidden ingredients in a myriad of popular remedies, including Alka-Seltzer, cold-and-allergy-relief medicines (many of which are not recommended during pregnancy anyway), and pain relievers, such as Anacin and Empirin. Read labels carefully—a good habit not only during pregnancy but all of the time.

Ibuprofen, the latest addition to the over-the-counter pain relief family (marketed under trade names like Advil and Nuprin), also shouldn't be used without medical approval anytime during pregnancy—and shouldn't be taken at all in the last trimester, when it could cause problems in the unborn baby and labor complications.

Headaches are extremely common during pregnancy. Often they are due to tension or other stresses on your body and to hormonal changes. Sinus headaches, too, may be more frequent because of the congestion of the mucous membranes caused by pregnancy hormones. But just because it isn't a good idea to find relief for your headaches in a pill doesn't mean you have to grin and bear them. There are many non-drug ways of overcoming (and preventing) headaches, many of which fit the cure to the cause:

Eat Regularly. Hunger often generates headaches.

Get Enough Rest. Lack of sleep, staying on the go all day without a break, can lead to headaches.

Seek Some Peace and Quiet. Stay away from loud music, noisy parties, crowded department stores.

Don't Get Stuffy. If overheated, smoke-filled, unventilated rooms trigger a headache, step outside for a stroll.

Relax. Most pregnancy headaches are—not surprisingly—of the tension variety. Ordinary relaxation (lying down in a dark, quiet room) may help. Even better are meditation, yoga, and other relaxation techniques. You can take a course or read a book on relaxation methods,

or simply try this: Sit with eyes closed. Relax muscles starting with feet and working up through legs, torso, neck, and face. Breathe only through the nose. As you breathe out, repeat the word "one" to yourself. Continue for 10 to 20 minutes.

For Relief from Sinus Headaches. Apply hot and cold compresses alternately to the aching area, 30 seconds each for 10 minutes, four times a day.

If your headache persists, returns very often, is very severe, or is accompanied by visual disturbances or puffiness of the hands and face, notify your practitioner about it.

GERMAN MEASLES (RUBELLA)

"I was exposed to German measles. Should I get an abortion?"

That's a question only one out of seven pregnant women need ever confront. The other six are, happily, immune to rubella, or German measles, having contracted it at some other time in their lives (usually during childhood) or because they were vaccinated (usually in early adolescence or when they were married). You may not know whether or not you are immune, but you can find out via a rubella antibody titer—a test which measures the level of antibodies to the disease in your blood and is performed routinely at the first prenatal visit by most practitioners. If a test was not performed, it should be now.

If it turns out you're not immune, you still needn't immediately consider drastic measures. Exposure alone cannot harm your baby. For the virus to do its damage, it has to infect you. And if you contract the illness after the third month, the risk is very slight.

Unfortunately, there is no way of actively preventing an exposed woman from coming down with rubella. Gamma globulin shots, which were once given routinely, have been found to be inconsistent in preventing infection. Should you contract rubella in the first trimester (this can be determined only through blood tests, since symptoms may be nonexistent), the chance of your baby developing serious congenital malformation is high—about 35% in the first month and 10% to 15% by the third. You should discuss this risk with your doctor; but in the end, it is you and your husband who must decide whether to continue the pregnancy.

If you are not immune and do not contract the disease, avoid this dilemma entirely in subsequent pregnancies by having your doctor vaccinate you after this delivery. As a precaution, you will be instructed not to become pregnant for two or three months following vaccination. But should you conceive accidentally during this time—or if you were vaccinated early in this pregnancy, before you knew you had conceived—don't worry. There have been no cases of congenital rubella reported in babies whose mothers were inadvertently vaccinated early in pregnancy or conceived right after vaccination.

SEXUAL DESIRE

"All of my pregnant friends say that they had an increased desire for sex early in pregnancy—some had orgasms and multi-orgasms for the first time. How come I feel so unsexy?"

P regnancy is a time of change in many aspects of your life, not the least of them sexual. Some women who have never had either orgasm or much of a taste for sex suddenly experience both for the first time when pregnant. Other women, accustomed to having a voracious appetite for sex and to being easily orgasmic, suddenly find that they are completely lacking in desire and are difficult to arouse. These changes in sexuality can be disconcerting, guilt-provoking, wonderful, or a confusing combination of all three. And they are perfectly normal.

As you will see by reading Making Love During Pregnancy (page 139), there are many logical explanations for such changes and for the feelings that they may provoke. Some of these factors may be strongest early in pregnancy, when nausea and fatigue make you feel understandably unsexy, when being able to make love without worrying about trying to get (or trying not to get) pregnant frees you of inhibitions and makes you sexier than ever, when guilt results because you're feeling sexy and you think you should be feeling motherly instead. Other factors, such as the physical alterations that make orgasm easier to achieve, more powerful, or more elusive, continue throughout gestation.

Most important is recognizing that your sexual feelings—and your husband's as well—during pregnancy may be more erratic than erotic; you may feel sexy one day and not the next. Mutual understanding and open communication will be needed to see you through.

ORAL SEX

"I've heard that oral sex is dangerous during pregnancy. Is this true?"

Cunnilingus is safe throughout pregnancy as long as your mate is careful not to blow any air into your vagina. Doing this could force air into your bloodstream and cause an embolism (an obstruction of a blood vessel), which might prove deadly to both mother and baby.

Fellatio, because it doesn't involve the female genitalia, is always safe during pregnancy and for some couples is a preferred substitute when intercourse isn't permitted.

CRAMP AFTER ORGASM

"I get an abdominal cramp after orgasm. Is this a sign that sex is hurting my baby? Will it cause a miscarriage?"

Cramping—both during and after orgasm, and sometimes accompanied by backache—is as harmless during a normal low-risk pregnancy as it is common. Its cause can be physical—a combination of the normal venous congestion in the area and the equally normal conges-

tion of sexual arousal and orgasm. Or it can be psychological—a result of anxiety that having intercourse and orgasm may injure your baby.

The cramping is not a sign that sex is hurting the fetus. Most experts agree that sexual relations and orgasm during a normal, low-risk pregnancy are perfectly safe and are not a cause of miscarriage. If the cramps bother you, ask your husband for a gentle low back rub. It may relieve not only the cramps but any tension that might be triggering them, too.[3] (For more about sexual relations, see Making Love During Pregnancy, page 139.)

BABY'S HEARTBEAT

"My friend's doctor picked up her baby's heartbeat at two and a half months. I'm a week ahead of her and my doctor hasn't heard my baby's yet."

It's possible to pick up the baby's heartbeat as early as the 10th or 12th week with a highly sensitive instrument called a Doppler (a hand-held ultrasound device which magnifies the sound). But an ordinary stethoscope isn't powerful enough to detect the heartbeat until the 17th or 18th week at the earliest. Even with sophisticated instruments, the heartbeat may not be audible this early because of the baby's position or other interfering factors, such as excess layers of maternal fat. It's also

---

3. Some women also experience crampiness in the legs after intercourse. See page 173 for tips on relieving such discomfort.

possible that a slightly miscalculated due date may be causing the delay. Wait until next month. By your 18th week, the miraculous sound of your baby's heartbeat is certain to be available for your listening pleasure.

WHAT IT'S IMPORTANT TO KNOW: WEIGHT GAIN DURING PREGNANCY

Put two pregnant women together anywhere—in a doctor's waiting room, on a bus, at a business meeting—and the questions are certain to start flying. "When are you due?" "Have you felt the baby kicking yet?" "Have you been feeling sick?" And, perhaps the favorite query of all, "How much weight have you gained?"

The comparisons are inevitable, and sometimes a little disturbing. Women who started off with a bang—enthusiastically eating their way to 10-pound first-trimester gains—wonder "what's too much?" Others who, appetites daunted by bouts with morning sickness, ended up with net gains which barely registered on the practitioner's scale (perhaps even with a slight weight loss) wonder "what's too little?" All wonder "what's just right?"

Total Increase. Though it was once in medical vogue to limit a woman's pregnancy weight gain to 15 pounds, it is now recognized that this was insufficient to guarantee good infant health. Babies whose mothers gain under 20 pounds are more likely to be premature, small for gestational age, and to suffer growth retardation in the uterus.

Almost as hazardous, however, is the present vogue: eat to your heart and soul's content and gain any amount of weight. There are serious risks in gaining too much weight: assessment and measurement of the fetus become more difficult; excess weight overworks muscles and results in backaches, leg pains, increased fatigue, and varicose veins; if the diet is high in fat and carbohydrates and low in protein, toxemia may result; the baby may become too large for a vaginal delivery; if surgery, such as cesarean section, is needed, it becomes more difficult, and postoperative complications more common; after pregnancy the excess weight may be hard to shed.

Though a woman with an enormous weight gain may have an oversized baby, the mother's weight gain and the weight of her infant don't always correlate. It's possible to gain 40 pounds and deliver a 6-pound baby, or to gain 20 and have an 8-pounder. The quality of the food that contributes to the weight gain is more important than the quantity.

The sensible and safe weight gain for the average woman is between 20 and 30 pounds, no more than 35. That would allow about 6 to 8 pounds for baby and 14 to 24 for placenta, breasts, fluids, and other by-products (see page 128). It also

Breakdown of Your Weight Gain

(All weights are approximate)

Baby	7 ½ pounds
Placenta	1 ½ pounds
Amniotic fluid	1 ¾ pounds
Uterine enlargement	2 pounds
Maternal breast tissue	1 pound
Maternal blood volume	2 ¾ pounds
Fluids in maternal tissue	3 pounds
Maternal fat	7 pounds
Total average	26 ½ -pound overall weight gain

assures a speedier return to prepregnancy weight for mom.

Women who begin pregnancy either extremely under- or overweight, who expect twins, or who have special medical problems will probably need to have this figure adjusted by their physician or nursemidwife.

Rate of Increase. The average-weight woman should gain approximately 3 to 4 pounds during the first trimester, and about a pound a week, 12 to 14 pounds in all, during the second trimester. Weight gain should continue at about 1 pound a week during the seventh and eighth months, and in the ninth month drop off to 1 pound or 2—or even none at all—for a total of 8 to 10 pounds during the third trimester.

Rare is the woman who can keep her weight gain tailored precisely to the ideal formula. And it's fine to fluctuate a little—¾ pound one week, 1 ¼ pounds the next. But the goal of every pregnant woman should be to keep weight gain as steady as possible, without any sudden jumps or drops. If you don't gain any weight for two weeks or more during the fourth to eighth months, or if you gain more than 3 pounds in any week in the second trimester, or more than 2 pounds in any week in the third, check with your doctor.

Beware of the practitioner who tells you at your first visit that you can eat all you like, and not to worry about your weight. When you then gain 30 pounds before the end of the sixth month, he or she may be the first to warn you to restrict your diet—at a time when your baby needs good nutrition most for optimal brain development. Monitor your weight carefully from the beginning, and you'll never have to put your baby on a diet to keep yourself from getting fat.

8
The Fourth Month

WHAT YOU CAN EXPECT AT THIS MONTH'S CHECKUP

This month you can expect your practitioner to check the following, though there may be variations depending upon your particular needs and upon your practitioner's style of practice:[1]

❖ Weight and blood pressure

❖ Urine, for sugar and protein

❖ Fetal heartbeat

❖ Size and shape of uterus, by external palpation, to see how it correlates to due date or estimated date of confinement (EDC)

❖ Height of fundus (top of the uterus)

❖ Hands and feet for edema (swelling), and legs for varicose veins

❖ Symptoms you've been experiencing, especially unusual ones

❖ Questions or problems you want to discuss—have a list ready

WHAT YOU MAY BE FEELING

You may feel all of these symptoms at one time or another, or only a few of them. Some may have continued from last month, others may be new. You may also have other, less common symptoms.

1. See appendix for an explanation of the procedures and tests performed.

PHYSICALLY:

❖ Fatigue

❖ A decrease in urinary frequency

❖ A decrease in, or end to, nausea and vomiting (in a few women, "morning sickness" will continue; in a very few it is just beginning)

❖ Constipation

❖ Heartburn and indigestion, flatulence and bloating

❖ Breasts continue to enlarge, but tenderness and swelling usually subside

❖ Occasional headaches

❖ Occasional faintness or dizziness, particularly with sudden change of position

❖ Nasal congestion and occasional nosebleeds; ear stuffiness

❖ Increase in appetite

❖ Mild edema (swelling) of ankles and feet, and occasionally hands and face

❖ Varicose veins of legs and/or hemorrhoids

❖ Slight whitish vaginal discharge (leukorrhea)

❖ Fetal movement near the end of month (but usually this early only if you are very thin or this is not your first pregnancy)

EMOTIONALLY:

❖ Instability comparable to premenstrual syndrome, which may include irritability, mood swings, irrationality, weepiness

❖ Joy and/or apprehension—if you have started to feel pregnant at last

❖ Frustration—if you don't really feel pregnant yet but are too big for your regular wardrobe and too small for maternity clothes

❖ A feeling you're not quite together. You're a scatterbrain, you forget things, drop things, have trouble concentrating

WHAT YOU MAY BE CONCERNED ABOUT

ELEVATED BLOOD PRESSURE AND PREECLAMPSIA

"My doctor said my blood pressure is up. Should I be concerned?"

A slight increase in blood pressure at one visit probably doesn't mean much of anything. Perhaps you were just nervous, or were late for your appointment and ran all the way, or were worrying about a report you had to finish at work. If your pressure were taken the next day, or even later that same day, it might very well have been normal. Because it is often difficult to determine the cause of an isolated elevated reading, your practitioner may advise you to take it easy until the next visit.

If your blood pressure remains slightly elevated, however, you may be among the 1% to 2% of pregnant women who develop transient high blood pressure during pregnancy (gestational hypertension). This type of hypertension is perfectly harmless, as far as is known, and disappears after delivery.

WHAT YOU MAY LOOK LIKE

By the end of the fourth month, the 4-inch fetus, now nourished by the placenta, is developing reflexes, such as sucking and swallowing. Body growth begins to outstrip that of the head; tooth buds appear; fingers and toes are well defined. Though human-looking, it cannot survive outside the uterus.

What is considered normal blood pressure in pregnancy varies somewhat over the course of nine months. A baseline pressure (what is normal for you) is obtained at the first prenatal visit. Generally the pressure drops a little over the next several months. But as delivery nears, somewhere about the seventh month, it usually begins to rise a bit.

During the first or second trimester, if pressure rises 30 mmHg systolic (the upper number) or 15 mmHg diastolic (the lower number) over the baseline reading (or by more than that in the third trimester) and stays up for at least two readings taken at least six hours apart, the pregnant woman's condition warrants close observation, and possibly treatment.

If increased blood pressure is accompanied by sudden weight gain (more than 3 pounds a week in the second trimester, or more than 2 pounds a week in the third), severe edema (swelling because of water retention), particularly in hands and face, as well as ankles, and/or protein in the urine,[2] the problem may be preeclampsia. In women who receive regular medical care, this disorder is generally diagnosed before it progresses to the more serious symptoms, of blurred vision, headaches, irritability, and severe gastric pain.

No one knows what causes preeclampsia in pregnancy, or why it develops most often in first pregnancies. (Some research ties it to poor nutrition, particularly inadequate protein, but the evidence is not conclusive.) It is known that it can progress to the much more serious eclampsia—characterized by convulsions and even coma—rather quickly. If preeclampsia is suspected, treatment at home may be tried first. But when a definite diagnosis of preeclampsia is established, partial or complete bed rest in the hospital, and medication if needed, is likely to be ordered.

If the pregnancy has not yet reached the 35th week, this conservative treatment may continue until the fetus gains sufficient matu-

---

2. See appendix for explanation of protein in the urine.

rity to survive outside the uterus. But because prolonged preeclampsia can lead to deteriorating environmental conditions in the uterus, permanent vascular damage to the mother, and also increases the risk of hazardous convulsions, induced delivery is desirable once the mother's condition has stabilized or improved. Thanks to modern medical treatment, the chances that both mother and baby will do well are excellent.

Women who begin pregnancy with hypertension (high blood pressure) are classified as high risk but usually do well with increased rest, a low-sodium diet, careful monitoring, and if needed, appropriate medication and bed rest.

SUGAR IN THE URINE

"At my last office visit the doctor said that there was sugar in my urine. She said not to worry, but I'm convinced I have diabetes."

Take your doctor's advice—don't worry. A small amount of sugar in the urine on one occasion during pregnancy does not a diabetic make. What is probably happening is that your body is doing just what it's supposed to do: trying to make sure that your fetus, which depends on you for its fuel supply, is getting enough glucose (sugar).

Since it is insulin that regulates the level of glucose in your blood and ensures that enough is taken in by your body cells for nourishment, pregnancy triggers *anti*-insulin mechanisms to make sure enough sugar remains circulating in your

bloodstream to nourish your fetus. It's a perfect idea that doesn't always work perfectly. Sometimes the anti-insulin effect is so strong that it leaves more than enough sugar in the blood to meet the needs of both mother and child—more than can be handled by the kidneys. The excess is "spilled" into the urine. Thus your "sugar in the urine"—a not uncommon occurrence in pregnancy, especially in the second trimester, when the anti-insulin effect increases.

In most women, the body responds to increased blood sugar levels with increased production of insulin, which will meet the challenge before the next office visit. But some, especially those who are diabetic or have diabetic tendencies, may be unable to produce sufficient quantities of insulin to handle the increase in blood sugar, or may have body tissues that are insulin-resistant. Either way, they continue to show high levels of sugar in both blood and urine. In women who were not previously diabetic, this is known as gestational diabetes.

If sugar appears in your urine at your next visit, your doctor may test your blood for sugar and may order a glucose-tolerance test, a procedure which accurately reflects the body's response to sugar in the bloodstream. Symptoms that may point to the development of diabetes in pregnancy include: excessive hunger and thirst, more frequent urination in the midtrimester, recurrent monilial infections of the vagina, and increase in blood pressure.

About 1% to 2% of pregnant women develop gestational diabetes, and the incidence increases with maternal age (diabetes is more common as we get older). This type of diabetes usually disappears after delivery, but it sometimes recurs later in life. Women who have developed gestational diabetes in a pregnancy should be aware of this possibility so that they can take measures in the future that may prevent this, such as maintaining ideal weight, cultivating good diet and exercise habits, and having regular medical checkups.

Though diabetic mothers-to-be and their fetuses were once at great risk, this is no longer the case. When blood sugar is closely controlled, diabetic mothers can have normal pregnancies and deliver healthy babies. (See page 37 for more on diabetes and pregnancy.)

ANEMIA

"A friend of mine became anemic during pregnancy. How can I tell if I am, and can I prevent it?"

Though nearly 20% of all pregnant women suffer from iron-deficiency anemia, it's a condition that can be easily avoided—in most cases simply by eating a good diet and swallowing one pill, or several, each day.

A blood test for anemia is administered at the first prenatal visit, but few women turn out to be iron-deficient at this time. Some may have come into pregnancy with the condition (common during the childbearing years because of monthly menstrual blood loss). But with conception and the cessation of menstruation, iron stores—if dietary intake is adequate—are replenished. It isn't until the 20th week (when the stores can deplete because of increased fetal requirements) that most cases of iron-deficiency anemia develop.

In a mild anemia, there may be no symptoms. But when iron deficiency is more severe, a woman may be pale, tired, weak, and suffer from palpitations, breathlessness, and even fainting spells. In either case, it's the mother who falls victim to the lack of iron, as her oxygen-carrying red blood cells are depleted. Since this is one of the few instances where the nutritional needs of the fetus are met first (at the expense of its mother), it rarely suffers.

While all pregnant women are susceptible to iron-deficiency anemia, certain groups are at particularly high risk: those who have had several babies in quick succession, those who vomit a lot or eat poorly because of morning sickness, those who are carrying more than one fetus, and those who are inadequately nourished before and/or during pregnancy.

To prevent iron-deficiency anemia, all expectant mothers should take a daily iron supplement of 30 to 60 mgs. In addition, your diet should include a variety of iron-rich foods (see the Best-Odds Diet, page 75). This same regimen will probably be prescribed by your practitioner if you become anemic.[3]

---

3. Iron supplements can cause diarrhea or constipation. Switching formulas may solve the problem; ask your practitioner.

NOSEBLEEDS AND NASAL STUFFINESS

"My nose has been congested a lot and sometimes it bleeds for no apparent reason. I'm worried because I know bleeding can be a sign of illness."

Nasal congestion, often with associated nosebleeds, is a common complaint in pregnancy. It is probably because the high levels of estrogen circulating in your body bring increased blood flow to the mucous membranes of your nose, causing them to soften and swell—much as your cervix does in preparation for childbirth.

You can expect the stuffiness to get worse before it gets better—which won't be until after delivery. You may also develop a postnasal drip, which can occasionally lead to nocturnal coughing or gagging. Don't use medication or nasal sprays to deal with the problem. But do be sure your fluid intake is adequate to compensate for any loss through sneezing or a runny nose. The congestion and bleeding are more common in winter, when heating systems force hot, dry air into the house, drying delicate nasal passages. Using a humidifier can help overcome this dryness.

Taking an extra 250 mg of vitamin C (with your practitioner's approval) along with your usual citrus fruits may help to strengthen your capillaries and reduce the chance of bleeding. (But don't take megadoses of the vitamin.) You might also try lubricating each nostril with a dab of Vaseline. Sometimes a nosebleed will follow overly energetic nose-blowing. Correct nose-blowing is an art, which you would do well to master: First, gently close one nostril with the thumb, and then carefully blow the mucus out the opposite side. Repeat with the other nostril, continuing to alternate until you can breathe through your nose.

ALLERGIES

"My allergies seem to have worsened since my pregnancy began. My nose is runny and my eyes tear all the time."

You may be mistaking the normal nasal stuffiness of pregnancy for allergy. Or, pregnancy—a major stress on the body—may have aggravated your allergies (though some lucky women find temporary relief from allergies during pregnancy). If your allergies worsen, you often can't rely on your usual medication. Check with your physician to see what you can safely use to relieve severe symptoms. Some antihistamines and other medications appear to be relatively safe for use in pregnancy. But, because no tests for safety are absolutely conclusive, drugs should be used only when all else fails. If your nasal discharge is heavy or you're sneezing a lot, increase your fluid intake to compensate for any loss and to thin secretions.

In general, however, the best approach to dealing with allergies in pregnancy is preventive—avoiding the offending substance or substances, assuming you know what they are:

❖ If pollens or other outdoor aller-gens trouble you, stay indoors in air-conditioned and air-filtered space during your susceptible sea-son as much as you can. Wash your hands and face if you've been out of doors, and wear big curved sunglasses to keep pollens from floating into your eyes.

❖ If dust is a culprit, try to have someone do the dusting and sweeping for you. A vacuum cleaner, damp mop, or a damp, cloth-covered broom kicks up less dust than an ordinary broom, and an absorbent cloth will do better than a feather duster. Stay away from musty places like attics and libraries full of old books. Have someone pack away things in your home that are dust collec-tors, like draperies and rugs.

❖ If you're allergic to certain foods, stay away from them, even if they are good foods for pregnancy. Consult the Best-Odds Diet (page 75) for equivalent substitutes.

❖ If animals bring on allergy at-tacks, let friends know of the problem in advance so that they can rid the room of both pets and their dander before you visit. And, of course, don't keep a pet in your own home, unless it has a completely separate living area.

❖ Tobacco-smoke allergy is easier to control these days since fewer people smoke and more smokers oblige if they are asked to refrain. To tame your allergy, as well as for the benefit of your baby, there should be no one smoking in any area you spend time in. Don't be embarrassed to say, "Yes, I mind very much if you smoke."

VAGINAL DISCHARGE

"I've noticed a slight vaginal discharge that is thin and whitish. I'm afraid I have an infection."

A thin, milky, mild-smelling dis-charge (called leukorrhea) is normal throughout pregnancy. It's much like the discharge many women have prior to their menstrual periods and/or at the time of ovula-tion. Since it increases until term and may become quite heavy, some women are more comfortable wear-ing sanitary pads during the last months of pregnancy.

Aside from the offense to your esthetic sensibilities (and possibly to your husband's—who may be turned off oral sex by the unusual taste and odor), the discharge should be of no concern. It is important to keep the genital area clean and dry; cotton, or cotton-crotched, under-wear may help to do this. Do *not* use a douche, however, unless it is pre-scribed by your doctor. (Even then, *do not use a bulb syringe,* such as the disposable variety. Use a douche bag or can, and hold it *no higher than 2 feet above the nozzle* to keep the water pressure low. The tip should not be inserted more than 1 inch past the entrance of the vagina, and the labia should be held open, allowing the fluid to run freely out. This procedure avoids the risk of a life-threatening air embolism.)

If you develop a vaginal discharge that is yellowish, greenish, or thick and cheesy, has a foul odor, or is accompanied by burning, itching, redness, or soreness—infection is likely. Notify your doctor or nurse-midwife so that the infection can be treated (probably with vaginal suppositories or gels, ointments, or creams inserted with an applicator). You may be able to hasten your recovery by maintaining scrupulous cleanliness, especially after going to the bathroom (always wipe from front to back), and by following the Best-Odds Diet—being especially careful to avoid refined sugars (which may help to create a breeding ground for infectious organisms). If the infection is a sexually transmittable one, avoiding intercourse until both you and your husband are infection-free is gener ally recommended. Unfortunately, though medication may banish the infection temporarily, it often returns. But simple vaginitis does not pose a risk to your baby.

If your vaginitis is caused by a yeast called monilia, your doctor will be careful to treat it with medication so you won't pass the infection on to your baby (in the form of thrush) during delivery.

FETAL MOVEMENT

"I haven't felt the baby moving yet; could something be wrong? Or could I just not be recognizing the kicking?"

Fetal movement may be the greatest source of joy in your pregnancy and, at the same time, the greatest cause of anxiety. More than a positive pregnancy test, an ex-

panding belly, or even the sound of the fetal heartbeat, its presence affirms that you've got a new life growing inside you. Its absence breeds terror that the new life is not thriving.

Though the embryo begins to make spontaneous movements by the seventh week, these movements do not become apparent to the mother until they are much stronger. That first momentous sensation of life, or "quickening," can occur anywhere between the 14th and 26th weeks, but generally closer to the average of 18 to 20 weeks. Variations on that average are common. A woman who's been pregnant before is likely to recognize movement earlier (because she knows what to expect) than one who is expecting her first child. A very slender woman may notice very early, weak movements, while an obese woman may not be aware of movements until they've become more vigorous.

Sometimes the first perception of movement is delayed slightly because of a miscalculated due date. Or because of the fetus's position in the uterus. Or sometimes it's delayed because a woman has failed to recognize fetal movement when she felt it.

Nobody can tell a first-time mother-to-be exactly what she can expect to feel; a hundred pregnant women may describe that first quickening in a hundred different ways. Perhaps the most common descriptions are "a fluttering in the abdomen" and "butterflies in the stomach." But early fetal movements have also been described as "a bumping or nudging," "a twitch," "a growling stomach," "someone hitting my stomach," "a bubble bursting," "the squirmies," "like being turned upside down on an amusement park ride." Often the first noticeable movements are mistaken for gas or hunger pains. And one woman recalls, "I thought a bug was on my shirt, but when I went to brush it off, I realized it was the baby moving."

Although it isn't unusual to be unaware of fetal movements until the 20th week or later, your practitioner may order a sonogram to check on the baby's condition if you haven't felt anything—and he or she hasn't been able to elicit fetal response—by the 21st week. If the fetal heartbeat is strong, however, and everything else seems to be progressing normally, he or she may hold off even longer on testing.

"I felt little movements every day last week, but for the last few days I haven't felt a thing. Could something have gone wrong?"

Anxiety over when the first movement will be felt is later replaced by other anxieties: that fetal movements don't seem frequent enough, or that they haven't been noted for a few days. While such anxieties are understandable, they're really unnecessary. At this stage of pregnancy, frequency of movement may vary a great deal, and there's no need to panic if the baby hasn't been heard from for three, four, even five days. Though the fetus is stirring almost continuously, only some of these movements may be strong enough for you

to feel. Others may be missed because of the fetal position (facing and kicking inwards, for instance, instead of outwards). Or because of your own activity (when you're walking or moving about a lot, the baby is usually rocked to sleep; and even if he or she isn't, you may be too busy to notice the movements). It's also possible that you're sleeping right through your baby's most active period—which is, for many fetuses, the middle of the night.

From the sixth month on, fetal activity becomes stronger and more regular, so that 24 hours without movement, while not automatically cause for alarm, is a reason to call your practitioner.

APPEARANCE

"I get depressed when I look in the mirror or step on a scale—I'm so fat."

In a society as obsessed with slenderness as ours, where those who can "pinch an inch" despair, the weight gain of pregnancy can often become a source of depression. It shouldn't. There's an important difference between pounds added for no good reason (other than willpower gone astray) and pounds gained for the best and most beautiful of reasons: your child and its support system growing inside you.

Yet in the eyes of many beholders, a pregnant woman isn't just beautiful inside but outside as well. Many women and their husbands consider the newly rounded pregnant reflection as the most lovely—and sensuous—of feminine shapes.

As long as you're eating right and not exceeding the recommended limits for pregnancy weight gain (see page 127), you needn't feel "fat"—just pregnant. The added inches you're seeing are all legitimate by-products of pregnancy and will disappear rapidly once the baby appears. If you *are* exceeding the limits, self-defeating depression won't keep you from getting fatter (and may even fuel your appetite), but careful scrutiny of your eating habits might. (See the Best-Odds Diet, page 75.)

REALITY OF PREGNANCY

"Now that my abdomen is swelling, the fact that I'm really pregnant has finally sunk in. Even though we planned this pregnancy, I suddenly feel scared, trapped by the baby—even antagonistic toward it."

E ven the most eager of expectant parents may be surprised (and guilt-ridden) to find themselves with second thoughts as their pregnancy starts to become a reality. An unseen little intruder has suddenly come between them, turning their lives upside down, depriving them of freedoms they'd always taken for granted, making more demands—both physically and emotionally—than anyone ever has before. Every aspect of the life they have become accustomed to—from how they spend their evenings, to what they eat and drink, to how often they make love—is being altered by this child even before it's born. And the knowledge that these changes will become still more imposing after delivery compounds their mixed feelings, deepens their apprehension.

Not only is a little ambivalence, a little fear, even a little antagonism, normal, it's healthy—as long as these feelings are confronted and acknowledged. And now is the best time to do that. Work out your resentments (over not being free to stay out late on Saturday nights, to pick up and go on a weekend trip when the spirit moves you, to work full time, or to spend your money any way you please) before the baby's born, and you won't find yourself venting them after he or she's arrived. Sharing your feelings with your partner is the best way to do this—and encourage him to do likewise.

It's true that your life is never going to be the same again once your "two" is turned to "three." But as some parts of your world become more constricted, others will open up. You may find yourself reborn with your baby's birth. And this new life may turn out to be the best yet.

UNWANTED ADVICE

"Now that everyone can see I'm expecting, everyone—from my mother-in-law to strangers on the elevator—has advice for me. It drives me crazy."

S hort of taking up a reclusive existence on a desert island, there's no way for a pregnant woman to escape the unsolicited advice of those around her. There's just something about a bulging belly that brings out the "expert" in all of us. Take your morning jog around the park and someone is sure to chide: "You shouldn't be running in your condition!" Lug home two bags of groceries from the supermarket and you're bound to hear: "Do you think you ought to be carrying such heavy bundles?" Or reach up for a subway strap and you may even be warned: "If you stretch that way the cord will wrap around your baby's neck and strangle it."

Between such gratuitous advice and the inevitable predictions about the sex of the baby, what's an expectant mother to do? First of all, keep in mind that most of what you hear is probably nonsense. Old wives' tales that *do* have foundation in fact have been scientifically substantiated and have become part of medical practice. Those that do not, though still tightly woven into the tapestry of pregnancy mythology, can be confidently dismissed. Those recommendations that leave you with a nagging doubt—"What if they are right?"—and are therefore impossible to dismiss are best checked with your doctor, nurse-midwife, or childbirth educator.

Whether it's possibly plausible or obviously ridiculous, however, don't let unwanted advice get your dander up. Neither you nor your baby will profit from the added tension. Instead, keeping your sense of humor handy, you can take one of two approaches. Politely inform the advice-giver that you have a trusted physician who counsels you on your pregnancy and that you can't accept suggestions from anyone else. Or, just as politely, smile, say thank you, and go on your way, letting their comments go in one ear and out the other—without making any stops in between.

But no matter how you choose to handle unwanted advice, you'd also do well to get used to it. If there's anyone who attracts a crowd of advice-givers faster than a pregnant woman, it's a woman with a new baby.

What It's Important to Know:
MAKING LOVE DURING PREGNANCY

Religious and medical miracles aside, every pregnancy begins with the sexual act. So why is it that what got you into this situation in the first place may now have become one of your biggest problems?

Whether sex suddenly becomes better than ever, virtually nonexistent, or just a little uncomfortable, almost every expectant couple finds that their sexual relationship undergoes some kind of change during the nine months of pregnancy.

Variations in sexual appetites and reactions before conception are wide to begin with. What is a satisfying sex life to one couple, "obligatory" relations once a week, for instance, would be completely unsatisfactory for another, for whom once a day might not always be enough. After conception, these variations may be even more exaggerated. And to further complicate matters sexual, physical and emotional upheaval may leave the once-a-day couple less in the mood for love than the once-a-week couple, and vice versa.

Though intensity differs from couple to couple, there is a general down-up-down pattern of sexual interest during the three trimesters of pregnancy. It's not surprising that diminution of sexual interest is common early in pregnancy (in one survey, 54% of women reported reduced libido in the first trimester). After all, fatigue, nausea, vomiting, and painfully tender breasts do make less than ideal bedfellows. In women with comfortable first trimesters, however, sexual desire often remains more or less the same. And a sizable minority of expectant women find it increases significantly—often because the early hormones of pregnancy leave the vulva engorged and ultrasensitive, and/or because the heightened breast sensitivity that is painful for other women is pleasurable for them. These women may experience orgasms or multi-orgasms for the first time.

Interest often—but not always— picks up during the midtrimester, when the couple is physically and psychologically better adjusted to the pregnancy. It usually wanes again as delivery nears, even more drastically than in the first trimester—for obvious reasons: first, the bulk of the abdomen is more and more difficult to "get around"; second, the aches and dis-

comforts of advancing pregnancy are capable of cooling even the hottest passion; and third, it's hard to concentrate on anything but that eagerly and anxiously awaited event.

Sexual pleasure, like sexual interest, seems to diminish in some—but certainly not all—couples. In one group of women, 21% received little or no pleasure from sex before conception. The percentage of these women finding sex not pleasurable rose to 41% at 12 weeks of gestation, and 59% going into the ninth month. The same study found that at 12 weeks, about 1 in 10 couples were not having sex at all; by the ninth month, more than a third were abstaining. But keep in mind also that the study found that more than 4 in 10 women were still enjoying sex at this point—more than half of these with *no* problems.

So you may find that sex during pregnancy is the best you've ever had. Or something you wish you could enjoy but find difficult. Or it may become an uncomfortable obligation. You may even abandon it altogether. "Normal" in pregnancy lovemaking, as in so many other aspects of pregnancy, is what is right for you.

UNDERSTANDING SEXUALITY DURING PREGNANCY

Unfortunately, some practitioners are as inhibited about sexuality as the rest of us. Often they don't tell expectant couples what to expect, or not to expect, in the intimate part of their relationship. And that leaves many couples uncertain how to proceed.

Understanding why making love during pregnancy is different than it is at other times can help ease fears and worries, and make having intercourse (or not having it) more acceptable and more pleasurable.

First of all, there are many physical changes that affect both interest and actual sexual pleasure. Some can be dealt with to minimize their interference in your sex life; others you may just have to learn to live with—and love with.

Nausea and Vomiting. If your morning sickness stays with you day and night, you may just have to wait its symptoms out. (In most cases, queasiness will start letting up by the end of the first trimester.) If it strikes just at certain hours, keep your schedule flexible, and put the good times to good use. Don't pressure yourself to feel sexy when you're feeling lousy; morning sickness is often aggravated by emotional stress. (See page 95 for tips on minimizing morning sickness.)

Fatigue. This, too, should pass by the fourth month. Until then, make love while the sun shines (when the opportunity presents itself), instead of trying to force yourself to stay up late for romance. If your weekend afternoons are free, cap off a nap with a lovemaking session. (See page 94 for more on fatigue.)

The Changing Shape. Making love can be both awkward and uncomfortable when a bulging belly seems to loom as large and forbidding as a Himalayan mountain. As pregnancy progresses, the gymnastics required to scale the growing abdomen may not seem, to some couples, worth the effort. (But there are ways to get around the mountain; see page 144.) In addition, the woman's full-figured silhouette may actually turn off one or both partners. This is a socially conditioned reflex you may be able to psych yourself out of by thinking: big (in pregnancy) is beautiful.

The Engorgement of Genitals. The increased blood flow to the pelvic area can heighten sexual response in some women. But it can also make sex less satisfying (especially later in pregnancy) when a residual feeling of uncomfortable, unrelieved fullness may persist after orgasm, leaving a woman feeling as though she didn't quite make it. For males, too, the engorgement of the pregnant woman's genitalia may increase pleasure (he feels pleasantly and snugly caressed), or reduce it (he feels the fit is too tight, and he loses his erection).

Breast Tenderness. In early pregnancy, the breasts may have to be avoided during love play because they are painfully tender. (Be certain to communicate this discomfort to your partner, rather than suffering, and resenting, his touch in silence.) However, as the tenderness diminishes toward the end of the first trimester, the extreme sensitivity of the breasts enhances sex for some couples. Others revel throughout in the fun of full-and-firm-for-the-first-time breasts.

Alterations in Vaginal Secretions.
These secretions increase in volume
and change in consistency, odor,
and taste. The increased lubrication
may make intercourse more enjoy-
able for the couple if the woman's
vagina has always been dry and/or
uncomfortably narrow. Or it might
make the vaginal canal so wet and
slippery that a man may have trouble
holding an erection. The heavier
scent and taste of the secretions may
also make cunnilingus unpleasant to
some men. Massaging scented oils
into the area may help disguise the
problem.

**Bleeding Caused by the Sensitivity
of the Cervix.** The mouth of the
uterus also becomes engorged during pregnancy—crisscrossed with
many additional blood vessels to accommodate increased blood flow to
the uterus—and much softer than
before pregnancy. This means that
deep penetration can occasionally
cause bleeding, particularly late in
pregnancy when the cervix begins
to ripen for delivery. If this occurs
(and possible miscarriage or any
other problem is ruled out by your
practitioner), simply avoid deep
penetration.

Leakage of Colostrum. This occurs
during sexual stimulation in some
women, and it can be disconcerting
in the middle of foreplay. It's nothing to worry about, of course, but if
it bothers you or your partner, it can
easily be avoided by refraining from
breast play.

There are also a full complement
of psychological hangups that can

interfere with sexual enjoyment
during pregnancy. These, too, can
be minimized.

**Fear About Hurting the Fetus or
Causing a Miscarriage.** In normal
pregnancies sexual intercourse will
do neither. The fetus is well cushioned and protected inside the amniotic sac, which is securely sealed off
from the outside world with a mucous plug.

**Fear That Having an Orgasm Will
Stimulate Miscarriage or Early Labor.** Although the uterus does contract following orgasm—and these
contractions can be quite pronounced in some women, lasting as
long as half an hour after
intercourse—such contractions are
not a sign of labor. Orgasm, particularly the more intense kind triggered
by masturbation, may be prohibited
in pregnancies at high risk for miscarriage or premature labor.

**Fear That the Fetus is "Watching"
or "Aware."** Though a fetus may
enjoy the gentle rocking of uterine
contractions during orgasm, it can
neither see nor understand what is
happening during intercourse, and
will certainly have no memory of it.
Fetal reactions (slowed movement
during intercourse, then furious
kicking and squirming and speeded-
up heartbeat after orgasm) are based
solely on hormonal and uterine activity.

**Fear That the Introduction of the
Penis into the Vagina Will Cause
Infection.** As long as the male does
not have a sexually transmittable

disease, there appears to be no danger of infecting either mother or fetus through intercourse during the first seven or eight months. The baby is safely sealed within the uterus in the amniotic sac, which can't be penetrated by either semen or infectious organisms. Most physicians believe this is true even during the ninth month—as long as the sac remains unbroken (the membranes haven't ruptured). But because they could rupture at any time, some suggest that a condom be worn during intercourse in the last four to eight weeks of pregnancy, as added insurance against infection.

Anxiety Over the Coming Attraction. Both the mother- and father-to-be are subject to mixed feelings over the blessed event; about the responsibilities and lifestyle changes to come; about the financial and emotional cost of bringing up a baby—all of which can inhibit relaxed lovemaking. This ambivalence, which many expectant parents experience, should be confronted and talked through openly rather than being brought to bed.

The Changing Relationship Between Husband and Wife. A couple may have trouble adjusting to the idea that they will no longer be just lovers, or husband and wife, but mother and father as well. The connection between parenthood and sex may be a difficult one for either or both partners to make. (After all, many of us still avoid associating our own parents with sex, though we are living proof that such an association exists.) On the other hand, some couples may discover that the new dimension in their relationship brings a new intimacy into bed with them—and with it, a new excitement.

Subconscious Hostility. Of the expectant father toward the expectant mother, because he is jealous that she has become the center of attention. Or of mom-to-be toward dad-to-be because she feels she is doing all the suffering (particularly if the pregnancy has been a rough one) for the baby they both wanted and will both enjoy. Such feelings must be talked out, but not in bed.

Belief That Intercourse During the Last Six Weeks of Pregnancy Will Cause Labor to Begin. It *is* true that the uterine contractions triggered by orgasm become stronger as pregnancy proceeds. But unless the cervix is "ripe," these contractions do not appear to bring on labor—as many overdue couples who have hopefully tried obligatory nightly sex can attest. However, since no one knows exactly what initiates labor, and because some studies do show an increase in premature births among couples having intercourse in the last weeks of pregnancy, abstinence is often prescribed for women with a tendency toward preterm delivery.

Fear of "Hitting" the Baby Once the Head Is Engaged in the Pelvis. Even couples who were relaxed about having intercourse earlier can tighten up now because the baby is too "close" for comfort. Many doctors suggest that though you can't really hurt the baby, deep penetration won't be comfortable at this time and should be avoided.

Psychological factors can also affect sexual relations for the better:

Switching from Procreational to Recreational Sex. Some couples who worked hard at becoming pregnant may be delighted at being able to have sex just for pleasure—free from thermometers, charts, calendars, and anxiety. For them, sex becomes fun for the first time in months, or even years.

Though sexual intercourse during pregnancy may be different from what you've experienced before, it is in most cases perfectly safe. In fact, in many ways it's good for you: it keeps you and your spouse close; it helps you get in shape, preparing your pelvic muscles for delivery; and it's relaxing—which is beneficial for everyone concerned, baby included.

Since lovemaking has so much to offer the expectant couple, it would be ideal if every couple could take advantage of it throughout pregnancy. Alas, for the exceptional few this isn't possible. In high risk pregnancies, intercourse may be restricted at certain times, or even throughout the nine months. For others, intercourse may be permitted without orgasm for the wife, or petting may be allowed as long as penetration is avoided. Knowing precisely *what* is safe and *when* is essential; if your doctor instructs you to abstain, ask why and whether he or she is referring to intercourse,

orgasm, or both, and whether the restrictions are temporary or meant for the entire gestation.

WHEN SEXUAL RELATIONS MAY BE LIMITED

❖ Any time unexplained bleeding occurs.

❖ During the first trimester if a woman has a history of miscarriages or threatened miscarriage, or shows signs of a threatened miscarriage during her current pregnancy.

❖ During the last 8 to 12 weeks if a woman has a history of premature or threatened premature labor, or is experiencing signs of it in this pregnancy.

❖ If fetal membranes (the bag of waters) have ruptured.

❖ When placenta previa is known to exist (the placenta is in an abnormal position, near or over the cervix, where it could be prematurely dislodged, threatening mother and baby).

❖ In the last trimester if multiple fetuses are being carried.

ENJOYING IT MORE, EVEN IF YOU'RE DOING IT LESS

Good, lasting sexual relationships—like good, lasting marriages—are rarely built in a day (or even a really terrific night). They grow with practice, patience, understanding, and love. This is true, too, of an already established sexual relationship that undergoes the emotional and physical assaults of pregnancy. Here are a few ways to "stay on top":

❖ Remember that the quality of lovemaking is always more important than the quantity—but never more so than during pregnancy. Never allow how frequently you have or don't have intercourse to interfere with other aspects of your relationship.

❖ Keep the emphasis on love, rather than lovemaking. If one or both of you don't feel like having intercourse, or if intercourse isn't fully satisfying, find alternative routes to intimacy. The possibilities are far more numerous than positions in a sex manual. For example: old-fashioned kissing and necking, hand holding, back rubs, foot massage, sharing a milkshake in bed (see page 87 for the recipe), reading love poems, watching television while cuddling under a blanket, taking a shower together, going out (or staying in) for a romantic candlelit dinner, meeting for a quiet lunch—or whatever else makes the lovebird in you coo.

❖ Recognize the possible strains that expectant parenthood may have placed on your relationship, and acknowledge any changes in the intensity of sexual desire that either or both of you may be feeling. Discuss the problems openly; don't hide them under the bedcovers. If the problems seem too big to handle by yourselves, seek professional help.

❖ When you start worrying that making love may be harmful, think positive: It's good physical preparation for labor and delivery. (Not many athletes have this much fun in training.)

❖ Think of having to try new positions during pregnancy as an adventure. But give yourselves time to adjust to each position you try. (You might even consider a "dry run"—trying out a new position fully clothed first, so that it'll be more familiar when you try it for real.) Usually comfortable positions include: male on top, but off to one side or supported by his arms (to keep his weight off the woman); woman on top (but avoid too-deep penetration); both partners on their side—front-to-front or front-to-back.

❖ Keep your expectations within reality's reach. Though some women achieve orgasm for the first time during pregnancy, at least one study showed that most women are less likely to achieve orgasm *regularly* during pregnancy—particularly in the last trimester, when only one out of four women reach climax consistently—than before conception. Your goal doesn't always have to be orgasm; sometimes just physical closeness can satisfy.

❖ If the doctor has ruled out sexual intercourse during any period of your pregnancy, ask if orgasm is okay—via mutual masturbation. If it isn't (if there is worry about potential miscarriage, orgasm through masturbation can cause more violent contractions than orgasm through intercourse), you might still get pleasure out of pleasuring your husband in this way.

❖ If the doctor has prohibited orgasm but not coitus, you might still want to enjoy lovemaking without your reaching climax. It's a way of feeling close to each other. Another possibility: intercourse between the thighs.

Even if the quality, or quantity, of your sexual relations isn't quite what it once was, understanding what is going on in the dynamics of a relationship during pregnancy can keep the relationship strong—even strengthen it—without spectacular or frequent coitus.

9
The Fifth Month

WHAT YOU CAN EXPECT AT
THIS MONTH'S CHECKUP

This month, you can expect your practitioner to check the following, though there may be variations depending upon your particular needs and upon your practitioner's style of practice:[1]

❖ Weight and blood pressure

❖ Urine, for sugar and protein

❖ Fetal heartbeat

❖ Size and shape of uterus, by external palpation

❖ Height of fundus (top of uterus)

❖ Feet and hands, for edema (swelling), and legs, for varicose veins

❖ Symptoms you have been experiencing, especially unusual ones

❖ Questions and problems you want to discuss—have a list ready

WHAT YOU MAY BE FEELING

You may feel all of these symptoms at one time or another, or only a few of them. Some may have continued from last month, others may be new. Still others may hardly be noticed because you've become so used to them. You may also have other less common symptoms.

PHYSICALLY:

❖ Fetal movement

❖ Increasing whitish vaginal discharge (leukorrhea)

❖ Lower abdominal achiness (from stretching ligaments)

---

1. See appendix for an explanation of the procedures and tests performed.

- ❖ Constipation

- ❖ Heartburn and indigestion, flatulence and bloating

- ❖ Occasional headaches, faintness or dizziness

- ❖ Nasal congestion and occasional nosebleeds; ear stuffiness

- ❖ Hearty appetite

- ❖ Leg cramps

- ❖ Mild edema (swelling) of ankles and feet, and occasionally hands and face

- ❖ Varicose veins of legs and/or hemorrhoids

- ❖ Increased pulse (heart rate)

- ❖ Easier—or more difficult—orgasm

- ❖ Backache

- ❖ Skin pigmentation changes on abdomen and/or face

EMOTIONALLY:

- ❖ An acceptance of the reality of pregnancy

- ❖ Fewer mood swings, but irritability still occasionally occurs; continued absentmindedness

WHAT YOU MAY LOOK LIKE

By the end of the fifth month, the activity of this 8- to 10-inch fetus is strong enough to be felt by its mother. Soft downy lanugo covers its body; hair begins to grow on its head; brows and white eyelashes appear. A protective vernix coating covers the fetus.

WHAT YOU MAY BE CONCERNED ABOUT

FATIGUE

"I get tired when I am exercising or doing heavy cleaning; should I stop?"

Not only should you stop when you get tired, you should, whenever possible, stop before then. Exerting yourself to the point of exhaustion is never a good idea. During pregnancy it's a particularly bad one, since overwork takes its toll not only on you but on the baby. Pay careful attention to your body's signals. If you become breathless when you're jogging, or find the vacuum suddenly feels as though it weighs a ton, take a break.

Instead of marathon activity sessions, pace yourself. Work or exercise a bit, rest a bit. Most of the time the work, or the workout, will get done, and you won't feel drained afterward. If occasionally something doesn't get done, you're getting good training for the days when the demands of parenthood will often keep you from finishing what you start.

FAINTNESS AND DIZZINESS

"I feel dizzy when I get up from a sitting or lying-down position. And yesterday I nearly fainted while I was shopping. Am I okay? Can this hurt my baby?"

On late-show movies, a fainting spell is a more reliable indicator of pregnancy than a dead rabbit. Screenwriters in the '40s were, however, misinformed. Though dizziness and fainting are fairly common in pregnancy, they are not likely to appear until the second trimester, when the mother's total blood volume increases dramatically.

The dizziness that occurs on rising from a sitting or prone position is called postural hypotension. It's a drop in blood pressure, caused by a sudden shifting of blood away from the brain. The cure is as simple as the explanation: Always get up very gradually. Jumping up quickly to answer the phone is likely to land you right back on the sofa.

You might also feel dizzy because your blood sugar has dropped. Generally this is caused by going too long without food and can be controlled by taking more frequent, smaller meals or eating snacks between your usual meal times. Carry a box of raisins, a piece of fruit, some whole-wheat crackers or breadsticks in your bag for quick blood-sugar lifts.

Dizziness can strike, too, in an overheated store or bus, especially if you are overdressed. The best way to handle such dizziness is to get out in the fresh air, or to an open window. Taking off your coat and loosening your clothes—especially around the neck and waist—should help, too. If you feel lightheaded and/or think you are going to faint, you should try to increase circulation to your brain. Lie down, if possible, with your feet (not your head) elevated, or sit down and put your head between your knees until dizziness subsides. If there's no place to lie or sit, kneel on one knee and bend forward as though you were trying to tie your shoe. Actual fainting is rare, but if you do faint, there is no need for worry or concern— although the flow of blood to your brain is temporarily being reduced, this will not affect your baby.[2]

Tell your practitioner about any faintness you experience when you see him or her next. Report actual fainting promptly. Frequent fainting—occasionally a sign of severe anemia or illness—needs to be evaluated by a physician.

---

2. First aid for mothers-to-be who've actually fainted is the same as the preventive measures.

SLEEPING POSITION

'I've always slept on my stomach. Now I'm afraid to. And I just can't seem to get comfortable any other way.''

G iving up your favorite sleeping position during pregnancy can be as traumatic as giving up your teddy bear was when you were six. You're bound to lose some sleep over it—but only until you get used to the new position. And the time to get used to it is now, before your expanding belly makes getting comfortable even more difficult.

Two common favorite sleeping positions—on the belly and on the back—are not recommended during pregnancy. The belly position, for obvious reasons: as your stomach grows, sleeping on it would be about as comfy as sleeping on a watermelon. The back position, though more comfortable, rests the entire weight of your pregnant uterus on your back, your intestines, and the inferior vena cava (a vein responsible for returning blood from the lower body to the heart). This can aggravate backaches and hemorrhoids, inhibit digestive function, interfere with breathing and circulation, and possibly cause hypotension, or low blood pressure.

This doesn't mean you have to sleep standing up. Curling up or stretching out on your side—preferably the left side—with one leg crossed over the other and with a pillow between them, is best for both you and the fetus. It not only allows maximum flow of blood and nutrients to the placenta, but also enhances efficient kidney function,

Sleep on your side.

which means better elimination of waste products and fluids and less edema (swelling) of ankles, feet, and hands.

Very few people, however, manage to stay in one position through the night. Don't be alarmed if you wake up and find yourself on your back or abdomen. No harm done—just turn back to your side. And don't be concerned if you feel uncomfortable for a few nights. Your body will soon adjust to the new position.

BACKACHE

"I'm having a lot of backaches. I'm afraid I won't be able to stand up at all by the ninth month.''

T he aches and discomforts of pregnancy are not designed to make you miserable. They are the side effects of your body's preparation for that momentous moment when your baby is born. Backache is no exception. During pregnancy, the usually stable joints of the pelvis begin to loosen up to allow easier passage for the baby at delivery. This, along with your oversized abdomen, throws your body off balance. To compensate, you tend to bring your shoulders back and arch your neck. Standing with your belly thrust forward—to be sure that no one who passes fails to notice you're pregnant—compounds the problem. The result: a deeply curved lower back, strained back muscles, and pain.

Even pain with a purpose, however, hurts. And without defeating the purpose, you can conquer (or at least subdue) the pain. The best approach, as usual, is prevention. Come into pregnancy with strong abdominal muscles, good posture, and graceful body mechanics. But if it's too late for that, there's still plenty you can do. In general, your goal will be to keep your pelvis from tilting forward and the small of your back from curving inward. Your pelvis should instead tip back and cra-

Take an anti-backache position.

dle the baby. The following should also help:

❖ Don't gain more than the recommended amount of weight. Excess poundage will only add to the load your back is struggling under.

❖ Don't wear very high heels, or even very flat ones without proper support. Some doctors recommend wide two-inch heels to help keep the body properly aligned.

Bend at the knees.

❖ Learn the proper way to lift heavy loads (packages, children, laundry, books, etc.). Don't lift abruptly. Stabilize your body first by assuming a wide stance (feet shoulder-width apart) and tucking your buttocks in. Bend at the knees, not at the waist, and lift with the weight on your arms and legs rather than on your back.

(See illustration.) If backache is a problem, try to limit the carrying you do.

❖ Don't stretch to put dishes back into the cupboard or to hang a painting. Instead, use a low, steady footstool. Stretching puts a strain on the back muscles.

Sit comfortably.

❖ Learn to walk, sit, lie, without putting stress on your back muscles. That means with buttocks tucked under and abdomen tilted inward.

❖ Do simple exercises that strengthen your abdominal muscles and tilt your pelvis the right way. (See the Pelvic Tilt, page 163.)

❖ Don't stay on your feet for long periods. If you must, keep one foot up on a stool, your knee bent. This will prevent your lower back from curving in. When standing on a hard-surfaced floor, as when cooking or washing dishes, put a small skid-proof rug underfoot as a cushion.

❖ Use a heating pad (wrapped in a towel) or warm (but not hot) baths to temporarily relieve muscle discomfort and spasm.

❖ Sleep on a firm mattress, or put a board under an oversoft one.

LATE MISCARRIAGE

"I know they say that once you pass the third month, you don't have to worry about miscarriage. But I know someone who lost her baby in the fifth month."

While it's essentially true that there's little reason to worry about miscarriage after the first trimester, it does occasionally happen that a fetus is lost between the 12th and 20th weeks. This is known as a *late* miscarriage, which accounts for fewer than 25% of all spontaneous abortions and is rare in an uneventful, low-risk pregnancy. After the 20th week, when the fetus usually weighs over 500 grams (17½ ounces) and there is the possibility that it can survive with special care, delivery is considered a premature birth and not a miscarriage.

Unlike the causes of early miscarriages, which are frequently related to the fetus, the causes of second-trimester miscarriages are usually related to either the placenta or the mother.[3] The placenta may separate

3. Many maternal causes of late miscarriage can be prevented by good medical care.

prematurely from the uterus, be implanted abnormally, or fail to produce adequate hormones to maintain the pregnancy. The mother may have taken certain drugs, or undergone surgery that affects the pelvic organs. Or she may suffer from serious infection, uncontrolled chronic illness, severe malnutrition, endocrine dysfunction, untreated Rh incompatibility with the fetus, myomas (tumors of the uterus), an abnormally shaped uterus, or an incompetent cervix that opens prematurely. Serious physical trauma, as in accidents, appears to play only a small role in miscarriage at any stage.

Early symptoms of a midtrimester miscarriage include a pink discharge for several days, or a scant brown discharge for several weeks. At this point, bed rest is often prescribed. If the spotting passes, this is an indication that it wasn't related to miscarriage, and resumption of normal activity is usually permitted. If, however, the cervix is found to have begun to dilate, a diagnosis of incompetent (or weak) cervix may be made and cerclage (the suturing closed of the cervix until a few weeks before the due date) performed. This can frequently prevent the threatened miscarriage. If, on the other hand, the spotting turns to heavier bleeding and is accompanied by cramping, a miscarriage is imminent, and probably inevitable. Hospitalization may be necessary to prevent hemorrhaging; continued cramping and bleeding following such a miscarriage indicate it is incomplete, and a D and C may be required to evacuate the uterus.

If the cause of a late miscarriage can be determined, it may be possible to prevent a repeat of the tragedy. If a previously undiagnosed incompetent cervix was responsible, future miscarriages can be prevented by cerclage early in pregnancy, before the cervix begins to dilate. If hormonal insufficiency was to blame, hormone replacement may allow future pregnancies to progress normally. Chronic disease, such as diabetes or hypertension, can be better controlled, and acute infection or malnutrition avoided. Rh incompatibility can be treated in utero, if necessary. And an abnormally shaped or myomatous uterus may, in some instances, be corrected by surgery.

ABDOMINAL PAIN

"I'm very worried about the pains I've been getting on the sides of my pelvis."

What you are probably feeling is the stretching of muscles and ligaments supporting the uterus—something most pregnant women experience. It may be crampy or sharp and stabbing, and often is most noticeable when you are getting up from a bed or chair, or when you cough. It may be brief, or last for several hours. As long as the pain is occasional and not persistent—and is not accompanied by fever, chills, bleeding, faintness, or other unusual symptoms—there's no cause for concern. Getting off your feet and resting in a comfortable position should bring some relief. You should, of course, mention the pain to your practitioner at your next visit.

FAST-GROWING HAIR AND NAILS—AND RED PALMS

"It seems to me that my hair and nails never looked so good. My palms, however, seem to be red all the time. Is it my imagination?"

T he bounteous circulation caused by pregnancy hormones is feeding your skin cells well. Two of the happy effects of this increased nourishment are nails that grow faster than you can manicure them, and hair that grows faster than you can secure appointments with your stylist. (Some pregnant women find hair flourishing everywhere, even on once smooth abdomens.)

A not-so-happy effect is redness and itching of the palms (and the soles of the feet), which gives the appearance of dishpan hands, even if you never wash a dish. All of these effects will disappear after delivery.

CHANGES IN SKIN PIGMENTATION

"In addition to the dark line down the center of my abdomen, I now have dark spots on my face. Is this discoloration normal, and will it remain after pregnancy?"

A gain, it's those pregnancy hormones at work. Just as they darkened the areola around your nipples, they are now coloring the linea alba—the white line you proba-

bly never noticed, which runs down your abdomen to the top of your pubic bone. From now on, it will be called the linea nigra, or black line.

Some women, usually those with darker complexions, will also find patches of darkened skin on their foreheads, noses, and cheeks. (In black women, these may appear as white patches.) These blotches, called chloasma, or the "mask of pregnancy," will fade after delivery. In the meantime, bleaching probably won't lighten chloasma, though cover-up makeups may disguise it. Sun can intensify the coloration, so use a sunblock containing PABA (para aminobenzoic acid) in sunny weather. Since there is some evidence that the excess pigmentation may be related to folic acid deficiency, be sure that your vitamin supplement contains folic acid and that you are eating enough green leafy vegetables, oranges, and whole-wheat bread or cereal daily.

DENTAL PROBLEMS

"My mouth suddenly seems to have become a disaster area. My gums bleed when I brush, and I think I have a cavity. But I'm afraid to go to the dentist because of the anesthesia."

W ith so much of your attention centered on your abdomen during pregnancy, it's easy to overlook your mouth—until it begins to scream for equal time, which it frequently does because of the heavy toll a normal pregnancy can take on teeth and gums.

Gums can take the worst

beating—swelling as a result of increased hormone production. (This swelling is similar to that which takes place in the nasal and vaginal mucous membranes during pregnancy.) Sensitive gums may become inflamed and bleed. And teeth, too, occasionally fall victim to the maternal condition.

You should see your dentist at least once during pregnancy, even if you don't experience any problems. If you do suspect a cavity or other incipient trouble, make an appointment right away. Sometimes there's actually more risk to the fetus in putting off necessary dental work than there is in having it done. For example, badly decayed teeth that are not taken care of can be a source of infection that spreads throughout the system, putting both mother and fetus in danger. And impacted wisdom teeth that are either infected or causing severe pain should also be attended to promptly.

However, special precautions must be taken when dental work is done during pregnancy to ensure that the supply of oxygen to the fetus is not compromised through the use of general anesthetics, and that no anesthetic is used that is known to cause harm to the fetus. In most cases a local anesthetic will suffice. If a general anesthetic is absolutely required, then it should be administered by an experienced anesthesiologist. Discuss the anesthesia with both your dentist and your physician to ensure safety.

If after the dental work you're left with chipmunk cheeks and can't chew solids, you're going to have to make some special dietary altera-tions. On a fluid-only diet you can obtain adequate nutrients (temporarily) by sipping high-protein-and-vitamin milkshakes (see Double-the-Milk Shake, page 87). Supplement the shakes with citrus juices (if they don't burn your gums) and homemade "creamed" soups made from vegetables puréed with cottage cheese, yogurt, or skim milk. Once you can manage soft foods, add puréed vegetables and meats, scrambled eggs, unsweetened yogurt, apple sauce, mashed bananas, mashed potatoes, and creamy cooked cereals enriched with non-fat dry milk.

Of course, for all dental difficulties, the best treatment is prevention. A program of preventive dental care that is carefully followed throughout pregnancy—and preferably throughout life—will avert most dental problems.

❖ See your dentist at least once during the nine months, preferably early on (be sure to inform him or her that you're pregnant). Have your teeth cleaned. Avoid x-rays unless they are absolutely necessary, and then take the special precautions suggested on page 63. Routine repair work requiring anesthesia should be postponed, because even a local anesthetic can enter your bloodstream, and thus the fetus's. If you've had gum problems in the past, you should also see your periodontist.

❖ Follow the Best-Odds Diet, eating little or no refined sugar, particularly between meals, and plenty of foods high in vitamin C. Sugar contributes to both decay and gum disease; vitamin C strengthens gums, reducing the possibility of bleeding. Also be sure to fill your calcium requirements daily (see page 82). Calcium is needed throughout life to keep teeth and bones strong and healthy.

❖ Floss and brush regularly, according to your dentist's prescription. (If your dentist does not instruct you in such preventive measures, you are probably going to the wrong dentist.)

❖ To further reduce bacteria in the mouth, brush your tongue when you brush your teeth. This will also help keep your breath fresh.

TRAVEL

"Is it safe for me to go ahead with the vacation my husband and I had planned for this month?"

For most women, travel during the midtrimester is not only safe, but the perfect chance to get away with their husband for a last fling (at least for a while) as a twosome. And with no diapers, no bottles, no jars of messy baby food to worry about, it'll certainly never be as easy to vacation with your baby again.

Of course, you will need your doctor's permission; if you have high blood pressure, diabetes, or other medical or obstetrical problems, you may not get the green light. (That doesn't mean you can't vacation at all. If you can't travel, pick a hotel or resort within an hour's drive of your doctor's office—and enjoy!) Even in a low-

risk pregnancy, traveling a great distance isn't a terrific idea in the first trimester, when the possibility of miscarriage is greatest and when your body is still making its initial adjustment to the physical and emotional strain of pregnancy. Likewise, travel is usually not recommended in the last trimester because, should labor begin early, you would be far from your doctor and hospital.

Travel to high altitudes isn't recommended at any time during pregnancy, since the adjustment to the decrease in oxygen may be too taxing for both mother and fetus. If you must make such a trip, you should plan on limiting exertion for several days after arrival, which may minimize the risk of acute mountain sickness (AMS).[4] If you are in your last trimester, your doctor may recommend you have a non-stress test on arrival, then daily for the next two days, then semi-weekly. Any signs of fetal distress will probably warrant the administration of oxygen and move to a lower altitude.

Once you have your doctor's permission, all you'll need is a little advance planning and a few precautions to ensure a safe and bon voyage for you and your baby:

Plan a Trip That's Relaxing. A single destination is preferable to a Grand Tour which takes you to nine cities in six days. A trip on which you set the pace is a lot better than a group tour that sets it for you. A few

---

4. Symptoms of AMS include: lack of appetite, nausea, vomiting, gassiness, restlessness, headache, lassitude, shortness of breath, scanty urine, and psychological changes.

hours of tiring sightseeing or shopping should be alternated with time spent sitting reading or napping.

Take Your Best-Odds Diet with You. You may be on vacation, but your baby is working as hard as ever at growing and developing, and has the same nutritional requirements he or she always has. Total self-sacrifice isn't required at mealtimes, but prudence is. Order carefully, and you will be able to savor the local cuisine while fulfilling your baby's requirements. (See Eating Out Best-Odds Style, page 159.) Don't skip breakfast or lunch in order to save up for a lavish dinner.

Don't Drink the Water if you're traveling to a foreign country—unless you're certain it's safe. (But do substitute fruit juices and bottled water to get your daily fluids.) In some regions, it may not be safe to eat unpeeled fresh fruit or raw vegetables. For complete information on such restrictions, on other foreign health hazards, and on immunizations, contact the American College of Obstetricians and Gynecologists, One East Wacker Drive, Chicago, IL 60601.

Pack a Pregnancy Survival Kit. Make sure you bring enough vitamins to last the trip; packets of dry skimmed milk if you're afraid you won't be able to find fresh milk; a small jar of wheat germ to enrich white bread or cereal in case whole grains aren't available; medication for traveler's stomach *prescribed by your doctor;* your favorite pregnancy book for reference; comfortable shoes roomy enough to accommodate feet swelled by sightseeing; and a spray disinfectant in case you have to sanitize a communal toilet.

Have the Name of a Reliable Local Obstetrician Handy. Just in case. Your doctor may be able to provide you with one. If not, contact the local medical association in the city you're traveling to or the International Association for Medical Assistance to Travelers, Suite 5620, Empire State Building, 350 Fifth Avenue, New York, NY 10001—which will, for a small donation, provide you with a directory of English-speaking physicians throughout the world. Some major hotel chains can also provide you with this kind of information. If for any reason you find yourself in need of a doctor in a hurry and can't find one, call the nearest hospital or head for its emergency room.

Head Off Traveler's Irregularity. Changes in schedule and diet can compound constipation problems. To avoid this, make sure you get plenty of the three most effective constipation-combators: fiber, fluids, and exercise. (See Constipation, page 120.) It may also help to eat breakfast a little early, so you'll have time to use the bathroom before you set out for the day.

When You've Got to Go, Go. Don't encourage urinary tract infection by postponing trips to the bathroom. Go as soon as you feel the urge.

If You're Traveling by Car: keep a bagful of nutritious snacks and a thermos of juice or milk handy; stop at least every 2 hours and walk for 5 or 10 minutes to revive circulation; wear your seat belt at all other times.

If You're Traveling by Plane: check with the airline in advance to see if it has special regulations concerning pregnant women (many airlines do). Arrange ahead of time for a seat in the front of the plane, or if seating is not reserved, ask for preboarding. *Do not fly in an unpressurized cabin.* All commercial jets are pressurized; but small private or feeder airline planes may not be, and changes in pressure may rob you—and your baby—of oxygen. Drink plenty of water, milk, and fruit juice to counter the dehydration caused by air travel, and bring along healthful snacks and fresh fruit to supplement starchy airline food. (Special-order ovo-lacto vegetarian meals are usually more nutritious.) Get up and stretch your legs for at least 5 or 10 minutes every couple of hours to keep your circulation going. Wear your seat belt comfortably fastened below your abdomen. If you're traveling to a different time zone, take jet lag into account. Rest up in advance, and plan on taking it easy for a few days once you arrive.

If You're Traveling by Train: check to be sure there's a dining car with a full menu. If not, bring adequate meals and snacks along. Take a stroll every couple of hours for circulation's sake. If you're traveling overnight, arrange for a sleeper. You don't want to start your vacation exhausted.

WEARING A SEAT BELT

"Is it safe to fasten my seat belt in the car or on an airplane?"

What's the major cause of death among pregnant women? Childbirth? Toxemia? Puerperal fever? Actually, none of the above. The most common way for a pregnant woman to lose her life is in an auto accident. And the best way to avoid such a fatality—as well as serious injury to you and your unborn child—is to always buckle up. Statistics prove conclusively that it is a lot safer to fasten your seat belt than not to fasten it.

For maximum safety and minimum discomfort, fasten your belt below your belly, across your pelvis. If there is a shoulder harness, use it. And don't worry that the pressure of the belt in a short stop will hurt the baby—he or she is well cushioned.

SPORTS

"I like to play tennis and swim. Is it safe to continue?"

In most cases, pregnancy doesn't mean giving up the sporting life—just living it with a little common sense and moderation. Most practitioners permit patients whose pregnancies are progressing normally to continue participating in sports they are proficient at for as long as is practical—but with several caveats. Among the most important: "Never exercise to the point of fatigue." Keeping fit is certainly recommended for anyone; for the pregnant

Eating Out Best-Odds Style

❖ **Best** are seafood; American; continental; and steak-house restaurants where broiled fish, poultry, and veal are served, along with fresh vegetables, salads, and potatoes.

❖ **Next Best** are ethnic restaurants where meats, fish, and poultry are featured rather than lost in stews, sauces, or casseroles. Included in this group are Italian (if pasta is eschewed for fish, chicken, and veal dishes); French (nouvelle is preferable to classic French); Jewish (if you avoid fatty meats and gravies, superfluous starches, and salty pickles); and Middle Eastern (if you order baked or grilled fish, meats, and poultry accompanied by bulgur wheat or brown rice). Health food restaurants can fit into this category, but they don't always. The items on their menus—cheese for example—are often low in protein and high in fat; desserts that boast "no sugar" usually contain hives-full of honey. Be discriminating.

❖ **Least Best,** restaurants to frequent infrequently during pregnancy, include: Chinese (when you do, make sure you get enough protein, request no MSG, don't order sweet-and-sour sauces or deep-fried dishes, skip the white rice, and forego adding soy sauce, which is very high in sodium); Japanese (sushi, as all uncooked fish and meat, is completely taboo, and teriyaki and sukiyaki dishes, soaked in soy sauce, should be avoided); German (steer away from empty calories in breading, dumplings, gravies, and the fat and nitrates in sausages and wursts); Mexican and Spanish (it's usually difficult to identify your protein in sauces and stews, and white rice, the starch of choice in these restaurants, is of little nutritional value); Southern American (poultry and fish are too often fried, vegetables overcooked, and pork fat ends up everywhere, whole grains nowhere).

A very occasional dining-out indiscretion won't upset the odds of your Best-Odds diet. But frequent ones will.

---

woman there are many bonuses. (See Exercise During Pregnancy, page 161.)

EATING OUT

"I try hard to stay on a proper diet, but with a business lunch nearly every day, it seems impossible."

For most pregnant women it isn't substituting Perrier for the two martinis that poses a challenge at business lunches (or when dining out after hours); it's trying to put together a meal that's nutritionally sound from a menu of cream sauces, elegant but empty starches, and tempting sweets. But with the following cues, it is possible to take the Best-Odds Diet to lunch or dinner:

❖ Push away the bread basket, unless it's filled with whole grains. Even whole grains should be restricted to whatever remains of your daily quota. Butter or margarine, too, should not exceed your allowance; when spreading, keep in mind that there may be other fats in your meal (for example, salad with dressing and vegetables with butter).

❖ Order salad as a first course, with the dressing on the side, or dress it yourself with oil and vinegar. Stay within the Best-Odds Diet guidelines for fat intake.

❖ If you're ordering soup, opt for a clear consommé or broth, or a vegetable-, milk-, or yogurt-based soup. Generally steer clear of cream soups (unless you know they're made with milk) and onion soup laden with cheese and white bread.

❖ Select a high-protein, low-fat main course. Fish, chicken, and veal are usually the best bets, as long as they aren't fried or drowned in butter or rich sauces. If everything comes with a sauce, ask for yours on the side. Often chefs will accommodate your request for fish broiled with little or no fat—wine is a good substitute (the alcohol evaporates).

❖ As side dishes, white or sweet potatoes (in any form but fried, heavily buttered, or candied), brown rice, kasha or groats, plus lightly cooked fresh vegetables are all appropriate.

❖ Desserts should be limited to unsweetened fresh or cooked fruits when you're eating out. (Indulge in sugar-free Best Odds treats when you get home; see pages 87–90.) Fruit or berries can be garnished with a dollop of unsweetened whipped cream or sour cream, but shouldn't be sugared or soaked in liqueurs.

MOTHERHOOD

"Will I be happy with the baby once I have it?"

Most people approach any major change in their lives—marriage, a new career, or an impending birth—wondering whether it will be a change they'll be happy with. And if they start out with unrealistic expectations, they may very well end up disappointed. If your visions of motherhood are filled with nothing but leisurely morning walks through the park, sunny days at the zoo, and hours coordinating a wardrobe of miniature, sparkling clean clothes, you're in for a heavy dose of reality shock. There'll be many mornings that will turn into evenings before you and your baby ever have the time to see the light of day, many sunny days that will be spent largely in the laundry room, and few tiny outfits that will escape unstained by spit-up puréed bananas and baby vitamins. And if you have images of bringing a cooing, enchanting Gerber baby home from the hospital, you are headed for certain postpartum disillusionment. Not only won't your newborn be smiling or cooing for many weeks, he or she may hardly communicate with you at all, except to cry—most particularly when you're sitting down to dinner, starting to make love, have to go to the bathroom, or are so tired you can't move.

What you *can* expect realistically, however, are some of the most wondrous, miraculous experiences of your life. The joy you will feel when cuddling a warm, sleeping bundle of

Carrying Baby, Fifth Month

Here are just three of the very different ways that a woman may carry near the end of her fifth month. The variations on these are endless. Depending on your size, your shape, the amount of weight you've gained, and the position of your uterus, you may be carrying higher, lower, bigger, smaller, wider, or more compactly.

baby (even if that cherub was a colicky devil moments before) is incomparable. That—along with that first toothless smile meant just for you—will be well worth all the sleepless nights, delayed dinners, mountains of laundry, and frustrated romance.

Can you expect to be happy with your baby? Yes, as long as you expect a real baby and not a fantasy.

WHAT IT'S IMPORTANT TO KNOW:
EXERCISE DURING PREGNANCY

Executives do it. Senior citizens do it. Doctors, lawyers, and construction workers do it. If they do it, pregnant women wonder, why shouldn't we?

"It," of course, is exercise. And

BASIC POSITION AND KEGEL EXERCISES

Lie on your back, knees bent, feet about 12 inches apart, soles flat on the floor. Your head and shoulders should be supported by cushions, and your arms resting flat at your sides. To do Kegels, firmly tense the muscles around your vagina and anus. Hold for as long as you can (working up to 8 to 10 seconds), then slowly release the muscles and relax. These also can be done in a standing position or while urinating (see page 318). Do at least 25 repetitions at various times during the day.

the answer for most women with normal pregnancies seems to be: you should. The concept of pregnancy as a state of ill health, and of the pregnant woman as an invalid, too delicate to climb a flight of stairs or carry a bag of groceries, is as dated as general anesthesia in routine deliveries. Though there still isn't a vast body of research on the subject of exercise during pregnancy, moderate physical activity is now considered not only thoroughly safe, but extremely beneficial for most expectant mothers and their babies.

As anxious as you might be to hit the jogging trail, however, there is one vitally important stop you must make first—at your doctor's office. Even if you're feeling terrific, you must obtain medical clearance before you start suiting up in your husband's extra-large sweat pants. Pregnant women who are in high-risk categories may have to curb exercise or even eliminate it entirely from their routines.

But if yours is among the great majority of normal pregnancies, and your doctor has given you the go-ahead, suit up and read on.

THE BENEFITS OF EXERCISE

I t appears that women who don't get any exercise during pregnancy become progressively less fit as the months pass by—particularly because they are becoming heavier and heavier. A good exercise program (which can be built right into your daily lifestyle) can counteract this trend toward decreasing fitness.

There are four kinds of exercise that can be useful during pregnancy: aerobics, specially-designed-for-pregnancy calisthenics, relaxation techniques, and Kegel exercises.

Aerobics. These are rhythmic, repetitive activities strenuous enough to demand increased oxygen to the muscles, but not so strenuous that demand exceeds supply (walking, jogging, bicycling, swimming, tennis singles). Aerobic exercises stimulate the heart and lungs, and muscle and joint activity—producing beneficial overall body changes, especially an increase in the ability to process and utilize oxygen, which is very important for you and your baby. Exercise too strenuous to be sustained for the 20 to 30 minutes necessary to reach this "training effect" (sprinting), or not strenuous enough (tennis doubles), is not considered aerobic.

Aerobic exercise improves circulation (enhancing the transport of oxygen and nutrients to your fetus while decreasing the risk of varicose veins, hemorrhoids, and fluid retention); increases muscle tone and strength (often relieving backache and constipation, making it easier to carry the extra weight of pregnancy, and facilitating delivery); builds endurance (making you more likely to be able to cope with a lengthy labor); burns calories (allowing you to eat more of the good food you and your baby need without gaining excessive weight, and promising a better postpartum figure); lessens fatigue and promotes a better night's sleep; imparts a feeling of well-being and confidence; and in general heightens your ability to cope with the physical and emotional challenges of childbearing.

Calisthenics. These are rhythmic, light gymnastic movements that tone and develop muscles and can improve posture. Calisthenics especially designed for pregnant women can be very useful in relieving backache, in improving physical and mental well-being, and in preparing your body for the arduous task of childbirth.

Relaxation Techniques. Breathing and concentration exercises (which relax mind and body) help conserve energy for when it's needed, assist the mind to focus on the task at hand, and increase body aware-

PELVIC TILT

Assume the basic position (see page 162). Exhale as you press the small of your back against the floor. Then inhale and relax your spine. Repeat this several times. The tilt can also be done standing up straight, with your back against a wall (inhale while pressing the small of your back into the wall). The standing version is an excellent way to improve your posture and a good alternative if your practitioner recommends that you do not lie on your back after the fourth month.

DROMEDARY DROOP

This exercise is useful throughout pregnancy and into labor, to relieve the pressure of the enlarged uterus on your spine. Get down on your hands and knees, with your back in a naturally relaxed position (don't let your spine sag). Keep your head straight, your neck aligned with your spine. Then hump your back, tightening your abdomen and buttocks, and allow your head to drop all the way down. Gradually release your back and raise your head to the original position. Repeat several times.

ness—all of which help a woman better meet the challenges of childbirth. Relaxation techniques are valuable in combination with more physical routines, or alone—especially in pregnancies when more active exercise is prohibited.

Pelvic Toning. Or Kegel exercise: a simple procedure for toning the muscles in the vaginal and perineal area, strengthening them in preparation for delivery. The increased elasticity will also aid recovery postpartum. This exercise is one virtually every pregnant woman can perform any time, any place.

DEVELOPING A GOOD EXERCISE PROGRAM

Get Started. The best time to get fit is before you get pregnant. But it's never too late to start—even if you're already pushing nine months.

Get Off to a Slow Start. Once you've decided to start exercising (and you've invested $50 in running shoes or $65 in leotards), it's always tempting to start off with a bang, running three miles the first morning or doing Jane Fonda's workout twice the first afternoon. But such enthusiastic beginnings lead not to fitness but to sore muscles, sagging resolve, and abrupt endings. They can also be hazardous.

Of course, if you've been following an exercise program before pregnancy, you can probably continue it—though possibly in a modified form (see Playing It Safe, page 167). If you're a fledgling athlete, however, build up slowly. Start with 10 minutes of warm ups followed by 5 minutes of more strenuous workout.

Stop sooner if you begin to tire. After a few days, if your body has adjusted well, increase the workout by a couple of minutes a day.

Get Off to a Slow Start Every Time You Start. Warm-ups can be tedious when you're anxious to get your workout started (and over with). But as every athlete knows, they're an essential part of any exercise program. They ensure that the heart and circulation won't be taxed suddenly, and that the muscles and joints, which are more vulnerable when "cold"—and particularly vulnerable during pregnancy—won't be injured. Walk before you run, stretch before you begin calisthenics, swim slowly before you start your laps.

Finish as Slowly as You Start. Collapse seems like the logical conclusion to a workout, but it isn't physiologically sound. Stopping abruptly traps blood in the muscles, reducing blood supply to other parts of your body and to your baby. Dizziness, faintness, extra heartbeats, or nausea may result. So finish your exercise with exercise: about 5 minutes of walking after running, paddling after a vigorous swim, light calisthenics or limbering exercises after almost any activity. Top off your cool-down with a few minutes of relaxation.

Watch the Clock. Too little exercise is not effective; too much can be debilitating. A full workout, from warm-up to cool-down, can take anywhere from 30 minutes to an hour. But the American College of Obstetrics and Gynecology recommends that the period of strenuous exercise—during which the pulse

NECK RELAXER

The neck is often a focus of tension, tightening under stress. This exercise can help to relax both your neck and the rest of you: Sit in a comfortable position (Tailor Sit might be best) with your eyes closed. Gently roll your head around, making a full circle, and inhaling as you do. Exhale and relax, letting your head drop forward comfortably. Repeat 4 or 5 times, alternating the direction of the roll and relaxing between rolls. Do this exercise several times a day.

Tailor Sit, Tailor Stretch

Sitting cross-legged is particularly comfortable during pregnancy. Sit this way often and do arm stretches: Place your hands on your shoulders, then lift both arms above your head. Stretch one arm higher than the other, reaching for the ceiling, then relax it and repeat with the other arm. Repeat 10 times on each side.

rate should not exceed 140—should be limited to 15 minutes. For healthy women who were entirely sedentary before pregnancy, working up to between 20 and 30 minutes of exercise every other day is a safe goal. The already active woman can, with her doctor's okay, do more.

Keep It Up. Exercising erratically (four times one week and none the next) won't get you in shape. Exercising regularly (three or four times a week, every week) will. If you're too tired for a strenuous workout, don't push yourself; but do try to do the warm-ups so that your muscles will stay limber and your discipline won't dissolve. Many women find that they feel better if they exercise every day.

Work Exercise into Your Schedule. The best way to be sure of doing your exercise is to allot a specific time for it: first thing in the morning; before going off to work; during a coffee break, if you have the place for it; or before dinner. If you have no regular block of free time for an exercise session, you can build exercise into your daily activities. Walk to work, if you can, or park your car or get off the bus a distance from the job and walk part of the way. Or walk an older child to school (or to a friend's) instead of driving. Do your vacuuming in a steady, 20-minute stretch after a few warm-ups, and you will exercise your body and clean the carpets at the same time. Instead of flopping down in front of the TV with your spouse after the dinner dishes are done, ask him to join you for a walk. No matter how busy your day, if there's the will, there's always a way to fit in some form of exercise.

Compensate for the Calories You Burn. Probably the best part of an exercise program is the extra eating you'll have to do. As always, make those calories count. Take this opportunity to add even *more* good-for-baby nutrients to your diet. You'll have to consume about 100 to 200 additional calories for every half hour of strenuous exercising, and at least a full glass of extra liquid to compensate for fluids lost through perspiration. You will need more in warm weather, or when you are perspiring profusely: drink before, during, and after exercising. The scale can give you a clue to how much fluid you need to replace: 2 cups for each pound lost during exercise.

If you Choose the Group Approach: take a class or join a health club program that is specifically designed for pregnant women. Be aware that not everyone who claims to be an expert, is; ask for the instructor's credentials before enrolling. Classes work better for some women than solo exercising (particularly if self-discipline is lacking) and provide support and feedback. The best programs maintain moderate intensity; meet at least three times weekly; individualize, and don't insist that every woman do the same routine; don't use fast-tempoed music, which may push participants into working too hard; have a network of medical specialists available for questions.

PLAYING IT SAFE

Don't Work Out on an Empty Stomach. Mother's rule about not swimming after a meal was valid. But exercising on an empty stomach could be just as hazardous. If you haven't eaten for hours, it's a good idea to have a light snack and a drink 15 to 30 minutes before beginning your warm-ups. If you're uncomfortable eating that close to exercising, have your snack an hour before.

Dress for the Occasion. Wear clothes that are loose or stretch when you're exercising. Fabrics should let your body breathe—right down to your underwear, which should be cotton. Well-fitting running shoes or well-cushioned sneakers will protect your joints when you're jogging or walking.

Do Everything in Moderation. *Never* exercise to the point of exhaustion when you're pregnant; the chemical by-products of overexertion are not good for the fetus. (If you're a trained athlete, you shouldn't even exercise to your fullest capacity, whether it exhausts you or not.) There are several ways of checking to see whether you're overdoing it. First, if it feels good, it's probably okay. If there's any pain or strain, it's not. A little perspiration is fine; a drenching sweat is a sign to slow down. A pulse that is still over 100 five minutes after completing a workout means you've worked too hard. So does needing a nap when you're finished. You should feel exhilarated, not depleted.

Know When to Stop. Your body will signal you when it's time. Sig-

Choosing the Right Pregnancy Exercise

Select the type of exercise that's right for you. Though you can probably continue a sport or exercise you are already proficient at, it's not advisable to undertake a new one during pregnancy. It is particularly important that you have a *high* degree of proficiency if you attempt such potentially dangerous sports as downhill skiing and horseback riding.

Exercises even a novice can embark on during pregnancy include:

* Walking, preferably at a brisk pace

* Swimming in shallow water

* Cycling on a stationary bike

* Calisthenics designed especially for pregnancy

* Pelvic toning

* Relaxation routines

Those that even an expert should avoid because of greater risks include:

* Scuba diving (diving gear may restrict circulation; decompression sickness is hazardous to fetus)

* Water skiing (water could be forced into the vagina in a fall)

* Diving and jumping into pools (this can force water into the vagina and cause injuries)

* Sprinting (too much oxygen is demanded too quickly)

* Skiing above 10,000 feet (the high altitude deprives both mother and fetus of oxygen)

* Bicycling on wet pavement or winding paths (falls are likely), and cycling in racing posture, leaning forward (which can cause backache)

* Contact sports, such as football and wrestling (they carry a high risk of injury)

* Calisthenics not designed for pregnancy, including those that pull on the abdomen (such as sit-ups or double straight leg lifts); that might force air into the vagina (such as upside-down "bicycling"); that stretch inner thigh or adductor muscles; that call for holding the soles of the feet together while sitting on the floor and bouncing or pressing down on your knees; that cause lordosis (an exaggerated inward curving of the spine); that require contortions or bridging; that call for knee-chest positions (avoid these in the first half of pregnancy only); that call for deep flexion or extension of joints for jumping, or for rapid changes in directions.

nals include: pain of any kind; a cramp or stitch; uterine contractions; light-headedness or dizziness; tachychardia or palpitations; severe breathlessness; bleeding; loss of muscle control; nausea; or headache. If symptoms aren't relieved by rest, check with your doctor (but call immediately if you have any bleeding). In the second and third trimester, you may notice a gradual decrease in performance and efficiency. It's best to slow down.

Stay Cool. Don't exercise in very hot or humid weather; don't use saunas, steam rooms, or hot tubs. Until research shows otherwise, exercise or environments that raise a pregnant woman's temperature more than 1½ to 2 degrees Fahrenheit should be considered dangerous (blood is shunted away from the uterus to the skin as the body attempts to reduce its temperature). So exercise at a cool time of day or in a cool setting.

Proceed with Caution. Even the most skilled sportswoman may lack grace when she's pregnant. As your center of gravity shifts forward with your uterus, a fall becomes an ever-increasing possibility. Be aware, and be careful. Late in pregnancy, avoid sports that require sudden moves or a good sense of balance, such as tennis.

Stay Off Your Back, and Don't Point Your Toes. After the fourth month, don't exercise flat on your back, as your enlarging uterus could compress a major blood vessel. Pointing your toes—at any point—may lead to cramping. Flex instead.

Taper Off in the Last Trimester. Though everybody has heard stories of pregnant athletes who have stayed in the pool or on the slopes right up until delivery, it is wise for most women to slack off during the last three months. This is especially true during the ninth month, when stretching routines and walking should provide adequate exercise. Serious athletics can be resumed at about six weeks postpartum.

IF YOU DON'T EXERCISE

Exercising during pregnancy can certainly do you a lot of good. It can relieve backaches, prevent constipation and varicose veins, and give you a general sense of well-being during gestation, make childbirth a little quicker and easier, and leave you in better physical shape postpartum. But sitting it out (whether by choice or by a doctor's prescription), getting most of your exercise from opening and closing your car door, won't do you or your baby any harm. In fact, if you're abstaining from exercise on doctor's orders, you're helping, not hurting, your baby and yourself. The doctor will almost certainly restrict exercise if you have a history of three or more spontaneous abortions or of premature labor, or if you have an incompetent cervix, bleeding, diagnosis of placenta previa, or heart disease. In some cases activity will be limited if you have high blood pressure, diabetes, thyroid disease, anemia or other blood disorders, are seriously over- or underweight, or have had an extremely sedentary lifestyle up until now. A history of precipitous (very brief) labor or of a fetus that didn't thrive in a previous pregnancy might also be a reason for a red light on exercise.

10
The Sixth Month

WHAT YOU CAN EXPECT AT THIS MONTH'S CHECKUP

This month you can expect your practitioner to check the following, though there may be variations depending upon your particular needs and upon your practitioner's style of practice:[1]

❖ Weight and blood pressure

❖ Urine, for sugar and protein

❖ Fetal heartbeat

❖ Height of fundus (top of uterus)

❖ Size of uterus and position of fetus, by external palpation

❖ Feet and hands, for edema (swelling due to fluid retention); legs, for varicose veins

❖ Symptoms you may have been experiencing, especially unusual ones

❖ Questions and problems you want to discuss—have a list ready

WHAT YOU MAY BE FEELING

You may feel all of these symptoms at one time or another, or only a few of them. Some may have continued from last month, others may be new. Still others may hardly be noticed because you've become so used to

them. You may also have other, less common symptoms.

PHYSICALLY:

❖ More definite fetal activity

❖ Whitish vaginal discharge (leukorrhea)

❖ Lower abdominal achiness (from stretching ligaments)

---

1. See appendix for an explanation of the procedures and tests performed.

❖ Constipation

❖ Heartburn and indigestion, flatulence and bloating

❖ Occasional headaches, faintness or dizziness

❖ Nasal congestion and occasional nosebleeds; ear stuffiness

❖ Hearty appetite

❖ Leg cramps

❖ Mild edema (swelling) of ankles and feet, and occasionally hands and face

❖ Varicose veins of legs and/or hemorrhoids

❖ Itchy abdomen

❖ Backache

❖ Skin pigmentation changes on abdomen and/or face

EMOTIONALLY:

❖ Fewer mood swings; continued absentmindedness

❖ A beginning of boredom with the pregnancy ("Can't anyone think about anything else?")

❖ Some anxiety about the future

WHAT YOU MAY LOOK LIKE

By the end of the sixth month, the fetus is about 13 inches long and weighs about 1¾ pounds. Its skin is thin and shiny, with no underlying fat; its finger and toe prints are visible. Eyelids begin to part, and the eyes open. With intensive care, the fetus may survive if born now.

WHAT YOU MAY BE CONCERNED ABOUT

PINS AND NEEDLES

"I frequently get a tingling sensation in my hands and feet. Does this indicate a problem with my circulation?"

As if it weren't enough to be on tenterhooks during pregnancy, some women occasionally experience the disconcerting tingling sensation of pins and needles in their extremities. Although it may feel as if your circulation is being cut off, this isn't the case. No one knows why this condition occurs or how to eliminate it, but it is known that it doesn't indicate anything serious. Changing your position may help.

If you are experiencing a great deal of swelling of your hands, you may also develop carpal tunnel syndrome, in which pressure on a nerve in the wrist causes burning of the palm next to your thumb and first two fingers. The pain and burning (and sometimes numbness and tingling) can radiate up your arm. The symptoms may worsen at night because, thanks to gravity, fluids have accumulated in your hands all day, making the swelling more severe. Ask your doctor about splinting and other possible treatment.

BABY KICKING

"Some days the baby is kicking all the time; other days he seems very quiet. Is this normal?"

Fetuses are only human. Just like us, they have "up" days, when they feel like kicking up their heels (and elbows and knees), and "down" days, when they'd rather take it easy. Most often, their responses are based on what you've been doing. Like babies out of the womb, fetuses are lulled by rocking. When you're on the go all day, your baby is likely to be pacified by the rhythm of your routine, and you're likely not to notice much kicking—partly because baby's slowed down, partly because you're so busy you overlook what movements there are. When you're relaxing, he or she is bound to start acting up. That's why most expectant mothers feel fetal movement more often in bed at

night, or in the morning before rising. Some pregnant women report increased fetal activity when they're excited or nervous: The baby may be stimulated by the increased adrenaline in mother's system.

Don't compare baby-movement notes with other pregnant women. Each fetus, like each newborn, has an individual pattern of activity and development. Some seem always active; others mostly quiet. The kicking of some is as regular as clockwork; that of others may exhibit no discernable pattern. As long as there is no radical slowdown in activity, all are normal.

After the 30th week, any 24-hour stretch of a significant decrease or of no noticeable activity should be reported to your practitioner immediately—though it is not necessarily an ominous sign. Until then, even if a full day goes by without your hearing from your baby, don't worry. Considering the often over-active imagination of the expectant mother, that may be easier for us to say than for you to do. If that's the case, you can try to elicit a fetal response by lying down (with a good book, not with your worries) for an hour or two. You might even poke your abdomen *gently.* Be aware, however, that this does not always work. Sometimes, you just have to wait until your baby's good and ready to communicate.

"Sometimes the baby pushes so hard it hurts."

As your baby matures in the uterus, he or she becomes stronger and stronger, and those once butterfly-like fetal movements pack more and more power. Don't be surprised if you get kicked in the ribs or poked in the abdomen or cervix with such force it hurts. When you seem to be under a particularly fierce attack, try changing your position. It may knock your little linebacker off balance and temporarily stem the assault.

"The baby seems to be kicking all over, and I'm very large. Could I be carrying twins?"

At some point in her pregnancy, just about every woman begins to think that she's carrying either twins or a human octopus. For most, of course, neither is true. Until a fetus becomes so large that his movements are restricted by the confines of his uterine home (usually at about 34 weeks), he's able to perform numerous acrobatics. So, while it may sometimes feel as if you're being pummeled by a dozen fists, it's more likely to be two fists that get around—along with tiny knees, elbows, and feet.

If your abdomen is unusually large and/or if there are fraternal twins in the family, if you have taken a fertility drug, or if you are over 35, your doctor may have already considered the possibility of twins. Sometimes twins are diagnosed when the examiner identifies two heartbeats; though in early pregnancy, ultrasound is more often needed to make the diagnosis. Later, the examiner may be able to palpate two or more fetuses through the abdomen with his or her hands. It does happen, however, that because of one fetus lying over the other or some other unusual positioning, twins occasionally arrive unannounced and unanticipated at delivery. To avoid such a surprise package, if you're suspicious that you're carrying twins, ask your practitioner about an ultrasound examination to explore the possibility ahead of time.

LEG CRAMPS

"I have leg cramps at night that interfere with my sleep."

Between your racing mind and your bulging belly, you probably have enough trouble sleeping without having to suffer from leg cramps. Unfortunately, these painful spasms, which occur most often at night, are very common among pregnant women in the second and third trimesters. Fortunately, however, there are ways of both preventing and alleviating them.

Since most leg cramps are believed to be caused by an excess of phosphorus and a shortage of calcium circulating in the blood, taking calcium tablets which do not contain phosphorus (calcium carbonate is most absorbable) is generally effective in alleviating them. It may be necessary—but only on your practitioner's advice—to reduce phosphorus intake by cutting down on milk and meat. (But be sure that you are getting your calcium and protein elsewhere. See the Best-Odds Diet, page 75, for substitutes.) Because fatigue and the pressure of the enlarging uterus on certain nerves are also thought to be possible contributing factors, wearing support hose during the day and alternating periods of rest with periods of physical activity may also be helpful in eliminating the problem of leg cramps.

If you do get a cramp in your calf, straighten your leg and flex your ankle and toes slowly up toward your nose. This should soon lessen the pain. (Doing this several times before retiring at night may even help ward off the cramps.) Standing on a cold surface is sometimes useful, too. If either technique reduces the pain, massage or local heat can then be used for added relief. If neither reduces it, don't massage your calves or apply heat. Do contact your doctor if the pain continues, as there is a slight possibility that a thrombus (blood clot) may have developed.

RECTAL BLEEDING AND HEMORRHOIDS

"I'm concerned about the rectal bleeding I've been having."

Bleeding is always a frightening symptom, especially during pregnancy—and particularly in an area so close to your birth canal. But unlike vaginal bleeding, rectal bleeding doesn't signal a possible threat to your baby. During pregnancy it's frequently due to external and, less often, internal hemorrhoids. Hemorrhoids, which are varicose veins of the rectum, afflict between 20% and 50% of all pregnant women. Just as the veins of the legs are more susceptible to varicosities at this time, so are the veins of the rectum.

Constipation often causes or compounds the problem.

Hemorrhoids (also called piles because of the resemblance these swollen veins sometimes bear to a pile of grapes or marbles) can cause itching and pain as well as bleeding. Rectal bleeding may also stem from fissures—cracks in the anus caused by constipation, which can accompany hemorrhoids or appear independently. They are generally extremely painful.

Don't try to self-diagnose hemorrhoids. Rectal bleeding is occasionally a sign of serious disease and should always be evaluated by a physician. But if you do have hemorrhoids and/or fissures, your role will be the most important in treating them. Good self-care can usually eliminate the need for more radical medical therapy.

❖ Avoid constipation. It is *not* a necessary component of pregnancy; see page 120. (Preventing constipation is, incidentally, frequently an excellent way to prevent hemorrhoids completely.)

❖ Sleep on your side to avoid putting extra pressure on the rectal veins; avoid long hours of standing or sitting.

❖ Don't strain at the toilet. Sitting with your feet on a stepstool may make evacuation easier.

❖ Do Kegel exercises: they improve circulation in the region. (See page 318.)

❖ Take warm sitz baths twice a day.

❖ Apply witch hazel soaks or ice packs to the area.

❖ Use topical medications or suppositories *only* if prescribed by the doctor. Do not take mineral oil.

❖ Keep the perineal area (from vagina to rectum) scrupulously clean. Wash the area with water after bowel movements, always wiping from front to back. Use only white toilet paper.

❖ If sitting is painful, get a special inflatable seat (it's shaped like an inner tube).

❖ Lie down several times a day—if possible, on your side. Watch TV, read, talk to your husband in this position.

With good care, hemorrhoids can be kept from becoming chronic and should disappear after delivery.

URINARY TRACT INFECTION

"I'm afraid I have a urinary tract infection."

Urinary tract infections (UTIs) are so common in pregnancy that 10% of pregnant women can expect to contract at least one. Most often it will be cystitis, a simple bladder infection. Even in cystitis, the symptoms (an urge to urinate frequently, and a burning sensation when the urine—often only a drop or two—is passed) can become quite uncomfortable. There may also be sharp lower abdominal pain. Cystitis should be treated promptly by a physician, with one of the antibiotics approved for use during preg-

nancy. Do not take medication previously prescribed for you or anyone else, even if it was prescribed for a urinary tract infection.

Untreated bladder infection may progress to kidney infection (pyelonephritis), which is more threatening to mother and baby. Symptoms are similar to those of cystitis but may also be accompanied by fever (often as high as 103 degrees), chills, blood in the urine, and backache (in the midback or on one or both sides). Should you experience these symptoms, notify your doctor *immediately.* Antibiotics can generally bring relief, but hospitalization for intravenous administration will probably be necessary.

Many physicians today try to head off kidney infection by screening pregnant women, at their first visit, for susceptibility. If a culture of the urine turns up bacteria (and it does in about 5% of pregnant women) antibiotics are administered to effectively prevent the development of cystitis or pyelonephritis.

There are some home remedies and preventives that may also help ward off UTI; used in conjunction with medical treatment, they may help speed recovery when infection occurs.

❖ Drink plenty of fluids, particularly water. Unsweetened citrus and cranberry juices may also be beneficial. But avoid coffee, tea (even the decaffeinated varieties), and alcohol.

❖ Empty your bladder just before and after intercourse.

❖ Every time you urinate, take time

to be sure your bladder is thoroughly emptied.

❖ Wear cotton-crotch underwear and pantyhose, and avoid wearing tight under or outer pants. Don't wear pantyhose under slacks. And sleep without panties on.

❖ Keep the vaginal and perineal areas meticulously clean. Wash daily and avoid perfumed soaps, sprays, and powders in the area. Always wipe from front to back after using the toilet.

❖ Eat plain yogurt containing active cultures when taking antibiotics to help restore bacterial balance in your intestines.

❖ Keep your resistance high by eating a nutritious low-sugar diet (see Best-Odd Diet, page 75), getting plenty of rest, not working to the point of fatigue, and not letting your life get too stressful.

ITCHY ABDOMEN

"My belly itches constantly. It's driving me crazy."

Join the club. Pregnant bellies are itchy bellies, and they can become progressively itchier as the months pass. Your skin is stretching, being pulled taut across your abdomen, and the result is dryness (more pronounced in some women than others) and itching. Try not to scratch, or at least keep scratching to a minimum. Keeping the area well softened with lotion may ease the itch but probably won't cure it.

TOXEMIA, OR ECLAMPSIA

"Recently a friend of mine was hospitalized for toxemia. How can you tell if you have it?"

Toxemia is a controversial term, abandoned by some because it is misleading—toxemia literally means blood poisoning, and this condition in pregnancy has nothing to do with blood poisoning. Yet it is still used by others as a blanket term to describe preeclampsia, which is characterized by a precipitate rise in blood pressure and generalized edema, and its more severe successor, eclampsia, in which convulsions occur.

Fortunately, even in its mildest form the condition is rare, occurring in only 7% of pregnant women, two-thirds of whom come into pregnancy with chronic hypertension (high blood pressure). It is most common beyond the 20th week, and in first pregnancies. In women who are receiving regular prenatal care, it is diagnosed and treated early, preventing needless complications. Though routine office visits sometimes seem a waste of time in a healthy pregnancy, it is at such visits that the earliest signs of preeclampsia can be picked up.

If you are seeing your practitioner regularly, haven't had a sudden rapid weight gain, severe swelling of your hands and face, headaches, or vision disturbances, you needn't worry about toxemia. See page 130 for tips on preventing and dealing with high blood pressure in pregnancy.

STAYING ON THE JOB

"I stand a lot on my job. I was planning to work up until I deliver, but is that safe?"

These days, when more first-time expectant mothers are working than are not, the question of how a mother-to-be's working affects an unborn fetus is an important one. The answer, at this point, however, isn't all that clear. We all know women who went from the office or the studio or the shop right to the hospital and delivered perfectly healthy babies. Some studies, on the other hand, are beginning to show that steady strenuous or stressful activity during the last half of pregnancy may result in babies that are smaller than average, and in placentas that have damaged areas in them. In a study of African women, hard physical labor during pregnancy retarded fetal growth and increased fetal and neonatal mortality— probably because the amount of exercise and the body positions assumed during work reduced blood flow to the placenta.

Whether this has any significance for American women, however, is not known because such heavy labor isn't common for females here. Studies do suggest that women who stand on the job after the 28th week—especially if they also have other children at home to care for— develop elevated blood pressure and deliver babies who weigh somewhat less than average. The risk increases if women stand at their work until term. No one yet knows, however, whether low birth weight and placental damage will later translate into physical or mental problems for the offspring. At the moment, it is believed they don't.

Should women who stand on the job—salespeople, cooks, waitresses, nurses, and so on—work past the 28th week? If they have hypertension, or have children at home to care for without help (and if they have the choice), probably not. The American Medical Association, in fact, recommends that women who work at jobs requiring more than four hours a day on their feet should quit by the 24th week, and that those who must stand for 30 minutes out of each hour should quit by the 32nd. But many physicians will permit women who feel fine to work a little longer. Standing on the job all the way to term, however, is not a good idea—especially considering the added discomfort of backache, varicose veins, hemorrhoids, and so on that may accrue.

It's also recommended that women not stay at jobs which require lifting, climbing (stairs, poles, or ladders), or bending below waist level past the 20th week if this kind of work is intensive, and past the 28th week if it is moderate.

On the other hand, you can probably plan on going straight from a desk job to the delivery room without any threat to you or your baby. A sedentary job that isn't particularly stressful may actually be less of a strain to you both than staying at home with a vacuum cleaner and mop. And doing a small amount of walking—up to an hour or two daily—on the job or off, is not only harmless, but may be beneficial (assuming you aren't carrying heavy loads as you go).

No matter how long you keep working, there are ways of reducing on-the-job stress during pregnancy:

❖ Wear support hose.

❖ Take frequent breaks. Stand up and walk around if you've been sitting; sit down with your feet up if you've been standing. Do some stretching exercises, especially for your back and legs.

❖ Stop working when you're fatigued.

❖ At your desk, keep your legs elevated (on a stool or carton) when possible.

❖ If you are standing for long stretches, keep one foot on a low stool, knee bent, to take pressure off your back. (See illustration, page 151.)

❖ Rest a lot when you are not working; cut down on strenuous activities such as running, tennis, climbing, and so on. The more strenuous your job, the more you need to cut down on other activities.

❖ Rest on your left side during your lunch hour, if possible. Sleep on your left side at night.

❖ Stay out of smoke-filled areas; they are not only bad for the baby, but can increase your fatigue.

❖ Avoid noxious fumes and chemicals.

❖ Avoid extremes in temperature.

❖ Empty your bladder at least every two hours.

❖ If you must stand or walk on the job, cut down on your hours, if possible, and increase your nap period.

PAIN OF CHILDBIRTH

"Now that pregnancy has become an unavoidable reality, I'm worrying about whether I will be able to tolerate the pain of childbirth."

Though almost every expectant mother eagerly awaits the birth of her child, very few look forward to the labor and delivery that precede it. Especially for those who've never experienced significant discomfort, the fear of this unknown is very real—and very natural. Unhappily, it's often compounded for these women by the horror tales of mothers, aunts, and friends whose footsteps to the labor room they dread to follow.

There's no point in dreading the pain—which may end up being worse than you bargained for or not so bad after all. But there's a lot to be said for being prepared for it. When women who anticipate that labor will be an incomparable, exhilarating, and ultimately fulfilling experience end up with 24 hours of excruciating back labor, they suffer as much from disappointment as from pain. And because the pain is unexpected, they have trouble dealing with it.

In general, both women who fear the worst pain and those who expect the least pain end up fearing and fighting the contractions of labor and are less well off during labor and delivery than women who are realistic in their expectations and prepared for any eventuality.

If you prepare both your mind and your body, you should be able to reduce your anxiety now, and at the same time help make your actual labor more comfortable and easier to tolerate.

Get Educated. One reason earlier generations of women found labor so unbearable was that they didn't understand what was happening to their bodies. Take a good childbirth education class with your husband if it's at all possible (see Childbirth Education, page 181); if it isn't, read as much on the subject of labor and delivery as you can (try to touch on all the major schools of thought), including the description beginning on page 238. What you don't know can hurt you more than it should.

Get Moving. You wouldn't think of running a marathon without the proper physical training. Neither should you consider going into labor (which is no less a Herculean feat) untrained. Work out faithfully with all the breathing and toning-up exercises your practitioner and/or childbirth educator recommends. (If they haven't recommended any, see page 161 for several basic exercises.)

Put Pain in Perspective. There are at least two good things to be said about the pain of childbirth, no matter how intense. First, it has a definite time limit. Though it may be difficult to believe at the time, you

will not be in labor forever. Average labor with a first child is between 12 and 14 hours—and only a few of those hours are likely to be very uncomfortable. (Rarely will a doctor allow labor to continue longer than 24 hours, after which point a cesarean is usually performed for the safety of both mother and child.) Second, it's a pain with a positive purpose: Contractions progressively thin and open your cervix, each contraction bringing you closer to the birth of your baby. Don't feel guilty, however, if you lose sight of that purpose during very hard labor and care little about anything but getting it over with. A low tolerance for pain does not reflect on the quality of your maternal love.

Don't Plan on Going Through It Alone. Even if you don't feel like holding hands with your mate during labor, it will be comforting to know he (or a close friend or relative) is there to mop your brow, to feed you ice chips, to massage your back or neck, to coach you through contractions, or just for you to curse at. Your coach should go through childbirth classes with you if possible, or if it's not, read up on the coach's role, starting on page 256.

Be Ready to Ask for Pain Relief If It's Needed. Asking for or accepting medication is a sign neither of failure nor of weakness, and it is sometimes absolutely necessary for you to be at your most effective. Keep in mind that you don't have to be a martyr to be a mother. (See page 198 for more on pain relief during labor and delivery.)

LABOR AND DELIVERY

"I'm getting very anxious about labor and delivery. What if I fail?"

Childbirth education has probably done as much as any of the miraculous medical advancements in the past decade to improve the experience of women in labor. However, by creating a mystique of the perfect labor and delivery, it has left some parents-to-be feeling pressured to achieve that ideal experience (much as the sexual revolution made multi-orgasmic sex obligatory). Childbirth becomes, in effect, the final exam for "prepared" parents, one in which they are expected to excel. It's not surprising many are afraid of flunking, and of thereby letting down not only themselves, but also their doctors, nurse-midwives, and childbirth educators.

But childbirth is not a test that you pass or fail. Nor is there one right way to experience it. Even forgetting, in the excitement, everything you're "supposed" to do won't change the outcome of the delivery.

Learn everything you can in your classes and from your reading, but don't become so obsessed with "natural childbirth" that you forget that childbirth is a natural process—one that women managed to stumble through successfully for thousands of years before Mrs. Lamaze gave birth to her son, the doctor.

"I'm afraid I'll do something embarrassing during labor."

The prospect of screaming or crying out, or of involuntarily emptying your bladder or bowel, might seem embarrassing now. During labor, however, avoiding humiliation will be the farthest thing from your mind. Besides, nothing you can do or say during labor will shock or disgust your birth attendants, who've doubtless seen and heard it all before. The important thing is to be yourself, to do what makes you feel most comfortable. If you are ordinarily a vocal, emotive person, don't try to hold in your moans. On the other hand, if you're normally very inhibited and would rather whimper quietly into your pillow, don't feel under an obligation to out-yell the woman in the next room.

"I dread losing control during labor and delivery."

To members of the take-charge-of-your-life generation, the thought of relinquishing control of your labor and delivery to the medical staff can be a little unnerving. Of course you want the doctors and nurses to take the best possible care of you and your baby. But you'd still like to maintain a modicum of control. And you can—by working hard now at your childbirth preparation exercises, becoming familiar with the birth process step by step (see page 256), and by having good rapport with a practitioner who respects your opinions.

WHAT IT'S IMPORTANT TO KNOW:
CHILDBIRTH EDUCATION

When your parents were expecting you, being prepared for childbirth meant that the baby's room was painted, the layette was ordered, and a suitcase packed with pretty nightgowns for the hospital was waiting at the door. It was the arrival of the child—not the childbirth experience—that was anticipated, planned for, and looked forward to. Women knew little of what to expect from labor and delivery; husbands knew even less. And since mother was likely to be unconscious during the birth, and father was likely to be absently thumbing through *Time* magazines in the waiting room, their ignorance was of little consequence.

Now that general anesthesia is relegated mainly to emergency cesareans, waiting rooms are for nervous grandparents, and mom and dad can go through childbirth together—ignorance is neither wise nor acceptable. Preparing for childbirth has come to mean preparing for the labor and delivery experience as much as for the new baby. Expectant couples devour stacks of books, magazine articles, and pamphlets. They participate fully in their prenatal visits, seeking answers to all their questions, reassurance for all their worries. And more and more often, they attend childbirth education classes.

Just what are these classes about, and why are they proliferating faster than stretch marks in the sixth month? The original, pioneering classes were intended to explain a new approach to childbirth—without medication and without fear—and were commonly known as classes in "natural childbirth." Since then, there has been a shift in emphasis from natural childbirth (though it's still considered the ideal) to education and preparation for all the possible eventualities of labor and delivery. So that whether the birth turns out to be medicated or unmedicated, vaginal or surgical, with an episiotomy or without one, parents will understand what is happening and will be able to participate as fully as possible.

Most curricula are based on the following:

❖ The imparting of accurate information, intended to reduce fears, improve the ability to cope with pain, and enhance decision-making skills.

❖ The teaching of specially designed techniques of relaxation, distraction, muscular control, and respiratory activity—all of which can increase a couple's sense of being in control, while contributing to the woman's endurance and a reduction in her perception of pain.

❖ The development of a productive working relationship between the laboring mother and her coach, which, if maintained during labor and delivery, may serve to provide a supportive environment which can, in turn, help her to minimize her anxieties and maximize her efforts during labor.

BENEFITS OF TAKING A CHILDBIRTH CLASS

Just how much a couple benefits from a childbirth course depends on the course, on the teacher, and on their own attitudes. These classes work better for some couples than for others. Some thrive in group situations and find sharing feelings natural and useful; others are uncomfortable in groups and find sharing difficult and unproductive. Some enjoy learning relaxation and breathing techniques and ultimately find them effective in the control of pain during labor; others feel that the rhythmic repetition of such exercises is forced and intrusive (tension-producing rather than tension-alleviating) and end up not using them. Just about every couple, however, stands to gain something from taking a *good* childbirth class—and certainly has nothing to lose. Some benefits include:

❖ The opportunity to spend time with other expectant couples: to share pregnancy experiences, compare progress, and swap tales of woes, worries, aches and pains. It'll also give you the chance to make friends-with-babies, for later. Many classes hold "reunions" once everyone has delivered.

❖ Increased involvement of the father in the pregnancy, particularly important if he isn't able to attend prenatal visits. Classes will familiarize him with the process of labor and delivery so that he can be a more effective coach, and allow him to meet other expectant fathers. Some courses even include a special session for fathers only, which gives them the chance to express and find relief for the anxieties they're reluctant to burden their wives with.

❖ A weekly chance to ask questions that come up between prenatal visits, or that you don't feel comfortable asking your practitioner.

❖ An opportunity to get hands-on instruction in breathing, relaxation, and coaching techniques, and to have an expert check how well you're performing them.

❖ An opportunity to develop confidence in your ability to meet the strenuous demands of labor and delivery, through increased knowledge (which helps banish fear of the unknown) and the acquisition of coping skills, which may enable you to feel more in control.

❖ A chance to learn coping strategies that may help to decrease your perception of pain, and hence increase your tolerance for it during labor and delivery—which may translate into less need for medication.

❖ The possibility of an improved, less stressful labor, thanks to better understanding of the birthing process and the development of coping skills. Couples who've had childbirth preparation generally rate their childbirth experiences as more satisfying overall than those who haven't.

❖ Possibly, a slightly shorter labor. Studies show that the average labor of women who have had childbirth education is somewhat shorter than that of women who haven't, probably because the training and preparation enables them to work with, instead of against, the work of the uterus. (There is no guarantee of a short labor, only the possibility of a *shorter* one.)

CHOOSING A CHILDBIRTH CLASS

In some communities where childbirth classes are few and far between, the choice is a relatively simple one. In others, the variety of offerings can be overwhelming and confusing. There are courses run by hospitals, by private instructors, by practitioners through their offices. There are "earlybird" prenatal classes—taken in the first or second trimester—which cover such concerns of pregnancy as nutrition, exercise, fetal development, hygiene, sexuality, dreams and fantasies; and there are down-to-the-wire 6- to 10-week childbirth classes, usually begun in the seventh or eighth month, which concentrate on labor, delivery, and postpartum mother and baby care.

If the pickings are slim, taking any childbirth class is probably better than taking none at all—as long as you keep your perspective and don't accept every word spoken in class as gospel. If there is a selection of courses where you live, it may help to consider the following when making your decision:

❖ Taking a class which is run either by your practitioner or in conjunction with your practitioner, or is recommended by him or her, often works out best. If the laboring and delivering philosophies of your childbirth education teacher vary greatly from those of the person who'll be assisting you during labor and delivery, you're bound to run into confusing contradictions and conflicts. If differences of opinion do arise, make sure you air them with your practitioner well before delivery.

❖ Small is best. Five or six couples to a class is ideal; more than 10 isn't recommended. Not only can a teacher give more time and individualized attention to an intimate group—particularly important during the breathing and relaxation technique practice sessions—but the camaraderie in a small group is more satisfying.

❖ Classes which set up unrealistic expectations can work against you. (If you're guaranteed that taking the class will make labor short or painless or glorious, for instance, beware.) There's no way to know for sure what a teacher's philosophy of childbirth will be until you take the class—

unless you're able to sit in on one in advance—but talking to him or her before signing up can give you some idea.

❖ What is the rate of drug-free labors among class "graduates"? This may be helpful information, but it can also be misleading. Does a low rate indicate that students were so well prepared in the various natural pain-reducing strategies that they rarely needed medication? Or were they so convinced that asking for medication was a sign of failure that they stoically withstood severe pain? Perhaps the best way to find the answer is to talk to some of the graduates.

❖ What is the curriculum like? Ask for a course outline, and if you can, sit in on a class. A good course will include a discussion of cesarean section (recognizing that 10% to 20% of students may end up having one) and of medication (recognizing that some will also need this, too). It will deal with feelings, as well as procedures.

❖ How is the class taught? Are films of actual childbirths shown? Will you hear from mothers and fathers who've recently delivered? Is there discussion, or just lecture? Will there be an opportunity for parents-to-be to ask questions? Is adequate time provided during class for practicing the various techniques that are taught? Is one particular philosophy followed—Lamaze or Bradley, for example?

THE MOST COMMON SCHOOLS OF THOUGHT

There are three major childbirth education philosophies, though many instructors combine elements of each.

Grantly Dick-Read. This psychophysical approach dates back to the '40s and '50s and was the first organized approach to childbirth preparation in the United States. Combining relaxation techniques and prenatal education to break the fear-tension-pain cycle of labor and delivery, it was the first to include fathers in the education process and to bring them into the labor room.

Lamaze. Also called the psychoprophylactic method, this approach is similar in some ways to the psychophysical approach in that its major weapons against pain are knowledge and relaxation techniques. In addition, Lamaze depends on conditioning, à la Dr. Pavlov, who conditioned dogs to salivate at the sound of a bell. The expectant mother is conditioned, through intensive training and practice, to substitute useful responses to the stimulus of labor contractions in place of counterproductive ones. In recent years, the father or other coach has trained with the mother to assist her during both labor and delivery.

Bradley. This approach, which originated the husband-coached delivery, emphasizes good diet and uses exercise to ease the discomforts of pregnancy and prepare muscles for birth and breasts for nursing. Women learn to imitate their sleeping position and breathing (which is deep and slow) and to use relaxation to make the first stage of labor more comfortable. Rather than the usual panting and contrived breathing patterns, the Bradley method employs deep abdominal breathing; instead of using distraction and a focus of concentration outside the body to take the mind off discomfort, Bradley recommends that the laboring woman concentrate within and work with her body. Medication is reserved for complications and cesareans, and about 94% of Bradley graduates go without it. Bradley-based classes begin as soon as pregnancy is confirmed and continue into the postpartum period in the belief that it takes a full nine months to get physically and emotionally prepared for labor and delivery.

11
The Seventh Month

What You Can Expect at This Month's Checkup

This month you can expect your practitioner to check the following, though there may be variations depending upon your particular needs and upon your practitioner's style of practice:[1]

❖ Weight and blood pressure

❖ Urine, for sugar and protein

❖ Fetal heartbeat

❖ Height of fundus (top of uterus)

❖ Size and position of fetus, by external palpation

❖ Feet and hands, for edema (swelling); legs, for varicose veins

❖ Symptoms you have been experiencing, especially unusual ones

❖ Questions and problems you want to discuss—have a list ready

What You May Be Feeling

You may feel all of these symptoms at one time or another, or only a few of them. Some may have continued from last month, others may be new. Still others may hardly be noticed because you've become so used to them. You may also have other, less common symptoms.

PHYSICALLY:

❖ Stronger and more frequent fetal activity

❖ Increasingly heavy whitish vaginal discharge (leukorrhea)

❖ Lower abdominal achiness

❖ Constipation, heartburn and indigestion, flatulence and bloating

---

1. See appendix for an explanation of the procedures and tests performed.

❖ Occasional headaches, faintness, or dizziness

❖ Nasal congestion and occasional nosebleeds; ear stuffiness

❖ Leg cramps

❖ Backache

❖ Mild edema (swelling) of ankles and feet, and occasionally hands and face

❖ Varicose veins of the legs and/or hemorrhoids

❖ Itchy abdomen

❖ Shortness of breath

❖ Difficulty sleeping

❖ Scattered Braxton Hicks contractions, usually painless (the uterus hardens for a minute, then returns to normal)

❖ Clumsiness (which makes it easier to take a fall—be careful)

❖ Colostrum, cither leaking or expressed, from breasts

EMOTIONALLY:

❖ Increasing apprehension about the baby, and about labor and delivery

❖ Continued absentmindedness

❖ Increased dreaming and fantasizing about the baby

WHAT YOU MAY LOOK LIKE

By the end of the seventh month, fat begins to be deposited. The fetus may suck its thumb, hiccup, cry; can taste sweet or sour; responds to stimuli, including pain, light, and sound. Placental function begins to diminish, as does the volume of amniotic fluid, as the 3-pounder fills the uterus. Good chance of survival if born now.

❖ Increased boredom and weariness with the pregnancy, the beginning of anxiousness to be over with it

WHAT YOU MAY BE CONCERNED ABOUT

INCREASING FATIGUE

"I've heard women are supposed to feel terrific in the last trimester. I feel tired all the time."

"Supposed to" is a phrase that ought to be stricken from a pregnant woman's vocabulary. There's no one way you're supposed to feel at any time in pregnancy.

Though some women may feel less tired in the third trimester than in the first and second, it can be perfectly normal to continue feeling fatigued or to feel even more fatigued. Actually, there are probably more reasons to feel tired in the last trimester than to feel terrific. First of all, you're carrying around a lot more weight than you were earlier. Second, because of your bulk, you may be having trouble sleeping. You may also be losing sleep to a constantly racing mind. Taking care of other children, a job, or both may be taking a toll on you—and so may preparing for the baby.

Just because your fatigue is a normal part of pregnancy doesn't mean you should ignore it. As always, it's a signal from your body that you should slow down. Take the hint: Rest and relax as much as you can. You'll need every bit of strength you can save up for labor, delivery, and—more important—what follows them.

Extreme fatigue that doesn't ease up when you get more rest should be reported to your doctor. Anemia sometimes strikes at the beginning of the third trimester, and many practitioners do a routine blood test for it in the seventh month. (See page 133.)

CONCERN ABOUT THE BABY'S WELL-BEING

"I worry all the time that something is wrong with my baby."

There probably isn't an expectant mother (or father) who hasn't been haunted by this same fear. Some will even put off buying baby clothes and furniture, or choosing the baby's name, until toes and fingers have been counted, the Apgars have been calculated, and the doctor has congratulated them on a healthy baby.

But the odds of having a completely normal baby have never been better. The U.S. infant mortality rate is the lowest in history, down to between 10 and 12 per 1,000 births. And most of the perinatal deaths occur in the newborns of indigent women living in inner cities and depressed rural areas who receive medical care late or not at all and who are inadequately nourished. A majority of the remainder occur in infants of high-risk women: those with a family history of genetic disease; with uncontrolled chronic illnesses; who drink heavily and/or smoke or take drugs; or who are carrying multiple fetuses. Even for these women, close medical supervision and good prenatal care has recently greatly increased the chances of having healthy babies.

Some experts had forecast that as the death rate fell—because more babies with birth defects would be saved by medical miracles—the rate of children with handicaps would rise. This hasn't happened; the percentage of birth defects, in fact, appears to be declining. And, again, these defects are more likely to occur in children born to high-risk women. Even when a child is born with a birth defect, he or she isn't necessarily permanently handicapped. Most minor, and many serious, defects are now correctable. If diagnosed in utero, some can be treated before birth through surgery or medication. Heart defects and other internal abnormalities can be mended with microsurgery shortly after birth; cleft palates and bone or limb abnormalities can be surgically repaired. Children who are intellectually disabled can, with early intervention, make remarkable strides.

So when worry strikes, strike back—with the knowledge that your baby couldn't have picked a better time to be born (and grow up) healthy.

EDEMA (SWELLING) OF THE HANDS AND FEET

"My ankles seem to be swollen, especially when the weather is warm. Is this a bad sign?"

Any degree of edema (swelling due to excessive accumulation of fluids in the tissues) was once considered a potential danger sign in pregnancy. Now doctors recognize that mild edema is related to the normal and necessary increase in body fluids in pregnancy. Some swelling of the ankles and legs without accompanying symptoms to suggest the development of preeclampsia (see below) is considered completely normal. In fact, 75% of women develop such edema at some point in their pregnancies.[2] It's particularly common late in the day, in warm weather, or after standing or

sitting a lot. Much of it should disappear however, after a good night's sleep.

Generally, edema is nothing but a little uncomfortable. To ease discomfort, elevate your legs or lie down when you can, preferably on your left side; wear comfortable shoes or slippers; avoid elastic-top socks or stockings. If the edema is really bothersome, put support panty-hose on before you get up in the morning, while the swelling is down. Help your excretory system to flush out waste products and excess fluids by drinking at least eight to ten eight-ounce glasses of liquids daily. Though it's no longer believed that salt restriction is wise during pregnancy, excessive salt intake isn't any smarter and could increase fluid retention.

If your hands and/or face become puffy, or if the edema persists for more than 24 hours at a time, you should notify your doctor. Such swelling may be insignificant, or—if accompanied by rapid weight gain, a rise in blood pressure, and protein in the urine—it could signal the beginning of preeclampsia. (See page 130.)

OVERHEATING

"I feel so warm most of the time, and I sweat a lot. Is this normal?"

With your basal metabolic rate (the rate at which your body expends energy at total rest) up about 20% during pregnancy, the heat's on. Not only are you likely to feel too warm in warm weather, you

---

2. One in four pregnant women never experience edema, and this can be completely normal, too. Others may not notice swelling.

may even feel overheated in the winter—when everyone else is cool. You will also probably perspire more, especially at night. This is a mixed blessing. While it helps to cool you off and rids your body of waste products, it is admittedly unpleasant.

To minimize discomfort: bathe often; use a good antiperspirant; and dress in layers—especially in the winter—so you can peel down to shirt-sleeves when you start heating up. And don't forget to take extra fluids to replace those lost through your pores.

MAKING LOVE AND THE BABY

"After I have an orgasm my baby usually stops kicking for about half an hour. Is sex harmful to him or her at this stage of pregnancy?"

B abies are individuals even while they're still in the womb. And their reactions to their parents' lovemaking vary. Some, like your baby, are rocked to sleep by the rhythmic motion of coitus and the uterine contractions that follow orgasm. Others, stimulated by the activity, may become more lively. Both reactions are normal; neither indicates any awareness of the proceedings on the fetus's part, or any kind of fetal distress.

Whether sexual intercourse is totally safe during the last two months of pregnancy, even in a normal pregnancy, is a matter of increasing controversy in the obstetrical community. Acquitted several years ago as an accessory to premature labor and perinatal infection, coitus in the final weeks of gestation is once again being implicated in such complications by researchers. To learn what is believed safe in sexual relations for expectant parents, see Making Love During Pregnancy, page 139.

PREMATURE LABOR

"Is there anything I can do to assure that my baby won't be born prematurely?"

F ar more babies are born late than early. Only about 7 in 100 deliveries in the United States are premature or preterm; that is, take place before the 37th week of pregnancy. And about three fourths of these involve women who are at high risk for premature delivery. The rate is lower for white women (fewer than 6 in 100) and higher for black women (nearly 13 out of 100), partly for socioeconomic reasons. Dramatic advances in preventing preterm labor, combined with better care, should go a long way in reducing the incidence of prematurity.

There are a wide variety of factors that are believed to be related to increased risk of preterm delivery. The more risk factors in a woman's history, the greater the chance that she will deliver prematurely. The risk factors that follow can be controlled, either partially or completely, greatly increasing the odds that a woman will carry to term:

Smoking. Quit as early as possible in pregnancy, or before.

Alcohol Consumption. Avoid regular drinking of beer, wine, and liquor (no one yet knows how much is too much, so it's safer to abstain).

Drug Abuse. Don't use unprescribed drugs during pregnancy.

Inadequate Weight Gain. If your prepregnant weight was normal, gain a minimum of 20 pounds; if you were significantly underweight before conceiving, gain closer to 30 pounds. (Overweight women, with excellent nutrition and their doctor's permission, may be able to gain less safely.)

Inadequate Nutrition. Follow a well-balanced diet (See the Best-Odds Diet, page 75) throughout pregnancy. Be sure that your vitamin supplement contains zinc; some recent studies have linked zinc deficiency with preterm labor.

Standing, or Heavy Physical Labor. If your job alone or your job plus housework require you to stand for several hours each day, stop working or cut down.

Sexual Intercourse (for Some Women). Expectant mothers who are at high risk for premature delivery are generally advised to abstain from intercourse and/or orgasm during the final two or three months of pregnancy. Or, to use a condom to prevent infection of the amniotic sac, which it is believed might trigger early labor.

Hormonal Imbalance. Just as it can trigger late miscarriage, an imbalance of hormones can sometimes trigger premature delivery; hormone replacement may prevent both.

Other risk factors are not always possible to eliminate, but their effects can sometimes be modified:

Infections (such as venereal disease, urinary tract and vaginal infections, and rubella). Avoid exposure whenever possible (see individual diseases), and seek prompt treatment if you do contract infection. In general, it helps to keep yourself in good health through adequate rest, optimal nutrition, exercise, and regular prenatal care.

Incompetent Cervix. This condition, in which a weak cervix opens prematurely, is often undiagnosed until after at least one instance of miscarriage or premature labor. When diagnosed, premature delivery can be avoided by suturing the cervix after the 14th week.

Placenta Previa (when the placenta is located low in the uterus, near or over the cervix). This condition may be diagnosed early through the use of ultrasound, or may be signaled by bleeding in mid or late pregnancy. Premature labor may be headed off by complete bed rest.

Chronic Maternal Illness (high blood pressure; heart, liver, or kidney disease; diabetes). Good medical care, sometimes necessitating bed rest, can often prevent premature delivery. (Premature babies of diabetic mothers, however, are rarely born with a low birth weight.)

Stress. Sometimes the cause can be controlled (by quitting a stressful job, getting counseling if your marriage is floundering); sometimes it cannot (as when your husband loses his job, you lose your husband through divorce or death, or you are pregnant and alone). But all kinds of stress can be reduced through education, relaxation techniques, good nutrition, a balance of exercise and rest, and talking out your problem—often in a self-help group.

Age Under 17. Optimal nutrition and prenatal care can help compensate for the fact that the mother, like her fetus, is still growing.

Age Over 35. Optimal nutrition, good prenatal care, reduction of stress, and prenatal screening for obstetrical problems specific to older women all reduce risk.

Low Educational or Socioeconomic Level. Again, good nutrition and medical care, and the elimination of all possible risk factors, can decrease the risk.

Structural Abnormalities of the Uterus. Once the problem has been diagnosed, surgical repair can frequently prevent future preterm births.

Multiple Gestations. Women carrying more than one fetus deliver an average of three weeks early. Meticulous prenatal care, bed rest and restrictions on activity as needed in the last trimester, and elimination of all other risk factors may help prevent a too-early birth.

History of Premature Deliveries. A diagnosed cause can be corrected; top-notch prenatal care, reduction of other risk factors, and limitations on activities may help to prevent a repeat.

When the cause of preterm labor cannot be prevented or modified, often the threatened labor itself can be postponed. Even a brief delay can be beneficial; each additional day the baby remains in the uterus (until term) improves its chance of survival. Only when the mother and/or child are endangered, such as when the placenta separates prematurely from the uterus (abruptio placenta), or there is fetal or maternal distress, is no attempt made to postpone early delivery.

Postponement (or the prevention of the onset of premature labor) can often be achieved through limitations on sexual intercourse and other physical activities, bed rest, and, if necessary, hospitalization and the administration of tocolytic agents (drugs which relax the uterine muscles and halt contractions). When treatment has successfully delayed labor, the expectant mother may be able to return home on oral medication and with orders to rest in bed.

But it is possible to postpone premature labor only if it is diagnosed early, before the cervix has effaced and dilated significantly and/or the membranes have ruptured. Since a premature baby is smaller than one at full term, the cervix does not have to dilate a full 10 centimeters before expulsion of the fetus; as a result, premature labor progresses quickly.[3]

So you can see it's important to be familiar with the signs of early labor, which follow, and to alert your practitioner if you've the slightest suspicion that labor is beginning. *Don't worry about bothering your doctor*—no matter what the day or hour.

❖ Menstrual-like cramps, with or without diarrhea, nausea, or indigestion.

❖ Lower back pain, or a change in the nature of lower backache.

❖ An achiness or feeling of pressure in the pelvic floor, the thighs, or the groin.

❖ A change in your vaginal discharge, particularly if it is watery or tinged or streaked pinkish or brownish with blood. The passage of a thick, gelatinous mucous plug may or may not precede this "bloody show."

❖ Rupture of membranes (you feel a trickle or rush of fluid from your vagina).

You can have all these symptoms and not be in premature labor, but only your practitioner can tell you for sure. If he or she suspects you're in labor, you will probably be examined promptly.

If premature labor does take place—despite steps to prevent or postpone it—your chances of taking a healthy, normal baby home from the hospital are excellent. (Of course, that trip home with the baby may have to be delayed days, weeks, or even months.) Top-grade medical care, utilizing the latest advances in neonatology (care of the newborn), often begins during labor with administration of the drug betamethasone, which speeds the maturity of the fetal lungs. Sometimes a woman will be moved early in labor into a regional perinatal center, so that the baby can be delivered directly into an intensive care nursery. With continued care in such units, even 2- and 3-pound premies have a nearly 100% chance of survival, and a very good chance of growing up without any handicapping aftereffects.

APPROACHING RESPONSIBILITY

"I'm beginning to worry that I won't be able to manage my job, my house, my marriage—and the baby, too."

You probably won't be able to manage if you attempt to be a full-time career woman, housekeeper, wife, and mother—seeking perfection in each. Many new mothers have tried to be "superwomen"; few have succeeded without sacrificing their health and sanity.

But it will be possible to survive if you reconcile yourself to the reality that you can't do it all—at least in the beginning. If job, husband, and baby are important, perhaps keeping the house immaculate will have to

---

3. If premature labor threatens and/or membranes rupture before significant dilatation occurs, and tests show the fetal lungs are immature, some physicians try to postpone delivery for two to three days. During that time, they administer a steroid drug to spur fetal lung maturation. Doctors differ on whether or not this is an effective course.

give way. If full-time motherhood appeals to you and you can afford to stay home for a while, maybe you can shelve your career temporarily. Or work part-time, as a compromise. It's just a matter of deciding in advance what your priorities are.

Whatever decision you make, your new life will be easier if you don't have to go it alone. Behind the most successful mom there's usually a cooperative dad, willing to share the workload. Don't feel guilty about asking him to change diapers and bathe the baby after a long day at the office. There's probably no better way for him to unwind and, at the same time, to get to know his child. If dad isn't available (all or part of the time), then you are going to need to think about other sources of assistance: mothers or other relatives, childcare or household workers, playgroups, day care centers.

ACCIDENTS

"I missed the curb today when I was out walking and fell belly-first on the pavement. I'm not worried about my skinned knees and elbows, but I'm terrified that I've hurt the baby."

A woman in the last trimester of pregnancy isn't exactly the most graceful creature on earth. A poor sense of balance, due to a shifting forward of her center of gravity, and looser, less stable joints contribute to her awkwardness and make her prone to minor falls—particularly belly-flops. So does her tendency to tire easily, her predisposition to preoccupation and day-dreaming, and the difficulty she may be having seeing past her belly to her feet.

But while a curb-side spill may leave you with multiple scrapes and bruises (particularly to the ego), it's extremely rare for a fetus to suffer the consequences of its mother's clumsiness. Your baby is protected by the world's most sophisticated shock-absorption system, comprised of amniotic fluids, tough membranes, a muscular uterus, and a sturdy abdominal cavity girded with muscles and bones. For this system to be penetrated, and for your baby to be hurt, you'd have to sustain very serious injuries—the kind that would very likely land you in the hospital.

Even though there's probably no harm done, you should let your practitioner know about a fall. You may be asked to come in so that your baby's heartbeat can be checked— mostly to set your mind at ease. Should you notice vaginal bleeding, a leaking of amniotic fluid, or that your baby is unusually inactive, however, medical attention should be sought immediately. Have someone take you to the emergency room if you can't reach your doctor.

BACK AND LEG PAIN

"I've been having pain on the right side of my back, that runs right down my hip and leg. What's happening?"

This is just another one of those occupational hazards of expectant motherhood. The pressure of the enlarging uterus, which has caused so many other discomforts, can also extend to the sciatic nerve—causing lower back, buttock, and leg pain. Rest, and a heating pad applied locally, may help.

FETAL HICCUPS

"I sometimes feel regular little spasms in my abdomen. Is this kicking, or a twitch, or what?"

Believe it or not, your baby's got hiccups. This phenomenon is very common in fetuses in the last half of pregnancy. Some get hiccups several times a day, every day. Others never get them at all. The same pattern may continue after birth.

But before you start holding a paper bag over your belly, you should know that hiccups don't cause the same discomfort in babies (in or out of the uterus) as they do in adults—even when they last as long as 20 minutes or more. So just relax and enjoy this little entertainment from within.

DREAMS AND FANTASIES

"I've been having so many vivid dreams about the baby that I'm beginning to think I'm going mad."

Though the many night- and day-dreams (both horrifying and pleasant) a pregnant woman can experience in the last trimester may make her feel as though she's losing her sanity, they're actually helping to keep her sane. Dreams and fantasies are both healthy and normal,

and help expectant women to sort out worries and fears in a non-threatening way.

Each of the dream and fantasy themes commonly reported by pregnant women expresses one or more of the deep feelings and concerns that might otherwise be suppressed:

❖ Being unprepared, forgetting or losing things—not feeding the baby; missing a doctor's appointment; going out to shop and forgetting you have a baby; being unprepared for the baby when it arrives; losing car keys, or even the baby—can express fear of not being adequate to the task of motherhood.

❖ Being attacked or hurt—by intruders, burglars, animals; falling down the stairs after a push or a slip—may indicate a sense of vulnerability.

❖ Being enclosed or unable to escape—trapped in a tunnel, car, a small room; drowning in a pool, a lake of snowy slush, a car wash—can signify fear of being tied down and deprived of freedom by the baby.

❖ Going off the diet—gaining too much weight, or gaining a lot of weight overnight; overeating; eating or drinking the wrong things (two hot fudge sundaes or a bottle of wine) or not eating the right things (forgetting to drink milk for a week)—is common among those trying to adjust to a restricted diet.

❖ Losing appeal—becoming unattractive or repulsive to her

husband; her husband finding another woman—expresses nearly every woman's fear that pregnancy will destroy her looks forever and drive her husband away.

❖ Sexual encounters—either positive or negative, pleasure- or guilt-provoking—may be an indication of the sexual confusion and ambivalence often experienced during pregnancy.

❖ Death and resurrection—lost parents or other relatives reappearing—may be the subconscious mind's way of linking old and new generations.

❖ Family life with the new baby—getting ready for the baby; loving and playing with the baby—is practice parenting, bonding mother with the baby prior to birth.

❖ What the baby will be like—can represent a wide variety of concerns. Dreams about the baby being deformed or unusual in size express anxiety about the health of the baby. Fantasies about the infant having unusual skills (like talking or walking at birth) may indicate concern about the baby's intelligence and ambition for his or her future. Premonitions that the baby will be a boy or a girl could signal a problem—your heart may be too set on one or the other. So could dreams about the baby's hair or eye color or resemblance to one parent or the other. Nightmares of the baby being born fully grown could be signaling another problem—your fear of having to handle a tiny baby.

Though dreams and fantasies in pregnancy are much more anxiety-provoking than they are at other times, they are also more useful. If you listen to what your motherhood fantasies are telling you—and heed their warnings—you can make the transition into real-life motherhood more easily.

WHAT IT'S IMPORTANT TO KNOW:
ALL ABOUT CHILDBIRTH MEDICATION

On January 19, 1847, Scottish physician James Young Simpson splashed a half teaspoonful of chloroform on a handkerchief and held it over the nose of a laboring woman. Less than half an hour later, she became the first woman to deliver while under anesthesia. (There was only one complication: When the woman—whose first baby had been born after three days of painful labor—awoke, Dr. Simpson was unable to convince her that she'd actually given birth.)

This revolution in obstetrical practice was welcomed by women, but fought by both the clergy and some members of the medical profession, who believed that pain in childbirth (woman's punishment for Eve's indiscretions in Eden) was a burden that women were born to carry. Relief of the pain would be immoral.

But opponents were doomed to failure. Once word got around that childbirth didn't have to hurt, obstetrical patients wouldn't take "no pain relief" for an answer. No longer was it a question of whether anesthesia had a place in obstetrics, but what kind of anesthesia would fill that place best.

The search for the perfect pain relief—a drug that would eliminate pain without harming either mother or child—was on. Enormous progress was made (and is still being made); analgesics and anesthetics became safer and more effective every year.

And then, in the 1950s and '60s, the love affair between childbirth medication and obstetrical patients began to get shaky. Women wanted to be awake for their deliveries and to experience every sensation, in spite of the discomfort. And they wanted their babies to arrive as alert as they were—instead of drugged from the effects of anesthesia.

In the 1980s, enlightened practitioners and patients alike are recognizing that, used prudently, childbirth medication plays a vital role in obstetrics. Though an unmedicated birth is considered the ideal, it's understood that there are times when it's not in the best interest of mother and/or child. This is particularly true when labor is long and complicated; when the pain is more than the mother can tolerate, or is interfering with her ability to push; in breech deliveries, and when outlet forceps are used; or, rarely, to slow down a precipitous (too rapid) labor. It can also be used to calm a woman who is so agitated that she is hindering the progress of labor.

Prudent use of any type of medication always requires a careful weighing of risk against benefit. In the case of obstetrical drugs, risks and benefits must be examined for both mother and baby, making the equation a more complicated one. In some instances, the risks of medications clearly outweigh the benefits they offer—as when the fetus doesn't appear strong enough to cope with the stresses of both labor and drugs because of prematurity or other factors.

Most experts agree that when childbirth medication is used, benefits can be increased and risks reduced by:

❖ Selecting a drug that has the fewest potential side effects or risks to mother and child and still provides effective pain relief (the goal, except in surgical deliveries, is not *total* elimination of pain), giving it in the smallest possible effective doses and at the optimum time.

❖ Having an expert anesthesiologist or anesthetist administer anesthesia. (You have the right to insist on this if you are to have general or spinal anesthesia.)

A major concern of careful medicating in obstetrics is not only the safety of the person receiving the medication (the mother), but that of an innocent bystander (the baby). Babies whose mothers have medication during delivery may be born drowsy, sluggish, unresponsive, and sometimes with breathing and sucking difficulties and an irregular heartbeat. Studies show, however, that when drugs have been properly used, these adverse effects largely disappear soon after birth. A fetus can handle a certain degree of the hypoxia (oxygen deprivation) that sometimes results from too much medication in labor or too much anesthesia during delivery; only very extreme cases of deprivation are hazardous. If a baby is so drugged that he doesn't breathe spontaneously at birth, quick resuscitation (a simple procedure) will prevent long-term damage. The problem is usually avoided in surgical deliveries by extracting the fetus very soon after anesthesia is administered, before the drug has a chance to cross the placenta and affect him or her.

WHAT KINDS OF PAIN RELIEF ARE MOST COMMONLY USED?

A variety of analgesics (pain relievers), anesthetics (substances that produce loss of sensation), and ataraxics (tranquilizers) may be given during labor and delivery. Which drug, if any, will be administered will depend on the situation, as well as upon the obstetrician's and/or anesthesiologist's preference and expertise, and—except in emergencies—the wishes of the mother. The efficacy will depend upon the woman, the dosage, and other factors. (Very rarely, a drug won't produce the desired effect, and will give little or no pain relief.) Obstetrical pain relief is most com-monly accomplished with the following drugs:

Analgesics. Meperidine hydrochloride, a powerful pain reliever commonly known under the trade name Demerol, is a frequently used obstetrical analgesic. It is most effectively administered intravenously (injected slowly into an IV apparatus, so that its effects can be gauged) or intramuscularly (one shot, usually in the buttocks). Demerol does not usually interfere with the contractions or their work, though with larger doses the contractions may appear to be less frequent. It may actually help normalize contractions in a dysfunctional uterus (one that is functioning abnormally). Like other analgesics, Demerol is not generally administered until labor is well established and false labor has been ruled out, but at least two to three hours before delivery is expected. A mother's reaction to the drug and the degree of pain relief achieved vary widely. Some women find it relaxes them and makes them better able to cope with contractions. Others very much dislike the drowsy feeling and find they are less able to cope. Side effects may, depending on a woman's sensitivity, include nausea, vomiting, depression, and a drop in blood pressure. The effect Demerol will have on the newborn depends on the dose and how close to delivery it is administered. If it is given too close to delivery, the baby may be sleepy and unable to suck; less frequently, respiration may be depressed and supplemental oxygen may be required. These effects are generally short-term and, if necessary, can be counteracted. Demerol may also be given postpartum, to relieve the pain of a cesarean.

Alphaprodine hydrochloride, trade-named Nisentil, is a less widely used analgesic (usually injected under the skin). It is more rapid and dramatic in its pain relief than Demerol, but is effective for a shorter time. It also appears to have less effect on the newborn.

Tranquilizers. These drugs (such as Phenergan, Vistaril, and Valium) are used to calm and relax an anxious woman so that she can participate more fully in childbirth. Tranquilizers can also enhance the effectiveness of analgesics, such as Demerol. Like analgesics, tranquilizers are usually administered once labor is well established, and considerably before delivery. But they are occasionally used in early labor if a first-time mother is extremely nervous. Women's reactions to the effects of tranquilizers vary. Some welcome the gentle drowsiness; others find it interferes with their control. A small dose may serve to relieve anxiety without impairing alertness. A larger dose may cause slurring of speech and dozing between contraction peaks—making use of prepared childbirth techniques impossible. Though the risks to a fetus from tranquilizers are minimal (except in cases of fetal distress), it's a good idea for you and your coach to try non-drug relaxation techniques before asking for medication.

Inhalants. Nitrous oxide is rarely used today, except in combination with other drugs to induce general anesthesia. Another inhalant, Penthrane (methoxyflurane), can be self-administered to relieve the discomfort of early labor, and in low concentrations does not cause fetal depression.

Regional Nerve Blocks. Anesthetics injected along the course of a nerve or nerves may be used to deaden sensation in that region. In childbirth, anesthetics may completely numb the area from the waist down for surgical delivery, or numb a smaller area partially or totally for a vaginal one. Regional blocks have an advantage over general anesthesia for surgical delivery, in that the mother is awake during the birth and is alert afterward. In a vaginal delivery, they have the possible disadvantage of inhibiting the urge to push. Occasionally, oxytocin may be administered to rev up contractions that have become sluggish because of the anesthetic effect. Often a catheter (tube) is inserted into the bladder to drain urine (because the urge to urinate is also suppressed). The most frequently used blocks are: pudendal, epidural, spinal, caudal, and paracervical.

A pudendal block, occasionally used to relieve early second-stage pain, is usually reserved for the vaginal delivery itself. Administered through a needle inserted into the perineal or vaginal area (while the mother lies on her back with her feet in stirrups), it reduces pain in the region, but not uterine discomfort. It is useful when outlet forceps (forceps used to ease the baby out once its head is visible at the vaginal outlet) are used, and its effect can last through episiotomy and repair. It is frequently used in combination with Demerol or a tranquilizer to provide excellent pain relief with relative safety—even when an anesthesiologist is not available.

The epidural block (or lumbar epidural) is becoming increasingly popular for both vaginal and cesarean deliveries, as well as for the relief of labor pain and to slow down very intense contractions. The major reason is its relative safety (less drug is needed to achieve the desired effect) and its ease of administration. The drug (usually bupivacaine, lidocaine, or chloroprocaine) is administered as needed during labor and/or delivery, through a fine tube which has been inserted through a needle in the back (after a local anesthetic numbs the area), into the epidural space between the spinal cord and the outer membrane, usually while the mother lies on her left side or leans over a table to steady herself. Blood pressure is checked frequently because the procedure can cause it to drop suddenly. Intravenous fluids, and possibly medication, may be given to counteract this reaction. Leaning the uterus to the left may also help. Because of the risk of a blood pressure drop, an epidural is generally not used when there is a bleeding complication, such as placenta previa, severe preeclampsia or eclampsia, or fetal distress.

Spinal blocks (for cesarean) and low spinal, or saddle, blocks (for vaginal delivery) are administered in a single dose just prior to delivery. The mother lies on her side (back arched, neck and knees flexed) and an anesthetic is injected into the fluid surrounding the spinal cord. There may be some nausea and vomiting while the drug is in effect, about 1 to 1½ hours. As with an epidural, there is a risk of a drop in blood pressure. Elevation of the legs, leaning the uterus to the left, intravenous fluids, and, occasionally, medication may be used to prevent or counteract this complication. After delivery, spinal-block patients must usually remain flat on their backs for about eight hours, and a few may experience post-spinal headache. As with epidurals, spinals are not usually used when there is placenta previa, preeclampsia or eclampsia, or fetal distress.

The caudal block is similar to the epidural, except that it blocks sensation in a more limited area, takes a larger dose to be effective, and requires greater skill on the part of the anesthesiologist. It also inhibits labor. Because of these potential risks, it is used less frequently today than it was in the past.

The paracervical block relieves the pain of labor, but not that of delivery. Because of potential hazard to the fetus, it is rarely used—except when no other anesthesia is suitable.

General Anesthesia. Once the most popular pain relief for delivery, general anesthesia—which puts the patient to sleep—is used today almost exclusively for surgical births, and occasionally for delivering the head in a vaginal breech. Because of ease of administration, it is most likely to be used in emergency cesareans, when there is no time for a regional anesthetic to be administered.

Inhalants, such as those used for analgesic effect, are used to induce general anesthesia—often in conjunction with other agents. This is done by an anesthesiologist in an operating/delivery room. The mother is awake during the preparations and unconscious for only a few minutes as the baby is delivered (and in the case of a cesarean, while the incision is sutured). When she comes to she may be groggy, disoriented, and restless. She may experience nausea and vomiting, and her bowels and bladder may be sluggish. A temporary drop in blood pressure is another possible side effect.

The major problem with general anesthesia is that as the mother is sedated, so is the fetus. Sedation of the fetus can be minimized, however, by administering the anesthesia as close to the actual birth as possible. That way the baby can be delivered before the anesthetic has reached him or her. Administering oxygen to the mother, and tilting her to the side (usually the left side), can also help reduce fetal sedation.

The other major risk of general anesthesia is that the mother may vomit and aspirate (inhale) the vomited material, which can cause complications, such as aspiration pneumonia. That's why you are asked not to eat when in active labor and why, if you do have general anesthesia, a tube will be inserted through your mouth into your throat to prevent aspiration. You may also be given oral antacids to neutralize the acids in your stomach.

Because it's important to keep doses of anesthetics moderate to avoid fetal sedation, the effect of general anesthesia is occasionally too weak to entirely block out the mother's awareness of the surgery. Supplementary use of potent inhalants can avoid this problem.

Hypnosis. Despite the somewhat disreputable image it's developed on the nightclub circuit, hypnosis, in qualified hands, provides a legitimate, medically acceptable route to pain relief. There's really nothing mysterious about hypnosis. Suggestion, and the power of mind over matter, are taught in every good childbirth preparation class. With hypnosis a very high level of suggestibility is achieved, which (depending on an individual's susceptibility and the type of hypnosis used) can do anything from making the patient more relaxed and comfortable to completely eliminating awareness of pain. Only about one in four adults is hypnotizable to some degree. (A very small percentage can even go through an unmedicated cesarean section without feeling any pain.)

Training of a subject in hypnosis for childbirth should start weeks or months in advance, under a physician certified in the subject or another practitioner recommended by your physician. You may use auto- or self-hypnosis, or you may depend upon the practitioner to make the suggestions. Either way, use caution.

MAKING THE DECISION

Women have more options in childbirth today than ever before. And, with the exception of certain emergency situations, the decision of whether or not to have medication during your labor and delivery will be largely yours. Here's how to make the best decision possible, for you and your baby:

❖ Discuss pain relief and anesthesia with your practitioner long before labor begins. Your practitioner's expertise and experience make him or her an invaluable ally in your decision-making process. Well before your first contraction, find out: what kinds of drugs or procedures he or she uses most often; what side effects may be experienced by mother and/or child; when he or she considers medication absolutely necessary; when he or she considers the option to be yours.

❖ Recognize that childbirth isn't supposed to be a trial by ordeal. Nor is it a test of your bravery, strength, or endurance. Medical technology has given women who are in pain during childbirth the option of relief through medication. Not only is it an acceptable option, it is, in certain cases, the best option. The pain of childbirth has been described by some as the most intense in the human experience. Seeking relief from such pain doesn't mean you've failed yourself, your coach, or your baby.

❖ Don't make up and close your mind in advance. Investigate and familiarize yourself with the various options in analgesia and anesthesia; think about what might be best for you; discuss it with your doctor and your coach. But don't try to make a final decision before the time comes. It's impossible to predict what kind of labor and delivery you'll have, and thus it would be foolhardy to decide in advance whether or not you'll want or need medication. Even if you're scheduled for a cesarean, you can plan only tentatively on an epidural or spinal; last-minute complications could necessitate general anesthesia.

❖ If during labor you feel you need medication, discuss it with your coach and the nurse or doctor. But don't insist on it immediately. Try holding out 15 minutes or so, and putting that time to the best possible use—concentrating extra-hard on your relaxation or breathing techniques; taking in all the comfort your coach can give you. You may find that with a little more support you can handle the pain, or that the progress you make in those 15 minutes gives you the will to go on without help. (If your physician decides that you need medication immediately, for your sake or your baby's, waiting may not be advisable.) If after waiting you find that you need the relief as much or even more, ask for it—and don't feel guilty.

❖ Remember that, as with all aspects of pregnancy, labor, and delivery, the well-being of you and your baby is your priority, and not some preconceived, idealized childbirth scenario. All decisions should be made on that basis, and on no other.

12
The Eighth Month

WHAT YOU CAN EXPECT AT THIS MONTH'S CHECKUPS

After the 32nd week, your practitioner may ask you to come in every two weeks, so your condition can be more closely monitored. You can expect the following to be checked, depending upon your particular needs and upon your practitioner's style of practice:[1]

❖ Weight and blood pressure

❖ Urine, for sugar and protein

❖ Fetal heartbeat

❖ Height of fundus (top of uterus)

❖ Size (you may get a rough weight estimate) and position of fetus, by palpation

❖ Feet and hands, for edema (swelling); legs, for varicose veins

❖ Symptoms you have been experiencing, especially unusual ones

❖ Questions and problems you want to discuss—have a list ready

WHAT YOU MAY BE FEELING

You may feel all of these symptoms at one time or another, or only a few of them. Some may have continued from last month, others may be new or hardly noticeable. You may also have other, less common symptoms.

PHYSICALLY:

❖ Strong, regular fetal activity

❖ Increasingly heavy whitish vaginal discharge (leukorrhea)

1. See appendix for an explanation of the procedures and tests performed.

❖ Increased constipation

❖ Heartburn and indigestion, flatulence and bloating

❖ Occasional headaches, faintness or dizziness

❖ Nasal congestion and occasional nosebleeds; ear stuffiness

❖ Leg cramps

❖ Backache

❖ Mild edema (swelling) of ankles and feet, and occasionally hands and face

❖ Varicose veins of legs and/or hemorrhoids

❖ Itchy abdomen

❖ Increasing shortness of breath as uterus crowds the lungs

❖ Difficulty sleeping

❖ Increasing Braxton Hicks contractions, abdominal achiness

❖ Increasing clumsiness

❖ Colostrum, either leaking or expressed, from breasts (though this premilk substance may not appear until after delivery)

EMOTIONALLY:

❖ Increasing anxiousness to be over with the pregnancy

WHAT YOU MAY LOOK LIKE

By the end of the eighth month, the baby is about 18 inches long and weighs 5 pounds. Growth, especially of the brain, is great in this period. Calcium, protein, and iron are more important than ever in the last weeks. Most systems are well developed, but the lungs may still be immature. Baby has an excellent chance of survival if born now.

❖ Apprehension about the baby's health, labor, and delivery

❖ Increasing absentmindedness

❖ Excitement at the realization that *it* won't be long now

WHAT YOU MAY BE CONCERNED ABOUT

SHORTNESS OF BREATH

"Sometimes I have trouble breathing. Could this mean that my baby isn't getting enough oxygen?"

Shortness of breath doesn't mean you—or your baby—are short of oxygen. Changes in the respiratory system during pregnancy actually allow women to take in *more* air, and to use it more efficiently. Still, most women experience varying degrees of difficulty breathing (some describe it as feeling a conscious need to breathe more deeply)—particularly in the last trimester, when the expanding uterus presses against the diaphragm, crowding the lungs. Relief usually arrives when lightening occurs (when the fetus settles back down into the pelvis, generally two to three weeks before delivery). In the meantime, you may find it easier to breathe if you sit straight up instead of slumped over, sleep in a semi-propped-up position, and avoid overexertion.

YOUR WEIGHT GAIN AND THE BABY'S SIZE

"I've gained so much weight that I'm afraid the baby will be very big and difficult to deliver."

Just because you've gained a lot of weight doesn't necessarily mean your baby has. Even a 35- to 40-pound weight gain can yield a 6- or 7-pound baby. On the average, however, a larger weight gain will produce a larger baby. Your baby's size may also be influenced by your own birth weight (if you were born large, your baby will tend to be) and by your prepregnancy weight (in general, heavier women have heavier babies). By palpating your abdomen and measuring the height of your fundus (the top of your uterus), your practitioner will be able to give you some idea of your baby's size, though such "guesstimates" can be off by a pound or more. A sonogram may more accurately gauge size, but it may be off, too.

Even if your baby is large, that doesn't automatically portend a difficult delivery. Though a 6- or 7-pound baby often slithers out faster than an 8- or 9-pounder, many women are able to deliver a bigger baby naturally and normally. The vital factor is whether the baby's head (its largest part) can fit through the mother's pelvis. If it can, delivery should be no problem. At one time, an x-ray was routinely ordered to try to determine whether or not a feto-pelvic disproportion existed. But experience and research have shown that the x-ray is not an accurate predictor of whether or not the baby can actually fit through the birth canal, partly because it can't foresee to what extent the fetal head will mold in order to squeeze through. Though the risk of the x-ray is slight, it is not recommended except in very unusual circumstances, when the benefits outweigh that risk.

More commonly today, when there is some suspicion of fetopelvic disproportion, the practitioner will allow a trial labor. If you progress, the labor will continue. If you don't, labor may get a boost with the administration of oxytocin. If labor still doesn't progress, a cesarean will usually be performed.

HOW YOU'RE CARRYING

"Everyone says I seem to be carrying small and low for the eighth month. Could it be that my baby isn't growing properly?"

Carrying Baby, Eighth Month

These are just three of the very different ways that a woman may carry near the end of her eighth month. The variations are even greater than before. Depending on the size and position of your baby, as well as your own size and weight gain, you may be carrying higher, lower, bigger, smaller, wider, or more compactly.

It would be a good idea to make earplugs and blinders a part of every pregnant woman's maternity wardrobe. Wearing them for nine months would enable her to avoid the worry generated by the misguided commentary and advice of relatives, friends—even strangers—and prevent invidious comparisons of her belly to those of other pregnant women, who are larger, smaller, lower, or higher.

Just as no two prepregnant figures are proportioned in precisely the same fashion, no two pregnant silhouettes are identical. How you carry, both in size and shape, is dependent on whether you started out tall or short, thin or not-so-thin, petite or voluptuous. And it is seldom an indication of *what* you're carrying. A petite woman carrying low and small may give birth to a larger infant than a bigger-boned woman carrying high and wide.

The only accurate assessments of your baby's progress and well-being are likely to come from your practitioner. When you're not in his or her office, keep your earplugs in and your blinders on—and you'll have a lot less to worry about.

PRESENTATION AND POSITION OF THE BABY

"My doctor says the baby is in a breech position. How will this affect my labor and delivery?"

It's never too early to prepare yourself for the possibility of a breech birth, but it's definitely too early now to resign yourself to one. Most babies turn and settle into a head-down position between the 32nd and 34th weeks, but a few keep their parents and doctors guessing until only a few days before delivery.

Some nurse-midwives recommend doing exercises in the last eight weeks, designed to encourage a breech baby to turn. There's no medical proof that these exercises work, but there's none to suggest that they hurt, either. When the fetus is still in a breech position near term, some physicians advocate fetal version—a turning of the breech fetus to the vertex, or head-down, position. The doctor, applying his or her hands to the mother's abdomen, gently, and often with ultrasound guidance, gradually shifts the position of the fetus. The fetal condition is monitored continuously to be sure that the umbilical cord isn't accidentally compressed or the placenta disturbed. Version is best done in very late pregnancy or very early labor, when the uterus is still relatively relaxed. Some doctors claim a successful turning rate of 75%, but

other physicians hesitate to use this procedure for fear of complications. Certainly, only an experienced obstetrician—who is ready to do an emergency cesarean if trouble arises—should attempt version.

Breeches are more common when the fetus is smaller than average and not cradled snugly in the uterus, when the uterus is unusually shaped, when there is an excess of amniotic fluid, when there is more than one fetus, and in women who have had babies before and whose uteri are more relaxed. If your baby is one of the 3% or 4% in breech position at term, you should discuss the delivery possibilities with your physician (nurse-midwives do not usually handle breech births). You may be able to have a normal vaginal delivery, or, depending on various conditions, you may indeed have to undergo a cesarean. (Which is *not* the end of the world, and for which eventuality every pregnant woman should be prepared anyway. See page 210.)

If your obstetrician routinely performs cesarean sections for breech presentations, don't ask for a vaginal delivery. Vaginal deliveries are perfectly safe in about one third to one half of breech births, but *only* if the doctor is experienced in the proper protocol. Some studies of vaginal breech deliveries show the potential risk is not always from the delivery itself, but from the reason for the breech: for example, the baby is premature or undersize, there are multiple fetuses, or there is some other congenital problem.

Experienced physicians will usually permit vaginal deliveries when all the following conditions are met:

❖ The baby is a frank breech (with the legs folded flat up against the face), the most common breech position.

❖ The baby is determined to be small enough (usually under 8½ pounds) for easy passage through the pelvis.

❖ The mother has no obstetrical or medical problem that would complicate a vaginal delivery.

❖ The presenting part is engaged, or descended into, the pelvis as labor begins.

❖ The fetal head is not hyperextended, but is tucked down toward the chest.

Breech labor is begun on a trial basis in a surgically equipped delivery room. If all goes well, it continues. If not, or if the cervix dilates too slowly, the doctor and surgical team are ready to perform a cesarean section in a matter of minutes. Continuous electronic fetal monitoring is absolutely essential. Often a pudendal nerve block (see page 199) is administered to prevent the mother from bearing down too hard before she is fully dilated (which might lead to the cord being compressed between the baby and the pelvis). Occasionally, a general anesthetic is administered to the mother when the baby is halfway delivered, to permit rapid completion of the birth by the physician. Forceps may be used to keep the head properly flexed, and to help deliver the head without pulling too much on the body or neck. A wide episiotomy is often routinely made to facilitate the birthing process.

How Does Your Baby Lie?

VERTEX

BREECH

About 96 out of every 100 babies present head first (vertex). The rest are usually in one or another breech position (buttocks first). The complete breech is illustrated here. The frank breech, in which the baby's legs are folded straight up, is the easiest breech to deliver vaginally.

"How can I tell if my baby is lying the right way for delivery?"

Playing "name that bump" (trying to figure out which are shoulders, elbows, and bottom) may be better evening entertainment than TV, but it's not the most accurate way of determining your baby's position. Your doctor or nurse-midwife can probably get a better idea than you, by palpating your abdomen with the flat of his or her trained hands, for recognizable baby parts. The baby's back, for instance, is usually a smooth, convex contour opposite a bunch of little irregularities which are the "small parts"— hands, feet, elbows. In the eighth month, the head has usually settled near your pelvis; it is round, firm, and—when pushed down—bounces back without moving the rest of the body. The baby's bottom is a less regular shape, and softer, than the head. The location of the baby's heartbeat is another clue to its position—if the presentation is head first, the heartbeat will usually be heard in the lower half of your abdomen; it will be loudest if the baby's back is toward your front. If there's any doubt, a sonogram will be used for verification.

ADEQUACY FOR DELIVERY

"I'm 5 feet tall and very petite. I'm afraid I'll have trouble delivering a baby normally."

Fortunately, when it comes to giving birth, it's what's inside, not what's outside, that counts. The size and shape of your pelvis is what determines whether your delivery will be easy and normal. And you can't always tell a pelvis by its cover. A short, slight woman can have a roomier pelvis than a tall, stocky woman. Only your practitioner can make an educated guess about its size—usually by measurements taken at your first prenatal exam. If there's some doubt whether your pelvis is adequate while you're in labor, a sonogram will be taken. (See Fetopelvic Disproportion, page 212.)

Of course, in general the overall size of the pelvis, as of all bony structures, is smaller in people of smaller stature. For example, Oriental women usually have smaller pelvises than Nordic women. Luckily nature, in its wisdom, rarely presents an Oriental woman with a Nordic-size baby—even if the father is a 6-foot fullback. Instead, all things being equal, babies are generally fairly well matched to the size of their mothers.

YOUR SAFETY DURING CHILDBIRTH

"I know medical science has taken most of the risk out of giving birth, but I'm still afraid of dying during delivery."

There was a time when mothers routinely risked their lives to have children; they still do in some areas of the world. In the United States today, the risk to maternal life in labor and delivery is virtually nonexistent. Just 1 in 10,000 women dies in childbirth. And this number includes not only women with chronic heart conditions and other serious illnesses, but those who give birth in backwoods shacks and dingy tenements, without medical assistance.

In short, even if your pregnancy falls into the highest-risk category—and certainly if it doesn't—you stand a lot better chance of surviving labor and delivery than you do a trip to the supermarket in your car, or a stroll across a busy street.

HAVING A CESAREAN SECTION

"My doctor just told me I will have to have a cesarean. But I'm afraid the surgery will be dangerous."

Though popular lore has it that the cesarean section got its name because Julius Caesar was born via abdominal delivery, that's virtually impossible. Julius might have survived such an operation, but his mother wouldn't have—and it is known that Mrs. Caesar lived for many years after his birth.

Today, however, cesareans are nearly as safe as vaginal deliveries for mother, and in difficult deliveries or when there's fetal distress, they are often the safest route for baby. Even though it is technically considered major surgery, a cesarean carries relatively minor risks—much closer to those of a tonsillectomy than a gall bladder operation, for instance.

Learning all you can about cesarean sections before delivery—from your doctor, in your childbirth class (a special class on cesareans is ideal), and through reading—will help to prepare you and to ease your fears.

"The doctor says I may have to have a cesarean section. I'm worried that this may be dangerous for the baby."

Chances are that if you have a cesarean, your baby will be at least as safe, and possibly safer, than if you had had a vaginal delivery. Every year thousands of babies who might not have survived the perilous journey through the birth canal (or might have survived impaired) are lifted from their mother's abdomen sound and unscathed.

Though there has been some speculation that cesareans are somehow harmful to babies, there's no hard evidence that this is so. Of course, a higher proportion of cesarean babies do have medical problems after birth—but most often because of the original distress that necessitated the operation, not because of the operation itself. Many of these infants would never have made it at all if left to a natural delivery.

In most ways, babies delivered via cesarean don't differ from those delivered vaginally—though cesarean babies do have the edge in appearance. Because they don't have to accommodate to the narrow confines of the pelvis, they usually have nicely unmolded heads. And because silver nitrate drops are not administered, their eyes will not become swollen or puffy.

Apgar scores (the rating scale used to evaluate an infant's condition one and five minutes after birth) on babies from both types of delivery are comparable. Cesarean-born babies do have the slight disadvantage of not having some of the excess mucus squeezed out of their respiratory tracts in the birthing process, but the mucus can be easily suctioned after delivery. Very, very rarely is there any serious damage done to a baby during cesarean delivery—much more rarely than during vaginal deliveries.

The most likely kind of damage a baby delivered abdominally might suffer is psychological—not from the delivery itself, but because of the mother's attitude toward it. Occasionally a mother who has had a cesarean will subconsciously resent the baby who she feels deprived her of her finest hour and brought such insult to her body.[2] She may allow the jealousy she feels toward mothers who've delivered vaginally, and the guilt she feels about failing, interfere with the establishment of a good relationship with her baby. Or she may incorrectly assume that the cesarean-born infant is unusually fragile (few are) and become overprotective. If such feelings develop, the mother should try to confront and deal with them and, if necessary, seek professional help in resolving them.

But often, destructive attitudes can be avoided right from the start. First, by recognizing that the method by which a baby is delivered in no way reflects on either the mother or the child. Second, by making sure that there is an opportunity for bonding with your baby at the earliest possible time (if this is important to you). Long before you go into labor, let your doctor know that if you have a cesarean you would like to be able to hold or even nurse the baby on the operating table, or if that's not possible, in the recovery room. If you wait until delivery day to state your case, you may not have the strength or opportunity to make it. Planning ahead also gives you the opportunity to challenge contrary hospital rules, such as those requiring every cesarean-delivered newborn, even healthy ones, to spend some time in the neonatal intensive care unit. If you present a strong argument in a rational, non-hysterical way, you may be able to effect a change in the rules.

If, good intentions notwithstanding, you turn out to be too weak to participate in any serious mother-baby bonding (and many women are, whether they've had abdominal or vaginal deliveries), or if your baby needs to be observed or cared for in the neonatal intensive care unit for a while, don't panic. There is no evidence, despite the hoopla the concept has aroused, that bonding *must* take place immediately after birth. It can, of course, but it can also take place weeks, even months, later (see page 288).

"I so much want a natural birth; but it seems like everybody is having a cesarean these days and I'm terrified I'll have to have one too."

Not quite "everybody" is having a cesarean these days—but far more women are than ever before.

---

2. Women who deliver vaginally may have a similar resentment, almost always temporary, because of the pain of delivery.

In the early 1960s your chances of having a cesarean would have been 1 in 20. Today they are at least 1 in 10, and if your pregnancy is in a high-risk category, as much as 1 in 5.

Why such a substantial increase? Many point an accusing finger at the medical community: at the occasional doctor who would prefer to schedule a cesarean during office hours than be awakened at 3 A.M. or who will, at the slightest medical pretext, jump at the chance to collect the higher fee a cesarean commands. (The fact that insurance carriers usually pick up the tab assuages the guilt.) And at the malpractice-shy physician, who will perform a cesarean to cover him- or herself when a vaginal delivery shows even the slightest potential for problems. (More suits against obstetricians are instituted for *not* performing a cesarean—and consequently getting a bad result—than for performing one.) Add the physicians who decide to do a cesarean the instant a negative reading is picked up on the fetal monitor (without double checking to be sure the baby, and not the fetal monitor, is in trouble), and it would appear that bad medicine is to blame.

But the major reason for the increase in cesareans is not bad medicine, but *good* medicine: Cesareans save the lives of babies who cannot be delivered safely via the vagina. Most doctors perform cesareans not for convenience, or more money, or because they are afraid of malpractice, but because they believe that in certain circumstances this surgery is the best, sometimes the only, way to protect the baby they are about to deliver. (The dramatic decrease in newborn deaths that has corresponded with the increase in cesareans suggests they may be right.)

Several changes in obstetrical practice have also contributed to the increase in cesareans. First of all, mid-forceps delivery is used less often than in the past (see page 253). Second, cesarean delivery has become extremely quick and safe—and in most instances mothers can be awake to see their babies born. Third, the fetal monitor, and a variety of fetal tests, can more accurately (though not infallibly) indicate when a fetus is in trouble and needs to be delivered in a hurry. In addition, thanks to better understanding and management of their problems, more women at high risk are able to have successful pregnancies, frequently aided by surgical deliveries. Finally, a major, and largely unnecessary, reason for the sizable number of cesareans is the repeat c-section.

Most women won't know whether or not they will have a cesarean until they are well into labor. There are, however, several advance indications that point to the possibility:

One or More Previous Cesarean Births. But only for reasons that may recur. Most women with prior c-sections can have normal vaginal deliveries.

Breech or Transverse (Crosswise) Presentation of the Fetus. Or other difficult-to-deliver presentations (see pages 207, 275).

Fetopelvic Disproportion. A mismatch between the baby's head and the mother's pelvic outlet, which will not permit vaginal delivery, is not usually apparent until labor fails to progress, but may be suggested in advance by ultrasound examination, or by previous difficult deliveries.

Preeclampsia or Eclampsia That Doesn't Respond to Treatment. In such cases the only way to protect both mother and baby is prompt delivery. If induction does not bring on labor, or if the fetus is very immature or in distress, a cesarean will put less stress on the baby than a vaginal delivery.

Placenta Previa (abnormally low positioning of the placenta). If the placenta partly or completely covers the cervical opening, cesarean delivery is absolutely essential. This may be determined by an ultrasound examination prior to labor, or by an internal exam once the cervix has begun to dilate. But vaginal delivery, with the help of fetal monitoring, can sometimes be attempted when the placenta is to the side and hasn't begun to separate from the uterus.

Abruptio Placenta (premature separation of a normally located placenta from the wall of the uterus). The separation before labor begins causes bleeding, and threatens the lives of both mother and baby if prompt delivery is not effected— either through induced vaginal delivery, if the separation is not extensive and there is no fetal distress, or through surgical delivery.

Rh Complications. When the baby has Rh disease, which is rare today

(see page 40), he or she may not be strong enough to tolerate vaginal delivery.

Active Maternal Herpes (within four weeks of delivery). Since a baby can contract herpes passing through the birth canal of a mother with an active infection, a cesarean is definitely indicated in such cases. (See page 41.)

A Dysmature Fetus (a fetus more than two weeks overdue, whose placental nourishment has begun to rapidly diminish).

Maternal Diabetes. Early delivery is often best for the babies of diabetic mothers, to prevent their becoming overly large and dysmature. Depending upon the condition of both fetus and mother, and on other factors, labor may be induced or cesarean performed.

Maternal Hypertension or Kidney Disease. Either of these may necessitate delivery by cesarean.

Preterm Fetal or Maternal Distress. When a mother or her fetus is suddenly in trouble and a speedy delivery seems necessary, a cesarean is usually the preferred route, both because it is faster than inducing labor and because it is less traumatic for the immature fetus.

It's during labor that most indications for a possible cesarean are first noted. They include:

Failure of Labor to Progress After 16 to 18 Hours. This may be due to

Cesarean Questions to Discuss With Your Doctor

❖ Will it be possible to try some other alternatives before cesarean is resorted to (except in emergency situations)? For example, oxytocin to stimulate contractions, or squatting to make contractions more effective?

❖ What kinds of anesthesia might be used? A general anesthesia that puts you to sleep is usually necessary when time is of the essence, but spinal or epidural anesthesia will allow you to be awake during a non-emergency abdominal delivery. (See All About Childbirth Medication, page 196.)

❖ Does he or she routinely use the low-segment, or "bikini," incision whenever possible, so that a vaginal delivery can be considered next time around?

❖ Can your coach be present if you are awake? If you are asleep?

❖ Can your nurse-midwife (if you have one) be with you, too?

❖ Will you and your husband be able to hold the baby immediately after birth (if you are awake and all is well), and will you be able to nurse in the recovery room? Will your husband be able to hold the baby if you're asleep?

❖ If the baby doesn't need special care, can he or she still room-in with you, possibly along with your husband, to help you out?

❖ After an uncomplicated cesarean birth, how much recovery time will you need both in and out of the hospital? What physical discomforts and limitations can you expect to experience?

❖ If the fetal monitor indicates the baby may be in distress, will other methods (such as checking the scalp pH) be used to verify the monitor readings before a cesarean is decided upon?

ineffective or weak contractions;[3] a fetus that is too large for the mother's pelvis; an unusually shaped pelvis that won't allow for the passage of the fetus; lack of pelvic flexibility, particularly in women over 40 who are having their first babies; and a fetus who is presenting face-first or "sunny-side up."

Fetal Distress. When the fetus is in trouble, prompt delivery is imperative. Fetal distress is most often diagnosed today through the use of an electronic fetal monitor. (Expert reading of the monitor printout is important to avoid misdiagnosis.)

Prolapsed Cord (an umbilical cord that comes down into the cervix or the vagina). The cord becomes wedged between the cervix and the baby, impairing blood flow to the fetus. An emergency cesarean is often necessary.

If cesareans are so safe, and sometimes lifesaving, why do most of us dread the prospect of having one?

---

3. The doctor may try to stimulate contractions with oxytocin, the drug used in the induction of labor, before resorting to cesarean in such cases.

Partly because major surgery, even when it's routine and almost risk-free, is still a little scary; but mostly because, although we spend months preparing ourselves for an idyllic natural childbirth, we usually enter the labor room utterly unprepared for the very real possibility—a 1 or even 2 in 10 chance—that we'll have a cesarean instead. For nine months, we block that unpleasant possibility out of our minds. We devour childbirth primers, but we bypass chapters on cesarean section. We ask dozens of questions about natural delivery in childbirth class, but not one about a surgical birth. We look forward to holding our husband's hand as we pant and push our baby into the world—not to lying passively, and possibly unconscious, as sterile instruments slice into our abdomen to extract him or her, like a hot appendix. When suddenly faced with a cesarean, we feel deprived of control over the birth of our baby. As we see it, medical technology has taken over, ushering in frustration, disappointment, anger, and guilt.

But that's not how it has to be. Not if you are as prepared for an abdominal delivery as for a vaginal one, if you start looking forward to the birth of your baby instead of to an idealized childbirth experience, and if you recognize that a cesarean birth can be beautiful, too.

Several steps taken now can make the prospect of cesarean less ominous and the reality more fulfilling. Even if you have no suspicion that you might need a cesarean, be sure at least one session on the subject is included in your childbirth preparation course. If you do have some reason to believe a cesarean section might be necessary, try to take a full preparatory course. Do some reading on your own, too.

Discuss the topic of a cesarean section with your doctor or the on-call physician your nurse-midwife uses. Don't be put off by assurances that you aren't likely to need one; explain that you want to be prepared, just in case. Let the doctor know that you would like to be part of the decision-making team if a cesarean seems to be necessary.

If your obstetrician decides in advance that a cesarean will be necessary, be sure to ask for a detailed explanation of why. Ask if there are any alternatives, such as a trial labor: Once in labor, you would be permitted to continue without a cesarean on the condition that the labor progresses normally. If you suspect the major reason a cesarean has been suggested is convenience, you can ask for, and get, another opinion.

Whether you're preparing for a scheduled cesarean or just for the possibility of one, there are a number of issues you should talk over with your physician (see Cesarean Questions to Discuss With Your Doctor, facing page).

Of course, few pregnant women would select cesarean as their delivery of choice; and almost 90% will have the vaginal delivery they've hoped for. But for those who don't, there's no reason for disappointment, or feelings of guilt or failure. Any delivery (vaginal or abdominal, medicated or unmedicated, with an episiotomy or without) that yields a healthy baby is an unqualified success.

PETS AND THE BABY

"We have a dog who's been like an only child. He's never been exposed to children, and we are very worried that there will be problems when we bring the baby home."

There's no bigger baby than the kind with four legs and a wagging tail—particularly when the affections and attentions of his "parents" (and possibly his place in their bed) are suddenly usurped by a noisy, red-faced, demanding, unfamiliar, and thoroughly unwelcome newcomer. To minimize the jealousy your pooch may feel when baby makes four, start his transition from "only child" to secondary sibling well in advance of delivery:

❖ If your dog isn't obedience-trained already, get him trained now. It's vitally important that his behavior be controllable and predictable (especially since the baby's won't be). Dogs who are obedience-trained feel more secure and stable, and are less likely to get out of hand.

❖ Expose your dog to babies and children now if he's never been around them before. It's good for him to be familiar with the sounds and erratic movements babies make.

❖ Bring a baby-sized doll home, and treat it like a baby. Put it in the baby's crib, cuddle it, sing to it, carry it around, take it into bed with you. If your dog's going to vent his jealous feelings, now is the time.

❖ If your dog has always slept with you but won't be allowed to once the baby comes home, get him used to a solitary sleeping arrangement now. Make up a comfortable doggie bed—perhaps with a favorite blanket or pillow for solace.

❖ Before you bring the baby home from the hospital, acquaint your dog with the baby's scent by sending home a piece of clothing that the baby has worn.

❖ Once the baby is home, don't make the mistake of being overly protective—which will only make the dog more jealous. Try to help the dog make friends with the baby, and make him feel that he's still part of the family. Pet him while you nurse the baby, walk him while you walk the baby, welcome him into the baby's room while you are there.

❖ If, despite all you've done, your dog shows hostility toward the baby, you may have to keep him tied up (inside or outside) until you are certain he has adjusted. It's dangerous to assume that a dog who's never bitten before isn't capable of causing harm.

TRAVEL SAFETY

"I've got an important business trip scheduled this month. Is it safe for me to travel, or should I cancel?"

If you can possibly avoid traveling in the last trimester, do. Not only is traveling in late pregnancy uncomfortable, it can be hazardous—

since you could suddenly go into labor (premature labor can't always be predicted) hundreds or thousands of miles from your doctor. The threat of labor occurring at thousands of feet in the air (and hours away from landing) is enough to keep airlines from allowing pregnant women in their ninth month to fly without a doctor's letter of permission. That letter may prove difficult to obtain, since most physicians don't recommend travel in the last trimester, particularly in the eighth and ninth months. If you must travel, refer to the tips on page 156. It's particularly important to secure the name of a local obstetrician.

DRIVING

"Should I still drive?"

Long car trips are too exhausting late in pregnancy, no matter who's driving. But as long as you're not experiencing any dizzy spells, and as long as you can still fit behind the wheel, you can safely drive short distances up to delivery day. Don't, however, try to drive yourself to the hospital while in labor. And don't forget: Fasten your seat belt.

BRAXTON HICKS CONTRACTIONS

"Every once in a while my uterus seems to bunch up and harden. What's going on?"

These are Braxton Hicks contractions, which usually begin to rehearse the pregnant uterus for la-

bor sometime during the latter half of pregnancy. Your uterus is flexing its muscles, practicing and preparing itself for the contractions which will soon push your baby out. You'll feel these contractions as a painless (but possibly uncomfortable) tightening of your uterus, beginning at the top and gradually spreading downward before relaxing. These contractions usually last about 30 seconds (ample time to practice your breathing exercises), but may last as long as 2 minutes or more.

As pregnancy draws to a close in the ninth month, Braxton Hicks contractions begin to get more frequent, intense—sometimes even painful—and thus more difficult to distinguish from true labor contractions (see Prelabor, False Labor, Real Labor, page 233). Though they're not efficient enough to deliver your baby, Braxton Hicks contractions may get the prebirth processes of effacement and dilation started, thereby giving you a leg up on labor before it ever begins.

BATHING

"My mother says she wasn't permitted to bathe after the 34th week. My doctor says it's okay. Why?"

This is one case where mother doesn't know best. Though well intentioned, she is misinformed. Her doctor, like most 20 or 30 years ago, believed that foreign substances, such as dirty bath water, could travel up the vagina to the cervix in pregnancy and cause an infection. But while further research remains to be done, doctors today believe that water does not enter the vagina unless it is forced, as in a douche; thus, worry about infection is not justified. Even if water does enter the vagina, the cervical mucous plug that seals the entrance to the uterus effectively protects the membranes that surround the fetus, the amniotic fluid, and the fetus itself from invading infectious organisms. Therefore, unless membranes have ruptured or the plug has been discharged, most doctors permit bathing in normal pregnancies.

Baths, however, aren't totally risk-free, particularly in the last trimester when ungainliness can lead to slips and falls. Bathe with care—and preferably with someone to help you in and out of the tub.

MAKING LOVE NOW

"I'm confused. I hear a lot of conflicting information about sexual intercourse in the last weeks of pregnancy."

The problem is that existing medical evidence on the subject is confusing and conflicting. It is widely believed that neither intercourse nor orgasm alone precipitate labor unless conditions are ripe (though many impatient-to-deliver couples have enjoyed trying). For that reason, many physicians and midwives allow patients with normal pregnancies to make love—assuming they're still interested—right up until delivery day. And most couples apparently can do so without complication.

There does, however, seem to be some risk of sexual intercourse triggering premature labor, at least in women at high risk for preterm delivery (such as those carrying multiple fetuses, those who start effacing and dilating early, and those with a history of premature labor). Premature rupture of the membranes (PROM), at term or preterm, may also be related to intercourse, particularly when there is also inflammation of the membranes. Some cases of chorion amnionitis (infection of the amniotic sac) and postpartum infection have been tentatively linked to late pregnancy intercourse, and may be prevented by the use of condoms in the last eight weeks.

Ease your confusion by checking with your practitioner to see what the latest medical consensus is. If you get a green light, then by all means make love—if you want to and feel comfortable about it. If the light is red (and it will be if you are at high risk, for premature delivery, have placenta previa or abruptio, are experiencing unexplained bleeding, or if your membranes have ruptured), then find your intimacy in other ways. Try a romantic rendez-vous at a candlelit restaurant, or walking hand-in-hand under the stars. Or try an evening at home snuggling in bed or under an afgan in front of the TV, hugging and kissing on the sofa, soaping each other in the shower, or using massage—of the neck, back, feet, and of course, belly—as the medium.

WHAT IT'S IMPORTANT TO KNOW:
FACTS ABOUT BREASTFEEDING

Thirty years ago, when the eldest of the authors had her first baby, she was the only woman in the maternity wing to breastfeed. Just recently, when the youngest had her first baby, there was only one woman in maternity who *wasn't* planning to nurse.

Today there is clearly a back-to-breast trend. At the turn of the century, nearly every baby was fed at the breast; there was no other choice. But in the early 1900s, women began to demand rights they'd never had—to vote, to work, to smoke cigarettes, to let down or bob their hair, to peel off confining undergarments, and to set their sights outside the kitchen and the nursery. Breastfeeding was old-fashioned, it was restricting, and it represented all that women sought freedom from. To be a modern woman was to bottle-feed. And by the 1950s, the only remaining breastfeeders (besides our senior author and an assortment of bohemian stragglers) were those with whom emancipation hadn't caught up.

Ironically, it was the revitalized women's movement of the '60s and '70s that brought breastfeeding back into vogue. Women wanted not only freedom, but control—control of their lives, control of their bodies. They knew that control came with knowledge, and knowledge told them that breastfeeding was best—for their babies and, on the whole, for themselves.

WHY BREAST IS BEST

There is no question but that given normal circumstances, breastfeeding provides your newborn with the most perfect food for human infants:

❖ Human breast milk contains at least a hundred ingredients that are not found in cow's milk and that cannot be perfectly duplicated in formulas. Breast milk is individualized for each infant; raw materials are selected from the mother's bloodstream as needed, altering from day to day, feeding to feeding, as the baby grows and changes. The nutrients are matched to infant needs. Variations from breast milk in cow's milk formulas can lead to nutritional deficiencies.

❖ Breast milk is more digestible than cow's milk. The proportion of protein in mother's milk is lower (1.5%) than in cow's milk (3.5%), making it easier for the infant to handle. The protein itself is mostly lactalbumin, which is more nutritious and digestible than the major protein component of cow's milk, caseinogen. The fat content of both milks are similar, but the fat in mother's milk is more easily digested by the baby.

❖ Breast milk is less likely to cause overweight in infants.

❖ No baby is allergic to breast milk (though some can have allergic reactions to a certain food or foods in their mothers' diets). Beta-lactoglobulin, a substance contained in cow's milk, can trigger an allergic response and, following the formation of antibodies, can even cause anaphylactic shock (a life-threatening allergic reaction) in infants—which some suspect could be a contributing factor in the sudden infant death syndrome (or crib death). The soy milk formulas, which are often substituted when an infant is allergic to cow's milk, stray even farther in composition from what nature intended.

❖ Nursed babies are never constipated, because of the easier digestibility of breast milk. They also rarely have diarrhea—since breast milk seems both to destroy some diarrhea-causing organisms and to encourage the growth of beneficial flora in the digestive tract, which further discourage digestive upset. On a purely esthetic note, the bowel movements of a breastfed baby are sweeter-smelling (at least until solids are introduced) and less apt to cause diaper rash.

❖ Breast milk contains one third the mineral salts of cow's milk. The extra sodium is difficult for immature kidneys to handle.

❖ Breast milk contains less phosphorus. The higher phosphorus content of cow's milk is linked to a decreased calcium level in the formula-fed infant's blood.

❖ Breastfed babies are less subject to illness in the first year of life. Protection is provided by the transfer of immune factors in breast milk and in the premilk substance, colostrum.

❖ Nursing at the breast, because it requires more effort than sucking on a bottle, encourages optimum development of jaws, teeth, and palate.

❖ Breast milk is safe. There is no risk of contamination or spoilage.

❖ Breastfeeding is convenient. It requires no advance planning or packing, no equipment; it is always available (in the car, on an airplane, in the middle of the night), and at just the right temperature. When mother and baby aren't together (if the mother works, for instance), milk may be expressed in advance and stored in the freezer for bottle feedings as needed. (Breast milk is so vital to the well-being of a premature infant that, if his mother can't nurse, human milk is often supplied by a donor (preferably a woman who delivered prematurely.)

❖ Breastfeeding is economical. There is no investment in bottles, sterilizers, or formula; there are no half-emptied bottles or opened cans of formula to waste. And a nutritious diet (such as the Best-Odds Nursing Diet, page 75), which enables a nursing mother to feed her infant well, probably costs less than a typical American diet—one saturated with empty but expensive fast-food calories.

❖ There is evidence that breastfeeding decreases a woman's risk of developing breast cancer later in life.

❖ Nursing helps speed the shrinking of the uterus back to its prepregnant size and decreases the flow of lochia (the postpartum vaginal discharge).

❖ Lactation suppresses ovulation and menstruation, at least to some degree. Though it shouldn't be relied on for birth control, it may postpone resumption of a woman's periods for months, or at least for as long as she nurses.

❖ Nursing can help burn off the fat accumulated during pregnancy. If a woman is careful to consume an adequate number of only quality calories, she can fill all of her infant's nutritional needs while losing weight.

❖ Breastfeeding enforces rest periods for the new mother—particularly important during the first six postpartum weeks.

❖ Nursing in public is becoming more acceptable. With a little discretion and a big napkin, both mother and baby can dine at the same restaurant table.

❖ Breastfeeding brings mother and baby together, skin to skin, at least six to eight times a day. The emotional gratification, the intimacy, the sharing of love and pleasure, can be very special and very fulfilling.

(A special note to mothers of twins: All the advantages of breastfeeding a single child are doubled for you. See page 301 for tips that make breastfeeding for two easier.)

WHY SOME PREFER THE BOTTLE

Just as there were hold-outs against bottle-feeding 30 years ago, however, there are women today who choose not to nurse. And though the advantages of bottle-feeding seem to be dwarfed by those of breastfeeding, they can be real and convincing for some women.

❖ Bottle-feeding doesn't tie the mother down. She's able to work, shop, go out in the evening, even sleep through the night—letting someone else feed the baby.

❖ Bottle-feeding allows the father to share the feeding responsibilities and the bonding benefits more easily. (Although he can also give baby a bottle of expressed mother's milk.)

❖ Bottle-feeding doesn't interfere with a couple's sex life (unless baby wakes up for a feeding at the wrong time). Breastfeeding, on the other hand, can. First, because lactation hormones can keep the vagina dry; and second, because leaky breasts are a turnoff to some couples during lovemaking. For bottle-feeding couples, the breasts can remain sensual instead of utilitarian.

❖ Bottle-feeding doesn't dictate your diet, cramp your eating style. You can eat all the garlic, spicy foods, and cabbage you want, and you don't have to drink even one glass of milk.

❖ Bottle-feeding may be preferable for a woman who is inhibited about her body, squeamish about having such intimate contact with her infant, and uncomfortable about the possibility of nursing in public. Or for a woman who feels she is too high-strung or impatient to breastfeed.

MAKING THE CHOICE

For more and more women today, no choice need be made. They know they will opt for breast over bottle long before they even decide to become pregnant. Others, who've never given it much thought before pregnancy, choose breastfeeding once they've read up on its many benefits. Some women teeter on the brink of indecision right through pregnancy, uncertain about their own feelings, uncertain about their husbands'. A few women, though convinced that nursing isn't for them, can't shake the nagging feeling that they ought to do it anyway.

For all of these women, we have one suggestion: Try it—you may like it. You can always quit if you don't, but at least you will have eased those nagging doubts. Best of all, you and your baby will have reaped the benefits of breastfeeding, if just for a brief time.

Give breastfeeding a fair trial, though. The first few weeks are always difficult, even for the most ardent breastfeeders. Some experts suggest that a full month of nursing

is needed to establish a successful feeding relationship.

WHEN YOU CAN'T OR SHOULDN'T BREASTFEED

Unfortunately, the choice of whether or not to breastfeed isn't open to every new mother. Some women can't or shouldn't nurse their newborns. The reasons may be emotional or physical, due to mother's health or the baby's, temporary or long-term—and the following are factors:

❖ Serious debilitating illness (such as cardiac or kidney impairment, or severe anemia) or extreme underweight.

❖ Serious infection, such as tuberculosis.

❖ Conditions that require medications which pass into the breast milk and might be harmful to the baby such as: antithyroid, anticancer, or antihypertensive drugs; lithium, tranquilizers, sedatives. If you take any kind of medication, check with your physician before beginning breastfeeding.[4]

❖ AIDS, which can be passed through any body fluids, including breast milk.

---

4. A temporary need for medication, such as penicillin, even at the time you begin nursing, need not necessarily eliminate the chances of breastfeeding. It may be possible to start the baby on formula temporarily, express milk to get your milk supply going, and, as soon as medication is halted, switch to breastfeeding.

❖ Drug abuse—including the use of tranquilizers, heroin, methadone, marijuana, cigarettes, and heavy use of caffeine or alcohol.

❖ A deep-seated aversion to the idea of breastfeeding.

Conditions in the newborn that interfere with breastfeeding include:

❖ A disorder such as lactose intolerance or phenylketonuria (PKU), in which neither human *nor* cow's milk can be digested.

❖ Cleft lip and/or cleft palate, or other mouth deformities that make sucking at the breast difficult.

❖ There have been some suggestions that breast cancer might be passed on from mother to daughter through a virus in the breast milk in families with a history of premenopausal breast cancer. This remains unsubstantiated; apparently women with such histories, or even who have had cancer in one breast, can safely and successfully breastfeed their babies.

MAKING BOTTLE-FEEDING WORK

Though breastfeeding is a good experience for both mother and child, there is no reason why bottle-feeding can't be, too. Millions of happy, healthy babies have been raised on the bottle. When you can't, or don't wish to, breastfeed, the danger lies not in the bottle, but in the possibility that you might communicate any guilt or frustration you feel to your baby. Know that, with a little extra effort, love can be passed from mother to child through the bottle as well as through the breast. Make every feeding a time to cuddle your baby, just as you would if you were nursing: Never feed baby in the crib with a propped bottle; make skin-to-skin contact by opening your shirt, when practical, and letting the baby rest against your bare breast while feeding.

13
The Ninth Month

WHAT YOU CAN EXPECT AT THIS MONTH'S CHECKUPS

After about the 36th week, you will see your practitioner weekly. Both the tenor and content of these examinations will be reminders that you are getting closer to D-day. In general, you can expect your practitioner to check the following, though there may be variations depending upon your particular needs and upon your practitioner's style of practice:[1]

❖ Weight (gain will probably slow down or cease) and blood pressure (it may be up slightly over what it was at mid-pregnancy)

❖ Urine, for sugar and protein

❖ Fetal heartbeat

❖ Height of fundus, to see if it's dropped

❖ Size (you may get a rough weight estimate), presentation (head or bottom first?), position of fetus (is presenting part engaged?)

❖ Feet and hands, for edema (swelling); legs, for varicose veins

❖ Your cervix, for effacement and dilatation, usually some time after the 38th week (by internal examination)

❖ Symptoms you have been experiencing, especially unusual ones

❖ Frequency and duration of Braxton Hicks contractions you may be having and which you may be noticing

❖ Instructions from your practitioner as to when to call if you think you are in labor

❖ Questions and problems you want to discuss, particularly those related to labor and delivery—have a list ready

---

1. See appendix for an explanation of the procedures and tests performed.

WHAT YOU MAY BE FEELING

You may feel all of these symptoms at one time or another, or only a few of them. Some may have continued from last month, others may be new. Still others may hardly be noticed because you are used to them and/or because they are eclipsed by new and more exciting signs indicating that labor may not be far off.

PHYSICALLY:

* Changes in fetal activity (more squirming and less kicking, as the uterus becomes a more cramped home)

* Vaginal discharge (leukorrhea) becomes heavier and contains more mucus, which may be streaked red with blood or tinged brown or pink after intercourse or a pelvic exam

* Constipation

* Heartburn and indigestion, flatulence and bloating

* Occasional headaches, faintness, dizziness

* Nasal congestion and occasional nosebleeds; ear stuffiness

* Leg cramps during sleep

* Increased backache and heaviness

* Buttock and pelvic discomfort and achiness

* Increased edema (swelling) of ankles and feet, occasionally hands and face

* Varicose veins of the legs and/or hemorrhoids

* Itchy abdomen

* Easier breathing after the baby "drops"

* More frequent urination after the baby drops

* Increased difficulty sleeping

WHAT YOU MAY LOOK LIKE

Final preparations are being made for birth, which can safely take place any time now. Lungs are mature. About 2 inches and 2½ pounds are added to baby's length and weight (the average baby will be 20 inches, 7½ pounds at term). More confined, and possibly engaged in the pelvis, the fetus may seem less active.

❖ Increasing and intensifying Braxton Hicks contractions (some may be painful)

❖ Increasing clumsiness and difficulty getting around

❖ Colostrum, either leaking or expressed from breasts (though this premilk substance may not appear until after delivery)

❖ Fatigue or extra energy, or alternate periods of each

❖ Increase in appetite, or loss of appetite

EMOTIONALLY:

❖ More excitement, more anxiety, more apprehension, more absent-mindedness

❖ Relief that you're almost there

❖ Irritability and oversensitivity (especially with people who keep saying: "Are *you* still around?")

❖ Impatience and restlessness

❖ Dreaming and fantasizing about the baby

WHAT YOU MAY BE CONCERNED ABOUT

CHANGES IN FETAL MOVEMENTS

'My baby, who used to kick so vigorously, isn't kicking at all now—just squirming.''

When you first heard from your baby, way back in the fifth month, there was ample room in the uterus for acrobatics—and lots of kicking and punching. Now that conditions are getting a little cramped, gymnastics are curtailed. In this uterine straightjacket, there is room for little more than turning, twisting, and wiggling. And once the head is firmly engaged in the pelvis, baby will be even less mobile.

It's not important what kind of fetal movement you feel at this stage—as long as you're conscious of activity every day. Should the rate of activity suddenly decrease dramatically, or movements cease altogether or become very weak, a call to your practitioner is warranted. He or she may ask you to try this test: Lie down and relax. Then over a period of half an hour or an hour, count the movements. Repeat, possibly two or three times during the day. Ten or more movements per hour during each test period will assure everyone that everything is okay. Fewer might suggest that further evaluation is needed, although even then there is no cause for alarm. Many babies who are relatively inactive in the womb turn out to be perfectly healthy. But if inactivity indicates fetal distress, prompt medical action is vital to the well-being of your baby.

"I've read that fetal movements are supposed to slow down as delivery approaches. My baby seems more active than ever. Could that mean he's going to be hyperactive?"

Before birth is too soon to start worrying about hyperactivity. Studies show that fetuses who are very active in the womb are no more likely than quiet fetuses to become hyperactive in childhood.

Recent research also contradicts the notion that the average fetus becomes lazy just before delivery. In late pregnancy, there is generally a gradual decline in movement (from about 25 to 39 movements an hour at 30 weeks to 18 to 28 at term), probably related to tighter quarters, a decrease in amniotic fluid, and improved fetal coordination. But unless they're counting, many women never notice a significant difference.

BLEEDING OR SPOTTING

"Right after my husband and I made love this morning, I began to bleed. Does this mean that labor is beginning—or is the baby in some kind of danger?"

Any new symptom in the ninth month immediately raises one of two questions—or both: Is it time? Is something wrong? Bleeding and spotting are two such anxiety-provoking events. What they indicate depends on the type of bleeding you experience and the circumstances that surround it:

❖ Pinkish-stained or red-streaked mucus appearing soon after, or brownish-tinged mucus or brownish spotting appearing about 48 hours after, intercourse or vaginal examination is probably just a result of the sensitive cervix being bruised or manipu-

lated. This is normal and not a danger sign—although it should be reported to your practitioner. He or she may advise abstinence from intercourse until delivery.

❖ Bright red bleeding or persistent spotting could be originating at the placenta and requires immediate medical evaluation. Call your practitioner at once. If he or she can't be reached, have someone take you to the hospital.

❖ Pinkish- or brownish-tinged or bloody mucus accompanied by contractions or other signs of oncoming labor (see Prelabor, False Labor, Real Labor, page 233) could be signaling the start of labor. The fact that this blood-streaked mucus appeared just after intercourse could be a coincidence. Put in a call to your practitioner.

LIGHTENING AND ENGAGEMENT

"If I'm past my 38th week and haven't dropped, does it mean I'm going to be late?"

"Dropping," also called "lightening," is the descent of the fetus into the pelvic cavity. In first pregnancies, lightening generally takes place two to four weeks before delivery. In women who have had children previously, it rarely occurs until they go into labor. But as with almost every aspect of pregnancy, exceptions to the rules are the rule. A first-time mother can drop four weeks before her due date and deliver two weeks "late," or she can go into labor without having dropped at all.

Often, lightening is quite apparent. The pregnant woman notes that her bulging belly seems to have dropped and tilted forward. As the uterus moves away from the diaphragm, she may find breathing less of an effort; with the stomach less crowded, she may be able to eat more at a sitting. These added comforts are offset by the discomfort of pressure on the bladder, the pelvic joints, and the perineal area—which results in increased frequency of urination, difficult mobility, the sensation of increased perineal pressure, and, sometimes, pain. Sharp little shocks or twinges may occur when the fetal head presses on the pelvic floor. Some women sense a rolling in their pelvis when the head turns. And often, because her center of gravity has again shifted, a pregnant woman feels off balance once lightening has occurred.

It is very possible, however, for lightening to occur without your ever realizing it. If, for instance, you carried low to begin with, the shape of your abdomen might not be altered significantly. Or if you never experienced difficulty breathing or urinated frequently throughout pregnancy, you might not notice any obvious change.

When the broadest diameter of the fetal head has reached the upper boundary of the bony pelvis, it is said to be "engaged." Only your practitioner knows for sure whether or not your baby's head is snugly engaged in your pelvis. He or she relies on two basic indicators: on internal examination, the presenting part (the part of the fetus closest to the exit, most commonly the head) is felt in the pelvis; on palpating the head externally, it is found to be fixed, no longer "floating."

How far the presenting part has progressed through the pelvis is measured in "stations," each a centimeter long. A fully engaged baby is at "zero (or 0) station"—that is, the fetal head has descended to the level of the ischial spines (prominent bony landmarks on either side of the midpelvis). A baby who has just begun to descend may be at -4 or -5 station. Once delivery begins, the head continues on through the pelvis past 0 to $+1$, $+2$, and so on, until it begins to "crown" at the external vaginal opening at $+5$. Though a woman who goes into labor at 0 station probably has less pushing ahead than the woman at -3, this isn't invariably true, since station isn't the only factor affecting the progression of labor.

Though the engagement of the fetal head suggests that the baby can probably get through the pelvis without difficulty, a fetus that is still floating going into labor is not necessarily going to have trouble. And in fact, a majority of them come through the pelvis smoothly.

WHEN YOU WILL DELIVER

"Can the doctor tell exactly how close I am to going into labor?"

No. And don't believe it if he or she tells you otherwise. There are clues that labor may soon begin, which your practitioner begins to look for in the ninth month. Has lightening or engagement taken place? What station (level in the pelvis) has the baby's presenting part reached? Have effacement (thinning of the cervix) and dilatation (opening of the cervix) begun?

But "soon" can mean anywhere from an hour to three weeks or more. Ask the woman whose euphoria at being told by her practitioner, "You'll be in labor by this evening," dissolves into depression as weeks of pregnancy proceed to pass with nary a contraction.

A practitioner's prognostication that, since effacement and dilatation haven't yet begun, labor is weeks away can be equally unreliable. As women will testify who, upon hearing such a prediction, have sagged home from the doctor's office resigned to another long month of pregnancy, only to give birth by the following morning.

The fact is that engagement, effacement, and dilatation can occur gradually over a period of weeks or even a month or more in some women. In others they can occur in a matter of hours. No one, no matter how well trained, can accurately predict the onset of labor—because no one knows exactly what triggers it. (That's why some practitioners are as loath to venture guesses on when you will deliver as on whether it's going to be a girl or a boy.)

So like every pregnant woman before you, you'll just have to play a waiting game, knowing for certain only that your day, or night, will come—sometime.

LABOR AND DELIVERY ROOMS

"I'm very uneasy about going into the hospital and having my baby in unfamiliar surroundings."

The labor and delivery floor is by far the happiest in the hospital. Still, if you don't know what to expect, you can be filled with trepidation. Most hospitals allow—in fact, encourage—tours of the labor and delivery suite by expectant couples. Inquire when you make your reservation. If tours aren't routine, ask your practitioner if he or she can arrange a visit for you. You can also stop in during visiting hours, and though you won't see the actual labor and delivery area, you can see what patient rooms look like in the postpartum section, and also take a good look at the nursery. Besides making you feel more comfortable, this will give you the opportunity to see what a newborn looks like before you hold your own in your arms.

Labor and delivery rooms vary from hospital to hospital. Some are very sterile and businesslike; others are more homey. Birthing rooms are becoming more and more common and boast the at-home look, with rocking chairs, bright pictures on the walls, curtains on the windows, and birthing beds that look more as if they came out of an Ethan Allen showroom than a hospital supply catalogue.

Though it's nice to be in pleasant surroundings, in the long run it won't be the talent of the hospital's interior designer but the skill and caring of the medical staff that will be important to your well-being and that of your baby.

THE OVERDUE BABY

"I'm a week overdue and my doctor's arranged to give me a non-stress test. Is it possible that I might never go into labor on my own?"

The magic date is circled in red on the calendar; every day of the 40 weeks that precede it is crossed off with great anticipation. Then, at long last, the big day arrives. And, as in the majority of pregnancies, the baby doesn't. Anticipation dissolves into discouragement. The baby carriage and crib sit empty for another day. And then a week. And then, in 10% of pregnancies, two weeks. Will this pregnancy never end?

Though women who have reached the 42nd week might find it hard to believe, no pregnancy on record ever went on forever—even before the advent of labor induction. (It's true an occasional pregnancy progresses to the 44th week or beyond, but today a large majority are induced before they go much past the 42nd.)

When a pregnant woman appears to be post-term (technically 42 weeks or more, though some doctors will take action sooner), the practitioner evaluates the situation, considering two major factors: One, is the estimated due date accurate? He or she can be reasonably sure that it is if the date corresponded throughout pregnancy with the fundal height and the size of the uterus, and if the timing of both the first fetal movements felt by the mother and the first fetal heartbeats detected by the examiner also correlated with it. Sometimes ultrasonography and urine and blood tests are used to verify the gestational age. It is estimated that about 70% of apparent post-term pregnancies are due to a miscalculation of the time of conception.

Two, is the fetus continuing to thrive? Many babies continue to grow and flourish well into the tenth month (although this can be a problem if the baby becomes too large to pass easily through the mother's pelvis). Occasionally, however, the aging placenta begins to deteriorate, and the fetus ceases to thrive. These "dysmature" babies may lose weight in the uterus and be born with long, thin limbs and dry, parchment-like skin that hangs loosely because of the depleted fat layers. Though the risk of distress during labor is greater for dysmature babies than for normal-term infants, they usually develop normally following birth.

There are several procedures which can determine the condition of the post-term fetus and its placenta. Such tests are performed at the discretion of the practitioner—either routinely, when the delivery is overdue by a week or more, or occasionally, because there is some sign of fetal or maternal difficulty.

The Non-Stress Test (NST) is simple and safe. The mother is hooked up to a fetal monitor so that the response of the fetal heart to fetal movements can be observed. Normally, the heart rate will accelerate immediately following each fetal movement. Two such accelerations in a 20-minute period indicate a reactive, and thus healthy, fetus.

The Stress Test, or Oxytocin Challenge Test (OCT), also evaluates the reactivity of the fetal heart, but to uterine contractions that simulate labor rather than to fetal movements. In this somewhat more complex and time-consuming test (it may take up to 3 hours), the mother is hooked up to a fetal monitor, just as she would be in labor. If contractions are not occurring frequently enough on their own, they are initiated via the intravenous administration of oxytocin, or by stimulation of the mother's nipples (with hot towels and, if necessary, manually by the mother). Fetal response indicates the probable condition of fetus and placenta, as well as whether or not they can safely meet the strenuous demands of labor.

Levels of Estriol (an estrogenic hormone produced by the fetal-placental unit) in the blood or urine of the mother may also be evaluated, sometimes in conjunction with a stress or non-stress test, or both. Normally, estriol levels rise from the 28th week of pregnancy until term. A series of estriol determinations that show a trend that is either stationary or decreasing is an indication that living conditions in the uterus are no longer optimal and prompt delivery is advisable. Several maternal factors are known to affect estriol levels (e.g., chronic disease, change in level of activity, medications), and results are interpreted accordingly. Low levels of HPL (human placental lactogen) may also indicate placental dysfunction.

If the fetus passes all its tests, the practitioner will probably allow the pregnancy to follow nature's course for a while longer. Tests will be repeated at least weekly. If at any point results indicate placental insufficiency (a fetal scalp pH may be taken to varify this), a decision will be made to remove the fetus from the deteriorating environment, by either induction of labor or cesarean.

MEMBRANES RUPTURING IN PUBLIC

"I live in fear of my membranes rupturing in public."

You're not alone in your fear. The idea of the "bag of waters" rupturing on a bus or in a crowded department store is as mortifying to most pregnant women as that of losing bladder control in public. One woman reportedly became so obsessed with her worry that she carried a jar of pickles in her handbag, ready to be dropped at the first telltale trickle of amniotic fluid.

But before you start rummaging through your cupboards for a jar of dills, there are two things you should know. First, the rupture of membranes before labor begins is uncommon—occurring in less than 15% of pregnancies. And once they do break, the flow of amniotic fluid is unlikely to be heavy except when you are lying down (something you aren't likely to do in public). When you are walking or sitting, the fetal head tends to block the opening of the uterus as a cork does in a wine bottle.

And second, should your membranes rupture and the amniotic fluid gush suddenly, you can be sure that those around you will not point, shake disapproving heads, or—worse—chuckle. Instead they will (as you would if you were a bystander) either offer you assistance or discreetly ignore you. Keep in mind, after all, that no one is likely to overlook the fact that you're pregnant or to mistake amniotic fluid for anything else.

Wearing a panty liner in the last weeks may give you a sense of security, as well as keeping you fresher as leukorrhea increases.

BREASTFEEDING

"My breasts are very small and my nipples are flat. Will I be able to breastfeed?"

As far as hungry babies are concerned, satisfaction comes in all kinds of packages. Breasts don't have to be centerfold-shaped or -sized, and they can come equipped with almost any kind of nipple—small and flat, large and pointy, even inverted. All combinations of breasts and nipples have the capacity to produce and dispense milk—the quantity or quality of which is not in the least dependent on outward appearance. Unfortunately, because so

many fallacies and old wives' tales exist about what kinds of breasts can and cannot satisfy a baby, many women are unnecessarily discouraged from breastfeeding.

Inverted nipples that don't become erect with sexual stimulation generally need some special priming prior to childbirth. The use of a breast shield is the best way to "pull out" an inverted nipple. Worn for as many hours as possible during the day in the last few months of pregnancy, the mild suction of the shield gently draws the nipple out. A manual breast pump used several times a day can also help to correct inverted nipples.

Some experts recommend that all women who expect to nurse try to prepare their breasts in advance by expressing a small amount of colostrum from the nipples daily from the eighth month on (though not every woman will be able to do this) and by pulling, twisting, or rolling the nipples between forefinger and thumb to toughen them. Others say that nursing comes naturally to nipples, without special preparation.

"My mother says she had milk leaking from her breasts by this time; I don't. Does this mean I won't have any milk?"

The thin, yellowish discharge that some pregnant women can express, or may notice leaking from their breasts, is not milk. It is a premilk fluid called colostrum. Richer in protein and lower in fat and milk sugar than the breast milk that comes in two or three days after delivery, it contains antibodies that may be important in protecting the baby against disease.

Many women, however, don't have any noticeable colostrum until after delivery. Even then, they may not be aware of it. This in no way predicts difficulty in breastfeeding.

MOTHERING

"Now that the baby's arrival is so close, I'm beginning to worry about taking care of it. I've never even held a newborn before."

Women are not born mothers, instinctively knowing how to rock a crying baby to sleep, change a diaper, or give a bath. Motherhood—or parenthood, for that matter—is a learned art, one that requires plenty of practice to make perfect (or even near-perfect). A hundred years ago, that practice commonly took place at an early age, when female children learned to care for younger siblings—much as they learned to bake bread and mend socks.

Today, a high percentage of fully grown women have never kneaded bread dough, taken a needle to a worn sock, or held—let alone taken care of—an infant. Their training for motherhood comes on the job, with some reading on the side. Which means that for the first week or two, the baby may do more crying than sleeping, the diapers may leak, and many a tear may be shed over the "no-more-tears" lather. Slowly but surely, however, the new mother begins to feel like an old pro. Her trepidation turns to assurance. The baby she was afraid to hold (won't it break?) is now cradled casually in her left arm while her right sets the table or pushes the vacuum cleaner. Dispensing vitamin drops, giving baths, slipping squirming arms and legs into sleepers, have ceased to be dreaded ordeals. They, like all the daily tasks of parenting, have become second nature. She's a mother, and—difficult though it may be to imagine—you will be one, too.

WHAT IT'S IMPORTANT TO KNOW: PRELABOR, FALSE LABOR, REAL LABOR

It always seems so simple on TV. Somewhere around 3 A.M., the pregnant woman sits up in bed, puts a knowing hand on her belly, and reaches over to rouse her sleeping husband with a calm, almost serene, "It's time, honey."

But how, we wonder, does this woman know it's time? How does she recognize labor with such cool, clinical confidence when she's never *been* in labor before? What makes her so sure she's not going to get to the hospital, be examined by the resident, and be found to be uneffaced, undilated, and nowhere near her time? That she won't be sent home—amidst snickers from the night shift—just as pregnant as when she arrived?

On our side of the TV, we're more likely to awaken at 3 A.M. with complete uncertainty. Are these really labor pains, or just some more Braxton Hicks? Should I turn on the light and start timing? Should I bother to wake my husband? Do I call the doctor in the middle of the night to report what might really be false labor? If I do, and it isn't time, will I turn out to be the pregnant woman who cried "labor" once too often, and will anybody take me seriously when it's for real? Or will I be the only woman in my class not to recognize labor? Will I leave for the hospital too late, maybe giving birth in a taxi cab? The questions multiply faster than the contractions.

The fact is that most women, worry though they might, *don't* end up misjudging the onset of their labor. The vast majority, thanks to instinct, luck, or no-doubt-about-it killer contractions, show up at the hospital neither too early nor too late, but at just about the right time. Still, there's no reason to leave your deliberations up to chance. Becoming completely familiar with the signs of prelabor, false labor, and real labor will help to allay the concerns and clear up the confusion.

No one knows exactly what triggers labor. Several theories have been suggested—none of which, in isolation, holds up under scientific scrutiny. Probably a combination of fetal, placental, and maternal factors are responsible for setting into motion the events of labor.

PRELABOR SYMPTOMS

The process of prelabor can precede real labor by a full month or more—or by only an hour or so. Prelabor is characterized by the beginning of cervical effacement and dilatation, which only your practitioner can confirm, as well as by a wide variety of related signs which you may notice yourself:

Lightening and Engagement. Usually somewhere between two and four weeks before labor begins in first-time mothers, the fetus begins to descend into the pelvis. This milestone is rarely reached in second or later births until labor has actually commenced.

Increasing Pressure Sensations in the Pelvis and Rectum. Crampiness and groin pain are particularly common in second and later pregnancies. Persistent low backache may also be present.

Loss of Weight or Cessation in Weight Gain. As labor approaches, some women lose up to 2 or 3 pounds; in general, weight gain slows in the ninth month.

Changes in Energy Levels. Some ninth-monthers find that they are increasingly fatigued. Others experience energy spurts. An uncontrollable urge to scrub floors and wash woodwork has been related to the "nesting instinct"—mom preparing the nest.

Changes in Vaginal Discharge. You may find that your discharge increases and thickens.

Loss of Mucous Plug. As the cervix begins to thin and dilate, the "cork" of mucus that seals the opening of the uterus becomes dislodged. This can happen a week or two before the first real contractions, or just as labor begins.

Pink, or Bloody, Show. As the cervix effaces and dilates, capillaries frequently rupture, tinting the mucus pink or streaking it with blood. This "show" usually means labor will start within 24 hours—but it could be as much as several days away.

Intensification of Braxton Hicks Contractions. These practice contractions may become more frequent and stronger, even painful.

Diarrhea. Some women experience loose bowel movements just prior to the onset of labor.

FALSE LABOR SYMPTOMS

Real labor probably has not begun if:

❖ Contractions are not regular and don't increase in frequency or severity.

❖ Pain is in the lower abdomen rather than the lower back.

❖ Contractions subside if you walk around or change your position.

❖ The uterus relaxes and contractions ease if you have an alcoholic drink.

❖ Show, if any, is brownish.[2] (This is usually a result of an internal exam or intercourse within the past 48 hours.)

❖ Fetal movements intensify briefly with contractions.

REAL LABOR SYMPTOMS

When contractions of prelabor are replaced by stronger, more painful, and more frequent ones, the question arises: "Is this the real thing or false labor?" It is probably real if:

❖ The contractions intensify, rather than ease up, with activity and aren't relieved by a change in position or by an alcoholic drink.

❖ Pain begins in the lower back and spreads to the lower abdomen; it may also radiate to the legs. Contractions may feel like a gastrointestinal upset and be accompanied by diarrhea.

❖ Contractions become progressively more frequent and painful, and generally (but not always) more regular. (This progression isn't absolute—not every contraction is more painful or longer than the previous one, but their general intensity does build up as real labor progresses. Nor does frequency always increase in regular, perfectly even intervals—but it does increase.)

❖ Show is present and pinkish or blood-streaked.

❖ Membranes rupture. In 15% of labors the membranes rupture—either as a gush of waters or a trickle—before labor begins.

---

2. Bright red blood requires immediate consultation with your practitioner.

What to Take to the Hospital

For the Labor or Birthing Room

❖ This book.

❖ A watch or clock with a second hand for timing contractions.

❖ A radio or a cassette player equipped with your favorite tapes, if music soothes and relaxes you.

❖ A camera, tape recorder, and/or video equipment, if you don't trust your memory to capture the moment completely (and if the hospital rules allow media coverage of births).

❖ Powder, lotions, or anything else you'd like to be massaged with.

❖ A small paper bag, to breathe into in case you begin to hyperventilate from breathing exercises.

❖ A tennis ball or plastic rolling pin, for firm counter-massage should backache be a problem.

❖ Sugarless lollipops to keep your mouth moist (though sugar-full candies are usually recommended, they will only make you thirstier and more dehydrated).

❖ Heavy socks, in case your feet become cold.

❖ A hairbrush, if having someone brush your hair is comforting.

❖ A washcloth for sponging down with, though the hospital may provide this (don't bring a white one which might accidentally end up in the hospital laundry).

❖ A sandwich or other snack for Dad (a coach who faints from hunger can't be effective).

❖ A bottle of champagne, wrapped and labeled with your name, for celebrating (your coach can ask the nurse to keep it in the fridge), though depending on the hour you deliver, you may be more in the mood for an orange juice toast.

For the Hospital Room

❖ A robe and/or nightgowns, if you'd rather wear your own than the hospital's. Be forewarned, however, that though pretty nightgowns can boost your spirits, they may get bled on and permanently stained. Ditto bathrobes. A good compromise might be a favorite bedjacket to wear over the hospital gown.

❖ Perfume, powder, or whatever else makes you feel fresh.

❖ Toiletries, including shampoo, toothbrush, toothpaste, lotion (your skin may be dry from a loss of fluids), a bar of soap in a carrying case, deodorant, hairbrush, hand mirror, makeup, and any other essentials of beauty and hygiene.

❖ Sanitary napkins, preferably the adhesive variety, though pads and a belt are usually provided by the hospital.

❖ Playing cards, books (including what-to-name-your-baby books if you're leaving that decision for the last minute), and other distractions.

❖ Packs of raisins, nuts, whole-wheat crackers, and other healthy snacks to keep you healthy and regular in spite of a hospital diet.

❖ A going-home outfit for you, keeping in mind that you'll still be sporting a sizable abdomen.

❖ A going-home outfit for baby—a kimono or stretch suit, T-shirt, booties, a receiving blanket, and a heavy bunting or blanket if it's cold; diapers will probably be provided by the hospital, but take along an extra, just in case.

WHEN TO CALL THE DOCTOR

When in doubt, call. Even if you've checked and re-checked the above lists, you may still be unsure of whether you're really in labor. Don't wait to find out for sure—unless you'd prefer a home birth. Call your practitioner. He or she will probably be able to tell from the sound of your voice, as you talk through a contraction, whether it's the real thing. (But only if you don't try to cover up the pain in the name of stoicism or good manners.) Fear of being embarrassed if it doesn't turn out to be labor shouldn't prevent your calling your practitioner. If it does turn out to be a false alarm, nobody's going to snicker. You wouldn't be the first patient to misjudge her labor signs—and you certainly won't be the last.

❖ Call anytime, night or day, if all signs indicate that you're ready to go to the hospital. Don't let an overdeveloped sense of guilt or politeness keep you from waking your practitioner up in the middle of the night, or disturbing his or her weekend at home. People who deliver babies for a living don't expect to work a 9-to-5 shift.

❖ Your practitioner has probably specified that you should call when your contractions have reached a particular frequency—say, 5, 8, or 10 minutes apart. Call when at least some of your contractions are that frequent. Don't wait for perfectly even intervals; they may never come.

❖ Your practitioner has probably also instructed you about when to call if your membranes rupture, or if you think they have ruptured, but labor has not begun. Some say: "If they break at 3 A.M., wait until morning." Others say to call immediately. Follow your practitioner's instructions, unless: your due date is still several weeks away; you know your baby is small or is not engaged in the pelvis; or the amniotic fluid is not clear, but is stained greenish brown. In these cases, call immediately since there is a risk of cord prolapse.

❖ Don't assume that if you're not sure it's real labor, it necessarily isn't. Err on the side of caution and call your practitioner.

14
Labor and Delivery

WHAT YOU MAY BE CONCERNED ABOUT

BLOODY SHOW

"I have a pink mucous discharge. Does it mean labor's about to start?"

Don't send your husband out for the cigars yet. Passage of "bloody show," a mucous discharge tinged pink or brown with blood, is a sign that your cervix is dilating and that the process that leads to delivery is beginning. But it's a process with an erratic timetable that will keep you in suspense until the first contractions. Labor could be one, two, or even three weeks away, with your cervix continuing to dilate gradually over that time. Or it could be less than an hour away.

If your discharge should suddenly become red or bloody, contact your practitioner immediately. Frank bleeding could indicate a premature separation of the placenta, which requires you to get prompt medical attention.

RUPTURE OF MEMBRANES

"I woke up in the middle of the night with a wet bed. Did I lose control of my bladder, or did my membranes rupture?"

A sniff of your sheets will probably clue you in. If the wet spot smells sort of sweet and not like ammonia, it's likely to be amniotic fluid. Another clue: You'll probably still be leaking the pale, straw-colored amniotic fluid (which won't run dry because it continues to be produced until delivery, replacing itself every three hours). If you stand up or sit down, however, the baby's head may act like a cork and slow down the leak.

Some women never experience a gushing of amniotic fluid when their membranes rupture—partly because of the cork effect, partly because there are no contractions to force the fluid out. All they notice is a constant trickle. (A leak that starts and then stops, particularly several weeks before term, probably indicates a tear in the membranes that healed itself.)

"My water just broke, but I haven't had any contractions. When is labor going to start, and what should I do in the meantime?"

If you're like the majority of pregnant women whose membranes rupture prior to labor, your labor will begin within the next 12 hours. If you're not, you'll probably be feeling the first contractions within 24 hours. About 1 in 10 women take even longer to go into labor. Because of the increasing risk of infection to baby and/or mother through the ruptured amniotic sac, most physicians will induce labor after 24 hours, though a few wait as little as 6 hours. When the membranes rupture before the 34th week, or if there is another reason to suspect fetal immaturity, some physicians recommend a carefully controlled delay of 48 to 72 hours, during which drugs are administered to accelerate the maturation of the fetal lungs. This approach, however, is still a matter of controversy.

If you think your membranes have ruptured, call your doctor or nurse-midwife. In the meantime, keep the vaginal area as clean as possible to avoid infection. Don't take a bath or have sexual relations; use sanitary napkins to absorb the flow of amniotic fluid; don't try to do your own internal exam; and wipe front to back at the toilet.

Rarely, in premature rupture of the membranes (more often in breech and premature births), when the presenting part is not engaged in the pelvis, the umbilical cord becomes "prolapsed"—swept into the neck of the uterus (the cervix) or even the vagina, with the gush of amniotic fluid. Because pressure on the cord can cut off the baby's oxygen supply, prolapse requires immediate medical attention. If a loop of cord appears at your vagina, get onto your hands and knees; this will reduce the pressure on the cord. If the cord still protrudes in this position, support it gently (do not compress it) with warm, wet gauze pads or a clean cloth. Have someone rush you to the hospital, or call an ambulance.

DARKENED AMNIOTIC FLUID (MECONIUM STAINING)

"My membranes ruptured, and the fluid is greenish-brown. What does this mean?"

Your amniotic fluid is stained with meconium, a foul-smelling, greenish-brown substance that comes from your baby's digestive tract. Ordinarily, meconium is passed after birth as the baby's first stool. But sometimes—particularly when there is some kind of fetal stress, and very often when the baby is postmature—it is passed prior to birth into the amniotic fluid.

Meconium staining alone is not a sure sign of fetal distress, but because it hints at the possibility, notify your practitioner immediately.

INDUCTION OF LABOR

"My doctor wants to induce labor. I'm upset because I had wanted a natural delivery."

Though some doctors 20 years ago believed it was safe to routinely induce labor in their patients so that birth would come at a convenient time, doctors today rarely induce without good cause. This has come about partly because the FDA has withdrawn approval of elective (not absolutely necessary) use of the drug oxytocin, with which labor is induced, and partly for fear of malpractice suits should something go wrong. But it has come about mostly because they recognize that, when possible, it's best to let nature take its time taking its course.

In certain circumstances, however, when labor hasn't begun on its own, or is weak or erratic, nature needs a little prodding. For example, when there is:

❖ Fetal distress—and there is time for a vaginal delivery.

❖ Premature rupture of membranes—to reduce the risk of getting an infection if labor has not begun spontaneously within 24 hours. (Some practitioners will wait longer, some not as long; some will suggest first trying to stimulate contractions "naturally" with mineral oil and/or nipple stimulation, under medical supervision in the hospital. See below.)

❖ Postmaturity—when the pregnancy has gone two or more weeks past a due date that is considered accurate, or when a stress or non-stress test shows that the placenta is no longer functioning optimally because of age.

❖ Arrested or inefficient labor—which could put both mother and child in jeopardy if delivery is delayed indefinitely.

❖ Maternal diabetes. Induced delivery of babies of diabetic mothers before the due date is often indicated because their placentas tend to deteriorate prematurely, and because, if carried to term, the babies are often oversized.

❖ Other maternal illness—such as high blood pressure or kidney disease, in which carrying a baby to term may present increased hazard.

❖ Severe Rh disease—when the fetus may not survive unless delivered early.

Though artificial rupture of the membranes (if they haven't already ruptured naturally) is sometimes indicated to try to bring on labor, oxytocin is much more commonly used for uterine stimulation.

Oxytocin is a hormone produced naturally by the maternal pituitary gland throughout pregnancy. As pregnancy progresses, the uterus becomes more and more sensitive to the hormone, although it isn't clear whether it plays a significant role in the triggering of labor. It is known that the hormone may be released by the pregnant woman when her nipples are stimulated, causing the uterus to contract. Some practitioners may, in fact, advise nipple self-stimulation to bring on, or speed up, contractions before resorting to less natural methods. The artificial administration of oxytocin, however, is a more reliable method of induction. When conditions are ripe, it is capable of initiating labor that mimics the naturally occurring variety, with contractions that may be a little more regular, and slightly different in quality.

The hormone (trade name Pitocin) can be administered intramuscularly (injected into a muscle), sublingually (placed under the tongue), or intranasally (sniffed)—but the intravenous (IV) oxytocin drip, utilizing an infusion pump, is the safest and easiest route to control. The IV is introduced via a needle in the arm or the back of the hand, and connected by tubing to two bottles of neutral (unmedicated) IV solution. The pump releases oxytocin into the primary bottle, one drop at a time. (The second bottle remains on standby.) Usually the induction begins slowly with very little oxytocin being released, and the reaction of the uterus and the fetus are carefully monitored. (A doctor or nurse must be in attendance at all times during induction.) The rate of infusion is increased gradually until effective contractions are established. Should the woman's uterus prove extremely sensitive to the drug, and be overstimulated into either too long or too powerful contractions, this method allows the infusion to be immediately reduced or halted entirely, with the IV being switched to the standby bottle.

If, after six to eight hours of oxytocin administration, labor hasn't begun or progressed, the procedure will probably be terminated in favor of an alternative. Treatment may also be terminated if contractions are well established and continue on their own.

Induction of labor is not considered appropriate when there is serious fetal distress; if there is any doubt the fetus can fit through the mother's pelvis; when a woman is judged to be in false labor; and, generally, in women who have had five or more previous births.

Some women find the sudden onset of hard labor that usually occurs with induction unpleasant; some even feel cheated by the short duration of their laboring experience. Others enjoy such down-to-business births. With their coaches at their side, they go through their induced labors otherwise naturally, using all the breathing exercises and other coping mechanisms learned in childbirth classes. And so can anyone who keeps in mind that labor (no matter how it started) is labor. There's no reason why a labor that doesn't begin "naturally" can't turn out to be a fully satisfying, memorable birth experience.

SHORT LABOR

"Can a short labor actually be harmful to the baby?"

Short labor isn't always as short as it seems. Often the expectant mother has been having painless contractions for hours, days, even weeks, which have been dilating her cervix gradually. By the time she feels the first contraction, she is often well into the transition stage of labor (see the stages of childbirth, beginning on page 256). This kind of slow-buildup, quick-resolution labor certainly places no extra strain on the fetus, and may be even less stressful than the average 12-hour labor.

Occasionally a cervix dilates very rapidly, accomplishing in a matter of minutes what most cervixes (particularly those of first-time mothers) take hours to do. But even with this abrupt, or precipitous, labor (one that takes three hours or less from start to finish), there is rarely any threat to the baby. There is no evidence to support the notion that an infant must go through a minimum amount of labor in order to arrive in good condition.

CALLING YOUR PRACTITIONER DURING LABOR

"I just started getting contractions and they're coming every three or four minutes. I feel silly calling the doctor, who said we should spend the first several hours of labor at home."

Most first-time mothers-to-be (whose labors often begin slowly, with a gradual buildup of contractions) *can* safely count on spending the first several hours at home. But if your contractions start off strong—lasting at least 45 seconds and coming more often than every five minutes—your first several hours of labor may very well be your last. Chances are that much of the first stage of labor has passed painlessly, and that your cervix has dilated significantly during that time. This means that not calling your doctor—and chancing a dramatic dash to the hospital at the last minute—would be considerably sillier than picking up the phone now.

Before you do, however, it is best to have timed several consecutive contractions. Be clear and specific about their frequency, duration, and strength when you report them. Don't try to minimize your discomfort when you describe it by trying to maintain a calm voice. (Your practitioner is used to judging the stage of labor in part by the sound of a woman's voice as she talks through a contraction.)

If you feel you're ready, but your practitioner doesn't seem to think so, don't take "wait" for an answer. Ask if you can go to the hospital and have your progress checked. (See Calling the Doctor, in Prelabor, False Labor, Real Labor, page 233.) You can take your suitcase along "just in case," but be ready to turn around and go home if you've only just begun to dilate.

BACK LABOR

"The pain in my back since my labor began is so bad I don't see how I'll be able to make it through delivery."

Technically, "back labor" occurs when the fetus is in a posterior (or occipitoposterior) position, with the back of its head pressing against the mother's sacrum—the rear boundary of the pelvis. It's possible, however, to experience back labor when the baby is not in this position, or after the baby has turned from a posterior to an anterior position—possibly because the area has become a focus of tension.

When you're having that kind of pain—which often doesn't let up between contractions and becomes excruciating during them—the cause is not really a crucial consideration. How to relieve it, even slightly, is. There are several measures that may help; all are at least worth trying:

❖ Stay off your back. Try to take the pressure off by changing your position—walk around (though this may not be humanly possible once contractions are coming fast and furiously), crouch or squat, get down on all fours, or do whatever is most comfortable and least painful for you. If you feel you can't move, and would prefer to be lying down, do it on your side, with your back well rounded.

❖ Your coach can apply heat (a hot water bottle wrapped in a towel, warm compresses, a heating pad) or cold (ice packs, cold compresses)—whichever soothes best.

❖ Apply counterpressure. Have your coach experiment with different ways of applying pressure to the area of greatest pain, or to adjacent areas, to find one or more that seem to help. He can try his knuckles, or the heel of one hand reinforced by pressure from the other hand on top of it, using direct pressure or a firm circular motion. Pressure can be applied while you are sitting or, to allow greater force, while you are lying on your side. The relief you may get from really intense counterpressure will be well worth any black-and-blue marks you find the morning after.

❖ Use acupressure. This is probably the oldest form of pain relief— and you don't have to be Chinese to try it. In the case of back labor, it involves applying strong finger pressure just below the center of the ball of the foot.

❖ Aggressively massage the area. This may spell relief either in place of counterpressure or alternated with it. A rolling pin or a tennis ball can be used for especially firm massage (although it will probably leave you aching afterwards). Oil or powder can be rubbed on periodically to avoid irritation.

IRREGULAR CONTRACTIONS

"In class we were told not to go to the hospital until the contractions were regular and five minutes apart. Mine are less than five minutes apart, but they aren't at all regular. I don't know what to do."

No two women have exactly the same fingerprints. And no two women have exactly the same labors. The labor described in books, in childbirth education classes, or by your practitioner is what is typical— close to what many women can expect. But far from every labor is

Emergency Home (or Office) Delivery

1. Call 911 (or your local emergency number) for the emergency squad; ask them to call your doctor or nurse-midwife.

2. The mother should start panting to keep from bearing down.

3. During all the preparations and during the delivery, comfort and reassure the mother.

4. If there's time, wash the vaginal area and your hands with detergent or soap and water.

5. If there's no time to get to a bed or table, place newspapers or clean towels or folded clothing under the buttocks, to give some height for delivering the baby's shoulders.

6. If there is time, place the woman onto the bed (or a desk or a table) sideways, with her buttocks slightly hanging off, her hands under her thighs to keep them elevated. A couple of chairs can serve as supports for her feet.

7. Protect delivery surfaces, if possible, with shower curtains, newspapers, plastic tablecloths, towels, and so on. A dish pan or basin can be used to catch the amniotic fluid and blood.

8. As the top of the baby's head begins to appear, instruct the mother to pant or blow (not push), and apply gentle counterpressure to keep the head from popping out suddenly. Let the head emerge gradually—*never* pull it out. If there is a loop of the cord around the baby's neck, hook a finger under it and gently work it over the baby's head.

9. When the head has been delivered, gently stroke the nose downward, the neck and under the chin upward, to help expel mucus and amniotic fluid.

10. Now take the head gently in two hands and press it very slightly downward, asking the mother to push at the same time, to deliver the frontward shoulder. As the upper arm appears, lift the head carefully, watching for the rearward shoulder to deliver.

11. Quickly wrap the baby in blankets, towels, or anything else that is available (preferably something clean; something recently ironed is relatively sterile). Place it on the mother's abdomen, or if the cord is long enough (don't tug at it), at her breast.

12. Don't try to pull the placenta out. But if it arrives on its own before the ambulance comes, wrap it in towels or newspaper, and keep it elevated above the level of the baby, if possible. Don't try to cut the cord.

13. Keep both mother and baby warm and comfortable until help arrives.

true-to-textbook, with contractions regularly spaced and predictably progressive.

If you are having strong, long, frequent (five minutes apart or less) contractions, even if they vary considerably in length and time elapsed between them, do not wait for them to become "regular" before calling your practitioner or heading for the hospital—no matter what you've heard or read. It's possible that your contractions are about as regular as they are going to get, and that you are well into the "active" phase of your labor. Waste no time in calling your practitioner and getting to the hospital; she who hesitates in a case like this could end up with an unscheduled home birth.

NOT GETTING TO THE HOSPITAL IN TIME

"I'm afraid that I won't get to the hospital in time."

Fortunately, most surprise deliveries take place in the movies and on television. In real life, deliveries rarely occur without ample warning. But once in a great while, a woman who has had no labor pains, or just erratic ones, suddenly feels an overwhelming urge to bear down; often she mistakes it for a need to go to the bathroom. If it happens to you, don't panic. Even if you don't know the first thing about delivering a baby, your lack of experience won't stop the baby from arriving. It is a good idea, however, for you and your husband to be familiar with a few basics (see boxes).

ENEMAS

"I've heard that enemas early in labor aren't really necessary, and that they interfere with natural birth."

Enemas were, until fairly recently, not a matter of choice. They were administered routinely in early labor, as part of the hospital admissions procedure. The theory was, and still is in many hospitals, that emptying the bowels before delivery prevents compression of the birth canal by hard fecal matter in

---

Emergency Delivery If You're Alone

1. Call 911 (or your local emergency number) for the emergency squad. Ask them to call your practitioner.

2. Find a neighbor or someone to help, if possible.

3. Start panting to keep from bearing down.

4. Wash your hands and the perineal area, if you can.

5. Spread some clean towels, newspapers, or sheets on a bed, sofa, or the floor, and lie down to await help.

6. If the baby starts to arrive before help does, gently ease it out by pushing each time you feel the urge, catching it with your hands.

7. Proceed with steps 9 to 13 on previous page, as best you can.

Emergency Delivery En Route to the Hospital

1. If you're in your own car and delivery is imminent, pull over. If you have a CB, call for help. If not, put your hazard warning lights or signal on. If someone stops to help, ask them to get to a phone and call 911. If you're in a cab, ask the driver to radio for help.

2. If possible, help the mother into the back of the car. Place a coat, jacket, or blanket under her. Then proceed as on page 244. As soon as delivery is completed, continue to the nearest hospital in a hurry.

---

the rectum (which would hinder the baby's descent) and contamination of the sterile birthing setup by involuntary evacuation during the pushing stage of labor. In addition, it spares the laboring woman "embarrassment" and lessens her inhibitions about pushing.

These theories are less in favor today. It is recognized that compression of the birth canal is not likely to be a problem if a woman has had a bowel movement in the past 24 hours, or if no hard fecal mass is felt in her rectum on internal examination. And the use during delivery of disposable sterile gauze pads to whisk away fecal matter virtually eliminates the threat of fecal contamination to mother and baby. (According to some studies, the possibility of neonatal infection from bowel organisms is highly remote to begin with.) For these reasons, some hospitals have abandoned the routine enema; others are certain to follow.

If your hospital isn't among these and the prospect of an enema is one you don't relish, discuss the question with your practitioner in advance of labor. If you feel strongly that you don't want an enema, he or she may agree to forgo it. (But be sure that the order is relayed to hospital staff.) On the other hand, if you're more uncomfortable with the prospect of moving your bowels on the delivery table (though an enema doesn't guarantee you won't), don't let anyone bully you into accepting the idea that enemas are unnatural and unnecessary.

You may be more comfortable taking care of the enema yourself at home, while you're in early labor. But whether it's given at home or in the hospital, a warm water enema may also provide the added benefit of boosting sluggish contractions and giving labor a little push.

The entire issue may be academic, however, if your labor begins, as many do, with loose or frequent bowel movements which effectively empty the colon; or if you arrive at the hospital in active labor, with contractions so close together that it's barely possible for hospital personnel to get you into a gown, much less give you an enema.

SHAVING THE PUBIC AREA

"The idea of having my pubic hair shaved is unpleasant to me. Is it obligatory?"

Though shaving of the pubic area is still a routine "prepping" procedure in some hospitals, it is being utilized less and less. It is most often done simply because it's always been done, not because it is necessary. It was once believed that pubic hair harbored bacteria which would infect the baby as it passed through the vaginal outlet. But since the entire area around the vagina is swabbed with an antiseptic solution prior to delivery, infection of this type is not likely. And in fact, some studies have shown a *higher* rate of infection among women who are shaved prior to delivery than those who aren't, probably because the small—sometimes microscopic—nicks which even very careful shaving can produce may serve as excellent breeding grounds for bacteria. From the woman's point of view, the humiliation of the shaving itself and the postpartum burning and itching as the hair grows back are additional reasons to object to the procedure.

Some doctors feel that shaving facilitates the episiotomy and repair, by providing a clearer area in which to work. Yet this, too, is more likely a matter of habit than conviction. An increasing number of physicians perform and repair episiotomies without shaving—either clipping the hair with scissors or pushing it back as they work.

Whether or not you will be shaved may depend on the flexibility of your practitioner and the hospital you are delivering at. Increasingly, it is one of the decisions of childbirth that you can, at the very least, be instrumental in making. Don't wait until you arrive at the hospital, however, to make your feelings about shaving known. Discuss them in advance of labor with your practitioner.

If your practitioner or the hospital insists on your being shaved, ask that they not shave any more than is absolutely necessary. A "mini-prep," which shaves only the hair in the area of any possible incision or tear, is usually sufficient. An alternative to being shaved at the hospital, which you may also discuss with your practitioner, is to have your mate shave or clip you at home.

ROUTINE IVs

"When we had our visit to the hospital, I saw a woman being wheeled from the delivery room with an IV attached. Is that necessary with a normal labor and delivery?"

It's difficult to associate an IV (intravenous setup), which we're used to seeing attached to the arms of mutilated GIs on reruns of *M*A*S*H,* with normal childbirth. Yet in many American hospitals, it is routine to set up an IV containing a simple solution of nutrients and fluid for a woman in labor. This is done partly to be certain that the woman does not become dehydrated from lack of fluids or weak from lack of food during labor, partly to allow ready access for medication should the need arise (it's injected right into the IV bottle or line, instead of into the patient). In these instances, the IV is precautionary.

Some doctors and midwives, on the other hand, prefer to wait until there is a clear need for the IV—for instance, because the labor is lengthy and the laboring woman is weakening. Ask your practitioner in advance what his or her policy is. If you strongly object to a routine IV, say so. It may be possible to hold off until the need for one arises.

If, however, it's your practitioner's policy to give IVs routinely, or if you end up needing one, don't despair. The IV is only slightly uncomfortable as it's inserted and thereafter should barely be noticed. When it's hung on a movable stand, you can take it with you to the bathroom or on a brief constitutional.

Though you can't always make the decision about whether or not you should have an IV, you do have a right to know what the IV is pumping into your veins. Ask the nurse or doctor who inserts it. Or have your labor partner check the label on the bottle. Occasionally medication you may not want is ordered without your being consulted. If so, ask to talk to your practitioner as soon as possible.

FETAL MONITORING

"My doctor believes in fetal monitoring at all births. I've heard that monitoring can lead to unnecessary cesareans and also makes labor more uncomfortable."

For someone who's spent the first nine months of his or her life swimming peacefully in a warm and comforting amniotic bath, the trip through the narrow confines of the maternal pelvis will be no joy ride.

Your baby will be squeezed, molded, compressed, and pushed with every contraction.

It is because there is an element of risk in this stressful journey (and not to promote maternal discomfort or unnecessary cesareans) that fetal monitors have come into such common use. In some hospitals, all labor and delivery patients are electronically monitored. In virtually every hospital, at least half of the patients—particularly those in high-risk categories, who have meconium staining of the amniotic fluid, who are receiving oxytocin, or who are having a difficult labor—are monitored electronically.

A fetal monitor gauges the baby's response, via its heart rate, to the contractions of the uterus. The reader of the monitor printout may be able to pick up signs of fetal stress and distress through variations from the normal reactions to labor. Sometimes an alarm is preset to go off if such variations occur. Fetal monitoring can be external or internal:

External Monitoring. In this type of monitoring, used most frequently, two devices are strapped to the abdomen. One, an ultrasound transducer, picks up the fetal heartbeat. The other, a pressure-sensitive gauge, measures the intensity and duration of uterine contractions. Both are connected to a monitor which displays or prints out the readings. This doesn't mean the laboring woman must be confined to bed, hooked up to a machine, like Frankenstein's monster, for hours on end. In most cases, monitoring will be required only intermittently, and you will be able to walk around between readings.

During the second (pushing) stage of labor, when contractions may come so fast and furiously that some women aren't sure when to push and when to hold back, the monitor may accurately signal the beginning of each contraction, so that pushing can be most effective. Or the use of the monitor may be all but abandoned during this stage, so as not to interfere with the mother's concentration. In this case, the fetal heart rate will be checked periodically.

Internal Monitoring. When more accurate results are required—often when fetal distress is suspected—an internal monitor may be used. Since the electrode that reads the fetal heartbeat is clipped, or otherwise attached, to its scalp through the cervix, internal monitoring is possible only once the cervix is dilated to at least 1 or 2 centimeters and the membranes have ruptured. Contractions can be measured either with the pressure gauge strapped to the maternal abdomen or with a fluid-filled catheter (tube) inserted into the uterus. Because an internal monitor can't be periodically disconnected and reconnected, mobility is somewhat limited—but changes in position are possible.

Sometimes internal monitoring employs telemetry, which reads and transmits vital signs via radio waves. This technique, pioneered in the space program, allows the patient to be monitored without being confined by equipment. With telemetry, the laboring woman is totally mobile—able to strike any position

she finds comfortable, to go to the bathroom, or even to take strolls.

Like any invasive medical procedure (one that enters or intrudes upon the body), internal fetal monitoring entails some risk—mostly of infection. In some instances the fetus may later develop a rash, or occasionally an abscess, on the site where the electrode was placed, or, very rarely, may even have a permanent bald spot. It may also be possible that the insertion of the electrode causes momentary pain or discomfort to the baby. Because of the risks, though they are slight, internal fetal monitoring is best used when its benefits are significant.

If your fetal monitor signals trouble, don't panic. The technology is far from perfect and the machine often produces false readings. Sometimes it just isn't working right; sometimes it is misread. Frequently the mother's position causes an undesirable change in the fetal heart rate, because pressure on the baby's cord or her vena cava is interfering with blood flow to the fetus. A change in position often rectifies the problem. If administration of oxytocin is causing the problem, reducing the dosage or terminating the infusion completely will generally eliminate it. Oxygen to the mother may also do the trick.

If the abnormal readings continue, several possible steps can be taken. If the danger to the fetus seems great, the physician may opt for an immediate abdominal delivery. If the reading is inconclusive, there will be a speedy check for other indications of distress, such as meconium in the amniotic fluid or an abnormal fetal blood pH (taken from a scalp sample). In order to make these determinations, the membranes must be ruptured, which will probably be accomplished artificially at this point, if it hasn't already occurred spontaneously. A check of the mother's medical and obstetrical history may be made to see if the fetal heartbeat abnormalities might be related to maternal medication, infection, or chronic disease. An experienced and knowledgeable obstetrician will take all factors into account before concluding that the baby is actually in trouble. If fetal distress is diagnosed, then an immediate cesarean is usually called for. If, in the physician's judgment, the baby is not threatened by labor, vaginal delivery will be allowed to continue.

It is estimated that fetal monitoring saves thousands of babies each year whose life-threatening difficulties in the birth canal would otherwise have gone unnoticed until it was too late. Yet because electronic monitoring has led to an increase in unnecessary cesareans in some hospitals (largely through misreadings), and because some view it as just another technological intrusion into the natural birthing process, its use remains controversial.

How expectant parents respond to the monitoring depends a great deal on their own attitudes. If they come into the labor or birthing room resentful and fearful of all that isn't "natural," they will probably find the fetal monitor objectionable. If they want the best of both worlds— the natural and the scientific—they will feel reassured and more in control at seeing their baby's heartbeats registering rhythmically on the bedside monitor.

THE SIGHT OF BLOOD

"The sight of blood makes me feel faint. What if I pass out while I'm watching my delivery?"

The sight of blood makes many people feel weak-kneed. But remarkably, though they might faint while watching a film of someone else's delivery, even the most squeamish women manage to get through their own without smelling salts.

First of all, there isn't all that much blood—not much more than you see when you're menstruating (though there can be some additional bleeding with an episiotomy or a tear). Second, you won't be a spectator at your delivery—you'll be a very active participant, putting every ounce of your concentration and energy into pushing your baby those last few inches. Caught up in the excitement and anticipation, (and, let's face it, the pain and fatigue), you are very unlikely to notice, much less be unsettled by, any bleeding. Few new mothers would be able to tell you just how much blood, if any, there was at their deliveries.

If you feel strongly that you don't want to see any blood, simply avert your eyes from the mirror (if one has been provided for you) during the episiotomy and at the moment of birth. Instead, just look down past your belly for a good view of the real thing as it emerges. From this vantage point, virtually no blood will be visible.

EPISIOTOMY

"My childbirth educator says we shouldn't have episiotomies—they aren't natural. My doctor says that's ridiculous. I don't know whether to have one or not."

To have or not to have an episiotomy? That is the question that has many obstetricians shooting it out with some childbirth educators and feminists—catching pregnant women in the crossfire.

The minor surgical procedure which is the center of this heated controversy was originated in Ireland in 1742 to help facilitate difficult births, but it wasn't commonly performed until the middle part of this century. Today, the episiotomy (a surgical incision made in the perineum to enlarge the vaginal opening just before the birth of the baby's head) is performed in 80% to 90% of first births, and in about 50% of subsequent deliveries.

There are two basic types of episiotomies: the median and the mediolateral. The median incision is made directly back toward the rectum. In spite of its advantages (it provides more space per inch of incision, heals well and is easier to repair, causes less blood loss, and results in less postpartum discomfort), it is less frequently used in the United States because it has a greater risk of tearing completely through to the rectum. To avoid this tearing, most physicians prefer the medio-lateral incision, which slants toward the side, away from the rectum.

Traditional medical wisdom supports the use of episiotomy for several reasons: Its straight edges are easier to repair than a ragged tear; timed well, it can prevent injury to the muscles of the perineum and vagina; it spares the fetal head from battering against the perineum; and it can shorten the pushing stage of labor by 15 to 30 minutes— especially useful in prolonged labors, when there may be fetal distress and/or maternal exhaustion.

Opponents (including many childbirth educators, nurse-midwives, and feminists) counter that episiotomies are an unnatural, largely unnecessary, technological intrusion into the birth process. They claim that the cuts made are often more extensive than tearing would be, and that they result in excessive bleeding, immediate postpartum discomfort, painful intercourse for months to come, and possible infection. Instead, they support the use of Kegel exercises and local massage to prepare and strengthen the perineum before delivery, and massage to gradually stretch the perineum during delivery, so that birth can take place without episiotomy and, hopefully, without tearing. (Results aren't always as desired. At birthing centers, where nurse-midwives are in charge, between 15% and 25% of women do have incisions, and 25% to 30% of the others tear badly enough to need repair. Another 3% or 4% have serious lacerations extending to the rectum.)

What hard-liners (those who routinely perform episiotomies, even when they're not needed, and those who routinely refrain from performing them, even when they are needed) fail to recognize is that "to have or not to have an episiotomy" is a question that shouldn't be answered in the classroom or the office—but in the delivery or birthing room, as the baby's head crowns. It is only then that an unbiased birthing attendant can make a realistic judgment as to whether or not the perineum can stretch sufficiently to accommodate the baby's head without tearing and without jeopardizing fetal or maternal well-being by prolonging labor. The prudent physician or nurse-midwife who has some doubt will generally opt for the controlled episiotomy rather than risk an uncontrolled tear.

What decision should the expectant mother make on episiotomies? None. She can form an opinion and can discuss this opinion with her doctor or nurse-midwife so that it can be taken into account at the time of childbirth. But the decision is going to be made, and should be made, by the birthing attendant, with the speedy and safe delivery of the baby and the well-being of the mother the prime considerations.

BEING STRETCHED BY CHILDBIRTH

"The thing that frightens me most is my vagina stretching and tearing. Will I ever be the same again?"

T he vagina is a remarkably elastic organ that is composed of accordion folds that open for child-

birth. It is normally so narrow that inserting a tampon may be difficult, yet it can expand to allow the passage of a 7- or 8-pound baby without tearing. After birth, it returns to almost its original size—though some women report a slight increase in roominess. For those who were unusually small before conception, this is a plus, because intercourse becomes more pleasurable. For most others, the widening is slight, even imperceptible, and does not interfere with sexual enjoyment.

The perineum, the area between the vagina and the rectum, is also elastic, but less so than the vagina. In some women, the perineum will stretch enough without tearing to allow the birth of a baby. But in others, it will tear unless an episiotomy is performed by the birth attendant. Stretching may leave the muscles a little slacker than will a carefully timed episiotomy, one in which the perineum wasn't allowed to stretch excessively before the incision was made.

But exercising the muscles of childbirth long before you get to the delivery room may enhance elasticity and certainly will hasten their return to normal tone. Kegel exercises, which strengthen the perineal area (see page 318), should be done regularly during pregnancy and for at least six months following childbirth.

Many couples report that sex after delivery is even more satisfying than it was before, thanks to the increased muscular awareness and control a woman may develop as a result of prepared childbirth training.

In other words, you may not be the same after childbirth—you may be even better!

BEING STRAPPED TO THE DELIVERY TABLE

"The idea of being strapped to a table terrifies me. Is this really necessary?"

The prospect of being bound, hand and foot, to a delivery table is a horrible one—particularly to women who wish to participate fully in childbirth. Fortunately, though it was once routine procedure, it is virtually unheard of today. Most birthing attendants will simply ask the woman to keep her hands above her waist, out of the sterile field; if she should forget this in the middle of a particularly consuming contraction, her coach and/or the nurse is there to remind her.

Whether or not the woman's feet are up in stirrups during delivery (there's no need for this during labor), and whether her legs are strapped to the stirrups, depends on hospital policy, practitioner preference, and, sometimes, the patient's wishes.

The use of stirrups in delivery evolved for several reasons. One, they kept the woman's legs elevated and out of the way so that the doctor had adequate work space. Two, they kept her from involuntarily kicking out during a powerful contraction (possibly interfering with the delivery). Finally, they kept her feet out of the sterile field.

One reason that stirrups are used less often in many hospitals—and hardly at all in birthing rooms, where special birthing beds have taken the place of delivery tables—is that a variety of birthing positions have replaced the standard woman-on-her-back-legs-up-and-spread attitude. Another is strong opposition from women who want to retain as much dignity and control as possible during their deliveries. In addition, because woman are now in general better prepared for childbirth, they aren't as likely to thrash around in pain and fear of the unknown.

Talk to your practitioner about this issue in advance, sharing your feelings and listening to his or hers. It is very likely that your wishes will be considered and that, at the very least, a compromise can be reached.

THE USE OF FORCEPS

"I've heard all kinds of horror stories about forceps. What if my doctor wants to use them?"

It was in 1598 that British surgeon Peter Chamberlen the Elder designed the first pair of forceps, using the tong-shaped instrument to ease babies out of the birth canal when a difficult delivery might otherwise cost both mother and infant their lives. Instead of writing himself up in the latest obstetrical journal, however, Dr. Chamberlen kept his discovery a secret—privy only to four generations of Chamberlen medical men and their patients, many of them royalty. Indeed, the use of forceps might have ended forever with the career of the last Chamberlen doctor had a hidden box of instruments not been uncovered beneath a floorboard in the family's ancestral home in the mid 1800s.

To the minds of some today, the use of forceps should have died with the Chamberlens. But that's not quite fair. Before safe cesarean sections became commonplace, forceps were the only way of delivering a baby stuck in the birth canal. The occasional serious damage they caused was considered a small price to pay for the countless lives they saved. The risks of using forceps clearly outweighed the benefits.

But the picture is more complicated. The high-forceps procedure to which most of the horror stories you've heard are probably linked, in which the doctor reaches up into the pelvis to extract a stuck baby, has been almost totally abandoned in favor of cesarean deliveries. But the American College of Obstetrics and Gynecology and most physicians still see a role for mid-, low-, and outlet forceps deliveries. Such deliveries, the most recent studies show, pose no more risk to mother and baby than cesareans when carried out properly by someone experienced in their use. Many physicians will try the judicious use of forceps when a baby's head is engaged and labor has stalled before resorting to a cesarean. In countries such as Great Britain where this is routine, the rate of cesarean deliveries is, as a consequence, relatively low.

Forceps should, however, be employed only when valid indications exist (fetal distress, maternal health, prolonged labor, prolonged second stage), never electively. And all should be in readiness for a cesarean

section should a trial of forceps fail.

When forceps are used, a local anesthetic (see page 199) is administered. Then the curved, blunt blades are cradled one at a time around the crowning head, at the temples, and the baby is gently delivered.

The vacuum extractor, an alternative to outlet forceps in which the infant is suctioned out of the birth canal via a metal or plastic cup (less traumatic) applied to the head, is popular in Europe but is used less frequently in the U.S.

If you have any concerns about the use of forceps or vacuum extraction during your delivery, discuss them with your practitioner now, before you go into labor. He or she should be able to allay your fears.

THE BABY'S CONDITION

"The doctor said the baby is okay, but her Apgar score was only 7. Is she really all right?"

Your doctor is right. Any Apgar score of 7 or over indicates the baby is in good condition. A score of under 4 indicates severe distress— but even most of these babies turn out to be normal and healthy.

The Apgar test was developed by the late Dr. Virginia Apgar, a renowned pediatrician, to enable medical personnel to quickly evaluate the condition of a newborn. At 60 seconds after birth, a nurse or doctor (usually not the person who assisted at the delivery) checks the infant's *A*ppearance (color), *P*ulse (heartbeat), *G*rimace (reflex), *A*ctivity (muscle tone), and *R*espiration.

APGAR TABLE

SIGN	POINTS		
	0	1	2
Appearance (color)*	Pale or blue	Body pink, extremeties blue	Pink
Pulse (heartbeat)	Not detectible	Below 100	Over 100
Grimace (reflex irritability)	No response to stimulation	Grimace	Lusty cry
Activity (muscle tone)	Flaccid (no or weak activity)	Some movement of extremities	A lot of activity
Respiration (breathing)	None	Slow, irregular	Good (crying)

*In non-white children, color of mucous membranes of mouth, of the whites of the eyes, of lips, palms, hands, and soles of feet will be examined.

Hence the acronym, APGAR. (See Apgar Table, above.) Those who score between 4 and 6 often need resuscitation—which generally includes suctioning their airways and administering oxygen. Those who score under 4 require more dramatic lifesaving techniques.

The Apgar test is administered once again at five minutes after birth. If the score is 7 or better at this point, the outlook for the infant is very good. Though it has long been believed that a low score at five minutes often indicates future neurological trouble, more recent studies show little correlation between a low Apgar and later problems.

WHAT IT'S IMPORTANT TO KNOW:
THE STAGES OF CHILDBIRTH

Few pregnancies seem as though they could have been lifted right from the pages of an obstetrical manual—with morning sickness that vanishes at the end of the first trimester, first fetal movements felt at precisely 20 weeks, and lightening that occurs exactly two weeks before the onset of labor. Likewise, few childbirth experiences mirror the textbook—commencing with mild regular contractions, widely spaced, and progressing at a predictable pace to delivery. Yet just as it's useful to have a general idea of what a typical woman can expect when she's expecting, it's valuable to know what an average childbirth is like—as long as you allow for the likelihood of variations that will make your experience yours alone.

Childbirth is divided (more loosely by nature, more rigidly by obstetrical science) into three stages. The first stage is labor, with its early, active, and transitional phases; the second stage is delivery, culminating in the birth of the baby; and the third is delivery of the placenta, or afterbirth. The whole process averages about 14 hours or less for first-time mothers, about 8

hours for women who have already had children.

All women who carry to term go through all three phases of labor, dilating from 0 to 10 centimeters in the process. Some, however, may not recognize that they are in labor until the second, or even the third, phase because their initial contractions were mild or painless. For a very few women, all of dilatation passes unnoticed; they don't realize they're in labor until they feel the urge to push that signals the second stage.

The timing and intensity of your contractions can help pinpoint where you are at any particular time. An internal exam, to check on the progress of dilatation, will confirm your progress.

THE FIRST STAGE OF CHILDBIRTH: LABOR

THE FIRST PHASE: EARLY OR LATENT LABOR

This is usually the longest and, fortunately, the least intense phase of labor. The dilatation (or opening) of the cervix to 3 centimeters and the accompanying effacement (thinning out) which characterize this phase can be reached over a period of days or weeks with no noticeable or bothersome contractions, or over a period of two to six hours (and, less commonly, up to 24 hours) of unmistakable labor.

Contractions in this phase (if they are felt) usually last 30 to 45 seconds. They are mild to moderately

strong, may be regular or irregular (between 5 and 20 minutes apart), and become progressively closer together, but not necessarily in a consistent pattern.

You will probably go to the hospital at the end of this phase or the beginning of the next.

What You May Be Feeling or Noticing. The most common signs and symptoms in this phase include backache (either with each contraction or constant), menstrual-like cramps, indigestion, diarrhea, a sensation of warmth in the abdomen, bloody show (a blood-tinged mucus discharge). You may experience all of these, or just one or two. Membranes may have ruptured before the

Labor Positions

Standing enlists gravity in the work of labor.

Try sitting almost completely upright, leaning back slightly in your coach's arms.

Talk to your practitioner in advance about the possibility of remaining at least partially upright during labor: perhaps standing, walking, or sitting (in a rocking or beanbag chair, or in your husband's arms). Studies show that upright positions can shorten labor by speeding dilatation and descent—though the position that works best and is most comfortable varies from woman to woman. Lying flat on your back can not only slow down labor, but can also compress important blood vessels (especially if you are on a firm surface), possibly interfering with blood flow to the fetus. If you are more comfortable lying down, lie on your side, switching sides and doing pelvic tilts periodically.

onset of contractions, but it is more likely that they will rupture sometime during labor itself. (If they don't rupture spontaneously, your practitioner may elect to rupture them artificially anytime after you've gone into active labor.)

Emotionally, you may feel excitement, relief, anticipation, uncertainty, anxiety, fear; some women are relaxed and chatty, others tense and apprehensive.

What You Can Do:

❖ Relax. Your practitioner has probably told you not to call until you are in more active labor. Or he or she may have suggested that you call early on if labor begins during the day or if your membranes have ruptured. Definitely call, however, if your membranes have ruptured and the amniotic fluid is murky or greenish, if you have any bright red bleeding, or if you feel no fetal activity (it may be hard to notice because you are distracted by contractions, so you might want to try the test on page 226). Although you may not feel like it, it's best if you, not your coach, make the call and talk to the practitioner. A lot can be lost in third-party translations.

❖ If it's the middle of the night, try to sleep (but not on your back; see page 150 for the recommended sleeping position). It's important to rest now, because you probably won't be able to later. And you needn't fear that you'll sleep through the next phase—the contractions will be too insistent. If sleep eludes you, don't just lie in bed timing contractions—that'll only make labor seem longer. Instead, get up and do things around the house that will distract you. Clean out a closet; put sheets on the baby's bed; finish packing your bag for the hospital (see page 236); make your coach a sandwich to take along; play solitaire.

❖ If you're laboring during daylight hours, go about your usual routine—as long as it doesn't take you far from home. If you have nothing planned, find something to keep you occupied. Try the distractions suggested above, take a walk (gravity aids the work of labor), watch TV, make and freeze a casserole or two for easy postpartum dining. Put your husband on alert, but it's not necessary for him to come running home—yet.

❖ Make yourself comfortable. Take a warm bath (only if your membranes haven't ruptured) or a shower; use a heating pad if your back is hurting—but *do not* take aspirin or lie on your back. A glass of wine may help you relax.

❖ Eat a light snack if you're hungry (broth, toast with apple butter, or fruit juice). Don't eat heavily, and avoid hard-to-digest foods, such as meats, dairy products, and fats. Not only will digesting a heavy meal compete with the birthing process for body resources, but a full stomach could cause problems if you should need anesthesia later on.

❖ Time contractions for a half-hour span if they seem to be getting

On to the Hospital

Getting to the Hospital. Sometime near the end of the early phase or the beginning of the active phase (probably when your contractions are five minutes apart or less, sooner if you live far from the hospital or if this isn't your first baby), your practitioner will tell you to pick up your bag and get going. Getting to the hospital will be easier if you've planned your route in advance, are familiar with parking regulations, and know which entrance will get you to the obstetrical floor most quickly. (If parking will be a problem, taking a cab may be more sensible.) You may be more comfortable if you stretch out in the rear seat with a blanket, if you've got chills, and a pillow for your head.

Hospital Admission. Procedures will vary, but you can probably expect something like the following:

❖ If you've preregistered (and it's best if you have), this procedure will be brief; if labor is active, your husband can take care of it.

❖ Once in the labor and delivery suite, you will be taken to a labor or birthing room by your nurse for this shift. Depending on hospital regulations, your husband and other family members may be asked to wait outside while you are being admitted and "prepped." (Note to the coach: This is a good time to make a few priority phone calls, to get a snack, and to arrange for stowing your wife's luggage in her room and for chilling the celebratory champagne. If you aren't called to join your wife within 20 minutes or so, remind someone at the nurses' station. You may be asked to change into a sterile outfit.)

❖ Your nurse will take a brief history, asking, among other things, when the contractions started, how far apart they are, whether your waters have broken, when it was that you last ate.

❖ Your nurse will ask you for your signature on routine hospital consent forms.

❖ Your nurse will give you a hospital gown to change into and will request a urine sample. She will check your pulse, blood pressure, respiration, and temperature; inspect your perineum for leaking amniotic fluid, bleeding, or bloody show; listen to the fetal heartbeat with a stethoscope, or hook you up to a fetal monitor; and, possibly, evaluate the position of the fetus and take a blood sample.

❖ Depending on the policies of your doctor and hospital, your pelvic area may be wholly or partially shaved, you may be given an enema, and/or an IV may be started.

❖ Your nurse, your practitioner, or a resident doctor will examine you internally to see how far dilated and effaced your cervix is. If your membranes haven't ruptured spontaneously and you are at least 3 or 4 centimeters dilated (many practitioners prefer to wait until at least 5 centimeters of dilatation), your membranes may be artificially ruptured—unless you and your practitioner have decided to leave them intact until later in labor. The procedure is painless; all you will feel is a warm gush of fluid. The intensity of contractions may increase; for this reason, artificial rupture of the membranes is often useful in stimulating sluggish labor.

If you have any questions that haven't been answered before, now is the time to speak your mind. Have your coach speak it for you, if you don't feel up to it.

closer than 10 minutes apart, and periodically even if they don't. But don't be a clock watcher.

❖ Urinate frequently to avoid bladder distention, which could inhibit the progress of labor.

❖ Use your relaxation techniques if they help, but don't start your breathing exercises yet, or you will be exhausted and bored long before you really need them.

What the Coach Can Do:

❖ Practice timing contractions. The interval between contractions is timed from the beginning of one to the beginning of the next. Time them periodically, and keep a record. When they are coming less than 10 minutes apart, time them more frequently.

❖ Be a calming influence. During this early phase of labor, your most important function is to keep the expectant mother relaxed. And the best way to do this is to keep yourself relaxed, both inside and out. Your own anxiety and tension can be transferred to her unwittingly, communicated not just through words but through touch. Relaxation techniques, a gentle, unhurried massage, or a glass of wine may be helpful. It's too soon, however, to begin using breathing exercises.

❖ Keep your sense of humor, and help her keep hers; time flies, after all, when you're having fun. It'll be easier to laugh now than when contractions are coming fast and hard.

❖ Help distract the expectant mother. Suggest activities that will help keep both your minds off her labor: reading aloud, playing board games or cards, viewing engrossing (and preferably light) television fare, taking short walks.

❖ Offer comfort, reassurance, and support. She'll need them all from now on.

❖ Keep up your own strength, so you'll be able to reinforce hers. Eat periodically, even though she can't. Prepare a sandwich to bring along to the hospital (but nothing with an overpowering odor that might make you, or your wife, feel queasy—such as salami or tuna).

THE SECOND PHASE: ACTIVE LABOR

The second, or active, phase of labor is usually shorter than the first, lasting an average of two to three-and-a-half hours (though variations on this average are great). The uterus's efforts are more concentrated now, accomplishing more in less time. With contractions becoming stronger and more frequent (generally three to four minutes apart and lasting 40 to 60 seconds), the cervix dilates to 7 centimeters. The pattern of contractions may still not be regular. Each contraction probably has a distinct peak (acme or apex) now, which constitutes from 40% to 50% of its total duration. There is less resting time between contractions.

You will probably be in the hospital by early in this phase.

What You May Be Feeling or Noticing. The most common signs and symptoms in this phase include increasing discomfort with contractions (you may be unable to talk through them now), increasing backache, leg discomfort, fatigue, increasing bloody show. You may experience all of these, or just one or two. Rupture of membranes may occur now if it hasn't earlier. (If they don't rupture spontaneously, your practitioner may elect to rupture them artificially sometime during this phase.)

Emotionally, you may feel restless and find it more difficult to relax; or your concentration may become more intense, and you may become completely absorbed in the work at hand. Your confidence may begin to waver, and you may feel it's never going to end; or you may feel that things are really starting to happen.

What You Can Do:

❖ Start your breathing exercises, if you plan to use them, as soon as contractions become too strong to talk through. (If you have never practiced exercises, some simple breathing suggestions from the nurse may help make you more comfortable.) If the exercises seem to make you less comfortable, or more tense, however, you don't have to use them. Women have given birth without them for centuries.

❖ Don't eat or drink anything, but suck on ice chips to replace the fluids you're losing and to keep your mouth moist.

❖ Make a concerted effort to relax between contractions. This will be increasingly difficult as they come more frequently, but it is also increasingly important as your energy begins to wane.

❖ Walk around, if possible, or at least change position frequently, experimenting to see which provides the most comfort. (See page 257 for useful labor positions.)

❖ Remember to urinate periodically; because of tremendous pelvic pressure, you may not notice the urge to empty your bladder.

❖ If you feel you need some pain relief, don't be afraid to discuss it with your attendant. He or she may suggest waiting for 20 minutes or half an hour before actual administration—at which point you may have made so much progress that you won't need it, or you may have renewed strength and no longer want it.

What the Coach Can Do:

❖ If possible, keep the door of the labor or birthing room closed, the lights low, and the room quiet to promote a restful atmosphere. Soft music, if permitted, may also help. Continue relaxation techniques between contractions. And stay as calm as possible yourself.

❖ Time the contractions. If your wife is on a fetal monitor, ask the practitioner or the nurse to show you how to read it so that later, when contractions are coming one on top of the other, you can warn your wife as each new contraction begins. (The monitor may detect them before she can feel them.) You can also encourage her by telling her when each peak is ending. If there is no monitor, learn to recognize the arrival and departure of contractions by placing your hand on your wife's abdomen. This will give both of you some sense of control over the labor.

❖ Breathe with her through difficult contractions, if that helps her. Don't pressure her to the exercises if she is uncomfortable with them, they make her tense, or they annoy her.

❖ If she shows any symptoms of hyperventilation (dizziness or lightheadedness, blurred vision, tingling and numbness of fingers and toes), have her exhale into a paper bag (the nurse will be able to supply one if you haven't brought one along) or into cupped hands. She should then inhale the exhaled air. After repeating this several times, she should feel better.

❖ Reassure your wife of her progress; praise, never criticize. Remind her to take her labor one contraction at a time, and that each pain brings her closer to seeing the baby.

❖ Massage her abdomen or back, or use counterpressure or any other techniques you've learned, to make her more comfortable. Take your cues from her; let her tell you what kind of stroking or touching or massage helps. If she prefers not to be touched at all (some women find it annoying), then it might be best to comfort her verbally.

❖ Don't pretend the pain doesn't exist; even if she doesn't verbalize it, tell her you know how uncomfortable she must feel. She needs your sympathy, not to have you avoid the subject.

❖ Remind her to relax between contractions.

❖ Remind her to urinate at least once an hour.

❖ Don't take it personally if she doesn't respond to—or even seems irritated by—your verbal comfort. A woman's moods during labor are mercurial. Stand by to offer support as she needs and wants it. Remember that your role is important, even if you sometimes feel superfluous.

❖ Be sure she has an ample supply of ice chips to suck on. From time to time ask her if she would like some.

❖ Use a damp washcloth to help cool her body and face; rechill it frequently.

❖ If her feet are cold, offer to get her a pair of socks and help her to put them on.

❖ Continue with distractions she finds useful (card games, conversation between contractions, reading aloud), encouragement, and support.

❖ Suggest a change of position;

walk around with her, if that's possible.

❖ Serve as her go-between with medical personnel as much as possible. Intercept questions that you can answer, ask for explanations of procedures, equipment, any medication, so you'll be able to tell her what's happening. Be her advocate when necessary, but try to fight her battles quietly, perhaps outside the room, so that she won't be disturbed. (One thing you might want to check on now is if a mirror will be provided so that she can view the delivery.)

❖ If she requests medication, transmit her request to the nurse or doctor, but suggest a waiting period before the administration. During that time, the practitioner will probably want to discuss the need for medication and to do an internal exam to check on the progress of labor. It's possible that a good progress report (or even just a brief period to think it over) may give your wife renewed strength to continue unmedicated. Don't be disappointed if she and the doctor decide that medication is needed. This isn't a test of endurance, and your wife hasn't failed if she needs some pain relief.

What Hospital Personnel Will Do:

❖ Provide a relaxed, comfortable, supportive environment, and answers to your questions and concerns.

❖ Continue monitoring the baby's condition with a stethoscope or electronic fetal monitor, and through observation of the amniotic fluid (greenish-brown staining is a sign of possible fetal distress). Fetal position may be assessed with external palpation.

❖ Continue checking your blood pressure.

❖ Periodically evaluate timing and strength of contractions and quantity and quality of bloody discharge. (Pads beneath your buttocks will be replaced as needed.) When there is an obvious change in the pattern or intensity of contractions, or the show becomes more bloody, an internal exam will be done to check the progress of your labor.

❖ Stimulate labor, if it is progressing very slowly, by the use of oxytocin, nipple self-stimulation, or artificial rupture of the membranes (if this wasn't done earlier).

❖ Possibly rupture your membranes, if they haven't ruptured spontaneously by the time you've reached the end of this phase.

❖ Administer sedatives and/or analgesics as needed and desired.

THE THIRD PHASE: ADVANCED ACTIVE OR TRANSITIONAL LABOR

Transition is the most exhausting and demanding phase of labor. Suddenly, the intensity of the contractions picks up. They become very strong, two to three minutes apart, and 60 to 90 seconds long—

If You Aren't Making Progress

Progress in labor is measured by the dilatation of the cervix and the descent of the fetus through the pelvis. Good progress is believed to require three main components: strong uterine contractions that effectively dilate the cervix; a baby that is small enough and in a position for easy exit; and a pelvis that is sufficiently roomy to permit the passage of the baby.

If one or more of these factors is not present, abnormal (or dysfunctional) labor, in which the progess is slow or nonexistent, generally occurs. There are several types of abnormal labor:

Prolonged Latent Phase—when little or no dilatation occurs after 20 hours of labor in a first-time mother, or after 14 hours in one who has delivered previously. Sometimes progress is slow because labor hasn't really begun, and the contractions felt are those of false—not real—labor. Sometimes the reason is overmedication before labor is well established. Sometimes, it is theorized, the cause may be psychological: a woman (almost always a first-time mother) panics when labor begins, triggering the release of chemicals in the brain that interfere with uterine contractions.

In general, the practitioner may suggest stimulating a slow first phase of labor with activity (such as walking) or the opposite (sleep and rest, possibly aided by the use of relaxation techniques or an alcoholic drink and, if the laboring woman is too agitated to relax naturally, the administration of a sedative). Such treatment will also help rule out false labor (the contractions of false labor will usually subside with activity, an alcoholic drink, or a nap). Once true latent phase labor is established, it may be speeded up with an enema or mineral oil, with nipple self-stimulation, or with the administration of oxytocin. (It is also a good idea to urinate periodically, as a full bladder could interfere with descent.) If these tactics are unsuccessful, the practitioner may explore the possibility of a disproportion in size between the fetus's head and the mother's pelvis (fetopelvic disproportion). A cesarean will usually be performed after 24 or 25 hours (sometimes sooner) if insufficient progress has been made by that time.

Primary Dysfunction of Active Phase—when the second, or active, phase of labor progresses very slowly (less than 1 to 1.2 centimeters per hour in women having their first babies, and 1.5 centimeters per hour in those with previous deliveries). When any progress, albeit slow progress, is being made, many practitioners will let the

with very intense peaks that last for most of the contraction. Some women, particularly women who have given birth before, experience multiple peaks. You may feel as though the contractions never completely disappear, and that you can't completely relax between them. The final 3 centimeters of dilatation, to 10 centimeters, will probably take place in a very short time: on average, 15 minutes to an hour.

What You May Be Feeling or Noticing. In transition, you are likely to feel strong pressure on the lower back and/or perineum. Rectal pressure, with or without an urge to push or move bowels, may cause you to grunt involuntarily. Body temperature may be erratic. You may feel either very warm and sweaty or chilled and shaky, or alternate between the two. Your bloody vaginal show will increase as capillaries in uterus set its own pace—on the theory that the woman will eventually deliver naturally, as two thirds of those who experience primary dysfunction do. (Most of the remaining one third will end up being delivered surgically because of a fetopelvic disproportion. Such a mismatch is frequently suspected when progress of labor ceases completely, and can often be confirmed by ultrasound and other examinations.) A laboring woman may be able to speed up the work of her uterus by walking, if possible, staying off her back, and keeping her bladder empty. Intravenous fluids will probably be administered during a lengthy labor.

Secondary Arrest of Dilatation—when, during active labor, there is no progress for two hours or more. In about half of these cases, it is estimated, fetopelvic disproportion exists, necessitating a cesarean delivery. In most other cases, oxytocin (sometimes along with artificial rupture of the membranes) will reestablish labor, particularly when a uterus is only suffering from exhaustion. Again, the woman may be able to make some contribution to the battle against sluggish labor by utilizing gravity (sitting upright, squatting, standing, when possible) and keeping her bladder empty.

Abnormal Descent of the Fetus—when the baby moves down the birth canal at a rate of less than 1 centimeter per hour in women having their first babies, or 2 centimeters per hour in others. In most such cases delivery will be slow, but otherwise uneventful. Trying to remove with forceps a baby that isn't already at the vaginal outlet, once common practice, is now considered dangerous and unnecessary. Today, stimulation with oxytocin and/or artificial rupture of the membranes are the preferred routes—once fetopelvic disproportion and a fetal position which would make vaginal delivery difficult have been ruled out.

Prolonged Second Stage—one that lasts longer than two hours in a first delivery, or slightly less in subsequent deliveries. Many physicians routinely use outlet forceps or perform a cesarean when a second stage goes beyond two hours; others allow the spontaneous vaginal delivery to continue if progress is being made and both mother and fetus (whose conditions are carefully monitored) are doing well. Sometimes the baby's head will be gently eased out those last few inches with outlet forceps. Rotation of the head (so that it faces front, providing for a better fit through the pelvis) may also be attempted, either manually or with outlet forceps. Gravity, again, can help; a semi-sitting or semi-squatting position is most effective for delivery.

the cervix rupture; your legs may be crampy and cold and may tremble uncontrollably. You may experience nausea and/or vomiting; and sleepiness may overcome you between contractions as oxygen flow is shifted from your brain to the site of the delivery. Not surprisingly, you may feel exhausted.

Emotionally, you may feel vulnerable and overwhelmed, as though you're reaching the end of your rope. In addition to frustration over not being able to push yet, you may feel irritable, disoriented, discouraged, restless, and have difficulty concentrating and relaxing (it may seem impossible).

What You Can Do:

❖ Hang in there. By the end of this phase, your cervix will be fully dilated, and it will be time to push your baby out.

❖ Instead of thinking about the work ahead, try to think about how far you've come.

❖ If you feel the urge to push, pant or blow instead, unless you've been instructed otherwise. Pushing against a cervix that isn't completely dilated can cause the cervix to swell, which can delay delivery.

❖ If you don't want anybody to touch you unnecessarily, if your coach's once comforting hands now irritate you, don't hesitate to let him know.

❖ If you find them useful, use breathing techniques you have learned (or ask the nurse for suggestions), adjusting them to the intensity of your contractions.

❖ Try to relax between contractions (if you find it humanly possible) with slow, rhythmic chest breathing.

What the Coach Can Do:

❖ Be specific and direct in your instructions, without wasting words. She may find small talk annoying. If she doesn't want your help at any point and wants to be left alone, take her cue without feeling helpless or rejected.

❖ Offer lots of encouragement and praise, unless she would prefer you to keep quiet. At this moment, eye contact may communicate more expressively than words.

❖ Touch her only if she finds it comforting. Abdominal massage may be offensive now, though counterpressure may be helpful if her back hurts.

❖ Breathe with her through every contraction, if it helps her through them.

❖ Remind her to take one contraction at a time. She may need you to warn her when each begins, and to tell her as it declines.

❖ Help her relax between contractions, touching her abdomen lightly to show her when a contraction is over. Remind her to use slow, rhythmic breathing.

❖ If her contractions seem to be getting closer and/or she feels the urge to push—and she hasn't been examined recently—tell the nurse or practitioner. She may be fully dilated.

❖ Offer her ice chips frequently, and mop her brow with a cool damp cloth often.

What Hospital Personnel May Do:

❖ Continue comfort and support.

❖ Continue monitoring your condition and that of the fetus.

❖ Continue checking duration and intensity of contractions, and the progress you are making.

❖ Prepare for delivery, ultimately moving you to a delivery room, if you are not delivering in a birthing or labor room.

❖ Administer anesthesia if planned or needed.

THE SECOND STAGE OF CHILDBIRTH: PUSHING AND DELIVERY

Your active participation in the birth of your child has been, up to this point, negligible. Though you've undeniably taken the brunt of the proceedings, your cervix and uterus (and baby) have done most of the work. But now that the task of dilatation has been completed, your help is needed to push the baby down, through the birth canal, and out. This generally takes between half an hour and an hour, but can be accomplished in 10 short minutes or in two to three very long hours.

The contractions of the second stage are more regular than the contractions of transition. They are still about 60 to 90 seconds long, but sometimes farther apart (usually about two to five minutes) and possibly less painful—though sometimes they are more intense. There now should be a well-defined rest period, although you may still have trouble recognizing the onset of each new contraction.

What You May Be Feeling or Noticing. Common in the second stage is an overwhelming urge to push (although not every woman has it). You may experience a burst of renewed energy (a kind of second wind) or fatigue; tremendous rectal pressure; very visible contractions, with the uterus rising noticeably with each; a possible increase in bloody show; a tingling, stretching, burning, or stinging sensation at the vagina as the head crowns; and a slippery wet feeling as the baby emerges.

Emotionally, you may feel relieved that you can now start pushing (though some women feel embarrassed or inhibited); you may also feel exhilarated and excited or, if the pushing stretches on for much more than an hour, frustrated or overwhelmed. In prolonged second stages, the woman's preoccupation is often less with seeing the baby than with getting the ordeal over with; this is a natural, and temporary, reaction, which in no way reflects on her capacity for motherly love.

What You Can Do:

❖ Get into a pushing position (which one will depend upon hospital policy, your practitioner's predilection, the bed or chair you are in, and hopefully, what is most comfortable and effective for you). A semi-sitting or semi-squatting position is probably the best because it enlists the aid of gravity in the birthing process and affords you more pushing power.

❖ Give it all you've got. The more efficiently you push, and the more energy you pack into the effort, the more quickly your baby will make that trip through the birth canal. But keep your work coordinated and rhythmical. Listen carefully to instruc-

A Baby Is Born

1. *The cervix has thinned (effaced) somewhat, but has not begun to dilate.* **2.** *The cervix has fully dilated and the baby's head has begun to press into the birth canal (vagina).* **3.** *To allow the narrowest diameter of the baby's head to fit through the mother's pelvis, the baby usually turns sometime during labor. Here the slightly molded head has crowned.* **4.** *The head, the baby's broadest part, is out. The rest of the delivery should proceed quickly and smoothly.*

tions. Frantic, disorganized pushing wastes energy and accomplishes little.

❖ Don't let inhibition or embarrassment break the pushing rhythm. Since you're bearing down on the whole perineal area, anything that's in your bowels may be pushed out, too; trying to control your bowels while you're pushing will impede your progress. A little involuntary evacuation is experienced by nearly everyone in delivery—even by some women who've had enemas. No one else in the room will think twice about it, and neither should you. Sterile pads will be used to whisk away any excretion immediately.

❖ Do what comes naturally. Push when you feel the urge, unless otherwise instructed. Take a few deep breaths while the contraction is building; take another and hold it. Then, as the contraction peaks, push with all your might until you can no longer comfortably hold your breath. You may feel as many as five urges to bear down with each contraction. Follow each urge, rather than trying to hold your breath and push through an entire contraction; breath-holding for long periods of time can exhaust you and may deprive the fetus of oxygen. Several deep breaths as the contraction wanes will help restore your respiratory balance. If nothing seems to be coming naturally— and it doesn't for every woman— your practitioner will help direct your efforts, and redirect them if you lose your concentration.

❖ Be sure your thighs and perineum are relaxed as you push. Tenseness works against your pushing efforts.

❖ Stop pushing when you're instructed to (as you may be, to keep the baby's head from being born too rapidly). Pant or blow instead.

❖ Rest between contractions, with the help of your coach and the attendants. If you are very exhausted, especially when the second stage drags on, your practitioner may suggest that you don't push for several contractions so you can rebuild your strength.

❖ Don't become frustrated if you see the baby's head crown, then disappear again. Birthing is a two-steps-forward, one-step-backward proposition.

❖ Remember to keep an eye on the mirror (if one is available). Seeing your baby's head crown (and reaching down and touching it, if your practitioner approves) will give you the inspiration to push when the pushing gets tough. Besides, unless your coach is videotaping, there won't be any replays.

What the Coach Can Do:

❖ Continue giving comfort and support, but don't feel hurt if your wife doesn't seem to notice you're there. Her energies are necessarily focused elsewhere.

❖ Guide her pushing and breathing, using the cues that you have both become familiar with during

Pain Risk Factors

Your perception of pain may be increased by:	It may be decreased by:
Being alone.	Having the company and support of those you love, and/or experienced medical personnel.
Fatigue.	Being well rested (try not to overdo things during the ninth month); trying to rest and relax between contractions.
Hunger and thirst.	Having light snacks during early labor; sucking ice chips throughout.
Thinking about and expecting pain.	Turning your mind to other thoughts and distractions; thinking of contractions in terms of how much they accomplish, rather than how much they hurt; and remembering that no matter how intense the discomfort, it will be of relatively brief duration.
Anxiety and stress; tensing up during contractions.	Using relaxation techniques between contractions; concentrating on your efforts during them.
Fear of the unknown.	Learning as much as you can about childbirth in advance; taking childbirth one contraction at a time; and not worrying about what's to come.
Self-pity.	Thinking about how lucky you are and about the wonderful reward to come.
Feeling out of control and helpless.	Having good childbirth preparation; knowing enough to feel some measure of control and confidence.

childbirth preparation; or relay instructions from the nurse or practitioner.

❖ Don't feel intimidated by the finesse and expertise of the professional medical team around you. Your presence is important, too. And in fact, your whispered "I love you" may be more valuable to her at this stage than anything their experience can offer.

❖ Help her to relax between contractions, with soothing words, a cool cloth applied to forehead, neck, and shoulders, and, if feasible, back massage or counterpressure to help ease backache

❖ Continue to supply ice chips to moisten her parched mouth, as needed.

❖ Support her back while she's pushing, if necessary; hold her hand, wipe her brow, stroke her arm—or do whatever seems to help her. If she slips out of position, help her back up.

❖ Periodically point out her progress. As the baby begins to crown, remind her to keep an eye on the mirror so she can have visual confirmation of what she is accomplishing; when she's not looking, or if there's no mirror, give her inch-by-inch descriptions. Take her hand and touch the head together for renewed inspiration (with the practitioner's okay).

❖ If you're offered the opportunity to "catch" your baby as it emerges or, later, to cut the cord, don't panic. Both are easy—and you'll get step-by-step directions, support, and backup from the attendants.

What Hospital Personnel May Do:

❖ Move you to the room in which you will deliver, if you aren't already there.

❖ Give support and direction to you as the delivery progresses.

❖ Continue to check the condition of the fetus periodically, usually by attaching the fetal monitor briefly.

❖ About the time the head crowns, prepare for the delivery—spreading sterile drapes and arranging instruments, donning surgical garments and gloves, dousing the perineal area with antiseptic.

❖ Perform an episiotomy just before the head is delivered, if necessary. (This will be painless if done at the height of a contraction, when the pressure of the baby's head naturally numbs the perineum, though the doctor may administer a local anesthetic.)

❖ Elect to use outlet forceps to ease the baby's head out if the second stage lasts more than two hours (some doctors will wait longer if mother and baby are doing well), if the baby shows signs of difficulty tolerating the stresses of labor, if your medical condition prohibits further pushing, or if progress is impeded because of a slightly irregular fetal presentation or a slight disproportion between fetus and pelvis. (See Forceps Delivery, page 254.) A regional anesthetic will be administered if an epidural or other block hasn't already been given, because forceps delivery can be painful. If forceps aren't feasible or don't work, a cesarean may be the safest route to delivery for baby and you.

❖ Once the head emerges, quickly suction the baby's nose and mouth to remove mucus, then assist the shoulders and torso out.

❖ Clamp and cut the umbilical cord, possibly with the newborn lying across your abdomen. Your husband may be asked to do the snipping. (Some practitioners prefer to wait until the placenta is deliv-

A First Look at Baby

Those who expect their babies to arrive as round and smooth and pink as a Botticelli cherub may be in for a shock. Nine months of soaking in an amniotic bath and a dozen or so hours of sausage-like compression in a contracting uterus and cramped birth canal take their toll on a newborn's appearance.

Fortunately, most of the less-lovely newborn characteristics which follow are temporary. One morning, a couple of months after you've brought your wrinkled, slightly scrawny, puffy-eyed bundle home from the hospital, you'll wake to find that the Botticelli cherub has taken its place in the crib.

An Oddly Shaped Head. At birth, the infant's head is, proportionately, the largest part of the body, as wide around as the chest. As the baby grows, the rest of the body will catch up. Often, the head has molded to fit through the mother's pelvis, giving it an odd, possibly pointed shape; pressing against an inadequately dilated cervix can further distort the head by raising a lump (called caput succedaneum). The caput will disappear in a day or two; the molded look within two weeks—at which point your baby's head will begin to take on a Botticelli roundness.

Newborn Hair. The hair that covers the head at birth may have little relationship to the hair the baby will have later. Some newborns are virtually bald; others have thick thatches. Either way, the newborn hair will eventually fall out and be replaced by new growth.

Vernix Caseosa Coating. The cheesy substance that coats the fetus in the uterus is believed to protect the skin from the long exposure to the amniotic fluid. Premature babies have quite a bit of this coating at birth, postmature babies have almost none, except in the folds of their skin and under their fingernails.

ered or the cord has stopped pulsating before cutting the cord.)

❖ Provide initial protective care for the newborn: evaluate his or her condition, and rate it on the Apgar scale at one minute and five minutes after birth (see page 255); give a brisk, stimulating, and drying rubdown; identify the baby by taking his or her footprints and your fingerprint for hospital records, and by attaching a bracelet with your name on it to the baby's wrist; administer non-irritating eyedrops, to prevent infection; weigh the baby, and wrap him or her for warmth. (In some hospitals additional procedures may be performed in the delivery room; in others they will be attended to later, in the nursery.)

❖ Show your now cleaned-up baby to you and your husband. Depending on the situation and hospital policy, you may be able to hold the baby briefly or for a longer period. If there's time, and if you wish to, you may be able to try breastfeeding (don't worry if you or your baby don't catch on immediately—see Getting Started Breastfeeding, page 294).

❖ Probably whisk baby off to the nursery (at least temporarily) and transfer you to your room.

Swelling of the Genitals. This is common in both male and female newborns, and is particularly pronounced in boy babies delivered via cesarean. The breasts of newborns, male and female, may also be swollen (occasionally even engorged, secreting a white substance nicknamed "witch's milk") due to stimulation by maternal hormones. The hormones may also stimulate a milky-white, even blood-tinged, vaginal secretion in girls. These effects are not abnormal, and disappear in a week to 10 days.

Lanugo. Fine downy hair, called lanugo, may cover the shoulders, back, forehead, and temples of full-term babies. This will usually be shed by the end of the first week. Such hair can be more abundant, and will last longer, in a premature baby.

Puffy Eyes. Swelling around the newborn's eyes is often caused by the eye drops that are used to protect the baby from infection, and disappears within a few days. Caucasian babies' eyes are almost always a slate blue, no matter what color they will be later on. In darker-skinned races, the eyes are brown at birth.

Birthmarks and Skin Lesions. A reddish blotch at the base of the skull, on the eyelid, or on the forehead is very common, especially in Caucasians. Mongolian spots, bluish-gray pigmentation of the deep skin layer that can appear on the back, buttocks, and sometimes the arms and thighs, are more common in Asians, Southern Europeans, and blacks. These markings will eventually disappear, usually by the time a child is four years old. Hemangiomas, elevated bright strawberry-colored marks, vary from tiny to about quarter-size. They will eventually fade to a mottled pearly gray, then disappear entirely. Coffee-with-cream-colored spots can appear anywhere on the body; they are usually inconspicuous, and don't fade. A variety of rashes, tiny "pimples," and whiteheads may also mar the newborn complexion, but all are temporary.

THE THIRD STAGE OF CHILDBIRTH: DELIVERY OF THE PLACENTA, OR AFTERBIRTH

The worst is over, the best has already come. All that remains is the tying up of loose ends, so to speak. During this final stage of childbirth (which generally lasts anywhere from five minutes to half an hour or more) the placenta, which has been your baby's life support inside the womb, will be delivered. You will continue to have mild contractions of approximately one minute's duration, though you may not feel them. The pressure these contractions exert separates the placenta from the uterus and moves it down into the lower segment of the uterus or into the vagina so you can push it out. Once the placenta is delivered, any necessary stitching up of episiotomy or tears will be taken care of.

What You May Be Feeling or Noticing. Now that your work is done, you may feel fatigue or, conversely, a burst of renewed energy. You are likely to be very thirsty and, especially if labor has been long, hungry.

Some women experience chills in this stage; all experience a bloody vaginal discharge (called lochia) comparable to that of a heavy menstrual period.

For many women, the immediate emotional reaction is a sense of relief. There may also be exhilaration and talkativeness; elation, tempered by a new sense of responsibility; impatience at having to push out the placenta or submit to the repair of the episiotomy or tear, though you may be too excited or tired to care. Some women feel a strong closeness to their husbands and an immediate bond with their new baby; others feel somewhat detached (who is this stranger at my breast?), even resentful (how he's made me suffer!), particularly after a difficult delivery. (See pages 160, 233, 288 for more on bonding and new mother love.)

What You Can Do:
❖ Help expel the placenta, by pushing as directed.

❖ Hold still and be patient while any repair of episiotomy or tears is being done.

❖ Nurse or hold the baby, though your husband may do the holding until the placenta is expelled. In some hospitals, and under some circumstances, the baby may be kept in a heated bassinette for a while.

❖ Take pride in your accomplishment, relax, and enjoy!

What the Coach Can Do:
❖ Give your wife some well-earned words of praise.

❖ Share in bonding with the new baby.

❖ Don't forget to do some husband-wife bonding, too.

❖ Ask the nurse for some juice for your wife; she'll be very dry. After she's been rehydrated, and if both of you are in the mood, break out the bubbly you've had the hospital staff keep chilled.

❖ Take pictures, if you've brought your camera, or tape the baby's first cries, if you have your tape recorder along.

What Hospital Personnel May Do:
❖ Help extract the placenta. The exact procedure will vary depending upon the practitioner and the situation. Some will pull the cord gently with one hand while pressing and kneading the uterus with the other; others will exert downward pressure on the top of the uterus. Many physicians will use oxytocin, by injection or IV, to encourage uterine contractions, which will speed expulsion of the placenta and minimize bleeding.

❖ Examine the placenta to be sure it is intact. If it isn't, the practitioner will inspect the uterus manually for placental fragments and remove any that remain.

❖ Cut the cord, if it wasn't cut earlier.

❖ Stitch an episiotomy or tear, if any. A local anesthetic (if none was previously given, or if it has worn off) will probably be used to numb the area.

❖ Check your vaginal bleeding.

❖ Sponge-bathe the lower part of your body, help you into a clean gown, and help you put on a perineal pad (sanitary napkin) held in place by a belt.

❖ Wheel you into the recovery room, or to your own room.

❖ Deliver the baby to the nursery for a bath and some additional protective measures. (If you have rooming-in, the baby will be returned as soon as possible.)

BREECH DELIVERY

As far as the mother and coach are concerned, labor and vaginal delivery of a breech baby don't differ much from that of a vertex (head-down) baby; tips for coping and comforting are virtually identical. The activities of the hospital staff will be different, however, and will vary further depending on the type of breech position and the delivery procedure that the practitioner elects to follow.

Up until the second stage, a vaginal breech delivery progesses about the same as a vertex delivery. But it is always considered a trial labor, allowed to proceed only as long as it progresses normally. Because of the ever-present possibility that a cesarean may become necessary, you will probably be transferred to a delivery/operating room at the end of the first stage. Depending upon your baby's exact breech position, your doctor will determine the safest and most effective way to proceed. (What is most advisable in such a case also depends on the practitioner's experience. Asking a doctor to perform a procedure for breech extraction that you've read or heard about, but with which he or she is not comfortable, is *never* in your or your baby's best interest.)

A common procedure is to allow the baby to deliver naturally until the legs and lower half of the torso are out. Then a local anesthetic is administered and the shoulders and head are delivered by the practitioner, with or without the aid of forceps.

A vaginal delivery is not likely to be attempted if the baby is in the complete breech (see page 207) or footling breech (with one leg dangling down) position, if the fetus is estimated to be oversized or the mother's pelvis inadequate, if the delivery is premature, or if there are signs of fetal distress.

A large episiotomy is often necessary with a breech, but occasionally it can be avoided. The delivery position for the vaginal breech birth will vary, again depending on the situation and on your practitioner's experience. Some find they have more control if the woman is flat on her back, legs up in stirrups. Others suggest that a woman may be more comfortable if she is placed in a sitting position.

Once the baby is delivered, the proceedings continue as with a vertex birth.

CESAREAN SECTION: SURGICAL DELIVERY

At a cesarean delivery, unlike a vaginal one, you won't be able to participate actively. And, in fact, your most important contribution to the comfort and success of your baby's cesarean birth can be made before you arrive at the hospital—possibly before you even know that you're having a cesarean. That contribution is preparation. Being prepared both intellectually and emotionally for a cesarean, in case it should become necessary, will minimize the disappointment many women feel and help make your surgical delivery experience a positive one.

Thanks to regional anesthesia and the liberalization of hospital regulations, most women (and often their husbands) are able to be spectators at their cesarean deliveries. Because they aren't preoccupied with pushing or discomfort, they are often able to relax and appreciate the birth—something women delivering vaginally can rarely do.

This is what you can expect in a typical cesarean birth:

❖ Your pubic and/or abdominal hair may be shaved, and a catheter (a narrow tube) will be inserted into your bladder to keep it empty and out of the surgeon's way.

❖ In the operating room, sterile drapes will be arranged around your exposed abdomen, which will be washed down with an antiseptic solution. If you are to be awake for the delivery, a screen will be put up at about shoulder level so that you won't see the incision being made.

❖ An IV infusion will be started to provide easy access if additional medication is needed.

❖ Either an epidural or a spinal block (which numb the lower part of your body but allow you to be awake) or a general anesthetic (which puts you to sleep—sometimes necessary when the baby must be delivered immediately) will be administered.

❖ If your coach is going to attend the delivery, he will be suited up in sterile garb. He will sit near your head, giving you support, holding your hand, and has the option of viewing the actual surgery. (Whether or not you know in advance you are going to have a cesarean, it's a good idea to discuss with your doctor ahead of time the possibility of your spouse being with you in case you do need surgery.)

❖ If yours is an emergency cesarean, things may move very quickly. Don't be upset by the seeming storm of activity around you. In such a situation, hospital policy, expediency, and concern for the safety of you and your baby may dictate that your husband leave during the delivery, which will only take about 5 or 10 minutes. You should both be prepared for this possibility.

❖ Once the physician is certain that the anesthetic has taken effect, an incision (a cut) is made in the lower abdomen. If you are awake, you may feel a sensation of being "unzipped," but no pain.

❖ A second incision is then made, this time in the lower segment of your uterus. The amniotic sac is ruptured and the fluid suctioned out; you may hear a sort of gurgling or swooshing sound.

❖ The baby is then eased out, either by hand or with forceps, usually with an assistant pressing on the upper end of the uterus. With an epidural (though not likely with a spinal block), you will probably feel some pulling and tugging sensations, as well as some pressure. If you're anxious to see your baby's arrival, ask the doctor if the screen can be lowered briefly, which will allow you to see the actual birth, but not the more graphic details.

❖ Your baby's nose and mouth are then suctioned; you'll hear the first cry, and if the cord is long enough, you will be allowed a quick glimpse.

❖ The cord will be quickly clamped and cut, and while the baby is getting the same routine attention as a vaginally delivered infant, the doctor manually removes the placenta.

❖ Now the doctor will check your reproductive organs quickly and stitch up the incisions that were made.

❖ An injection of oxytocin may be given intramuscularly or into your IV bottle, to help contract the uterus and control bleeding.

❖ Depending upon your condition and the baby's, as well as hospital rules, you may or may not be able to hold the baby right there in the delivery room. If you can't, perhaps your husband can. If the infant has to be whisked away to the ICU nursery, don't fret. This is standard in many hospitals and doesn't indicate a problem with the baby's condition. As far as bonding is concerned, later can be just as good as sooner.

Part 3

LAST BUT NOT LEAST:

Postpartum, Fathers, and the Next Baby

15
Postpartum: The First Week

WHAT YOU MAY BE FEELING

PHYSICALLY:

❖ Bloody vaginal discharge (lochia), turning pinkish toward week's end

❖ Afterpains in abdomen after first 24 hours

❖ Exhaustion

❖ Perineal discomfort and/or pain and numbness, if you had a vaginal delivery (especially if you had stitches); worse with sneezing and coughing)

❖ Incisional pain and, later, numbness in the area, if you had a cesarean (especially a first one)

❖ Discomfort sitting and walking if you had an episiotomy or a cesarean

❖ Difficulty urinating for a day or two; difficulty and discomfort with bowel movements for the first few days; constipation

❖ General soreness, especially if pushing was difficult

❖ Bloodshot eyes; black-and-blue marks around eyes, cheeks, elsewhere, from vigorous pushing

❖ Sweating, possibly profuse, after the first couple of days

❖ Breast discomfort and engorgement about the third or fourth day postpartum

❖ Sore or cracked nipples, if you are breastfeeding

EMOTIONALLY:

❖ Elation, depression, or swings between the two

❖ Feelings of inadequacy and trepidation about mothering, especially if you're breastfeeding

❖ Frustration, if you're still in the hospital and would like to leave

❖ Little interest in sex or, less commonly, increased desire (intercourse won't be okayed until at least three weeks postpartum)

WHAT YOU MAY BE CONCERNED ABOUT

BLEEDING

"I'd been told to expect a bloody discharge after delivery, but when I got out of bed for the first time and saw the blood running down my legs, I was really frightened."

Don't be alarmed. This discharge of leftover blood, mucus, and tissue from your uterus, known as lochia, is normally as heavy as (sometimes even heavier than) a menstrual period for the first three postpartum days. And though it'll probably seem more copious than it really is, it may total up to two cups before it begins to taper off. A sudden gush on getting out of bed in the first few days is common, and no cause for concern. And since blood and an occasional blood clot arc the predominant ingredients of lochia during the immediate postpartum period, your discharge will be quite red for two or three days, gradually turning to a watery pink, then to brown, and finally to a yellowish white over the next week or two. Sanitary napkins, not tampons, should be used to absorb the flow, which may continue on and off for as long as six weeks.

Breastfeeding and the intramuscular or intravenous administration of oxytocin (routinely ordered by some doctors following delivery) may both reduce the flow of lochia by encouraging uterine contractions and helping to shrink the uterus back to normal size more quickly.

The contraction of the uterus after delivery is important because it pinches off exposed blood vessels at the site where the placenta separated from the uterus, thus preventing hemorrhage. If the uterus is too relaxed and doesn't contract, excessive bleeding occurs. This can happen for several reasons: a long, exhausting labor; a traumatic delivery; a uterus that was overdistended because of multiple births, a large baby, or excess amniotic fluid; an oddly placed placenta, or one that separated prematurely; fibroids that prevent symmetrical contraction of the uterus; or generally weakened condition of the mother at the time of delivery (due to, for example, anemia, preeclampsia, or extreme fatigue).

Postpartum hemorrhage can also occur because of lacerations to the genital tract, or because fragments of the placenta have been retained in the uterus. (In the latter case, bleeding may not occur until a week or two after delivery.) Occasionally internal bleeding causes swelling and severe pain over the site. Rarely, hemorrhage is caused by a previously undetected bleeding disorder. Infection can also cause postpartum hemorrhage, right after delivery or weeks later.

Most postpartum hemorrhages occur about 7 to 14 days after delivery, without any warning. Since this relatively rare complication of childbirth can be life-threatening, prompt diagnosis and treatment are vital. Any of the following signs of abnormal bleeding (some of which are also signs of postpartum infection) should be reported immediately to your practitioner:

❖ Bleeding that saturates more than one pad an hour for more than a few hours.

❖ Frank (bright red) bleeding any time after the fourth day; but don't worry about an occasional blood-tinged discharge.

❖ Lochia that has a foul odor (it should smell like a normal menstrual discharge).

❖ Large clots in the lochia.

❖ Pain or discomfort in the lower abdominal area, beyond the first few days after delivery.

❖ A temperature of over 100 degrees for more than a day.

AFTERPAINS

"I've been having cramp-like pains in my abdomen, especially when I'm nursing."

These are probably "afterpains," which are believed to be caused by the contractions of the uterus as it makes its normal descent back into the pelvis following birth. The contractions are more likely to be felt by, and be more intense in, women whose uterine musculature is flaccid (lacking in tone) because of previous births or excessive stretching (as with twins).

Afterpains can be more pronounced during nursing, when contraction-stimulating oxytocin is

released. Mild analgesics may be prescribed if necessary, but the pain should subside naturally within four to seven days. If analgesics don't relieve the symptoms, or if they persist for more than a week, see your practitioner to rule out postpartum infection.

PAIN IN THE PERINEAL AREA

"I didn't have an episiotomy, and I didn't tear. Why am I so sore?"

You can't expect some 7 pounds of baby to pass by the perineum unnoticed. Even if the perineum was left intact during the baby's arrival, the area has still been stretched, bruised, and generally traumatized; and discomfort, ranging from mild to not-so-mild, is the very normal result.

"My episiotomy site is so sore, I'm afraid my stitches are infected. But how can I tell?"

The perineal soreness experienced by all vaginal deliverees is likely to be compounded if the perineum was torn or surgically cut. Like any freshly repaired wound, the site of an episiotomy or laceration will take time to heal—usually 7 to 10 days. Pain alone during this time, unless it is very severe, is not an indication that an infection has developed.

Infection is possible, but very unlikely if good perineal care has been practiced. While you're in the hospital, a nurse will check the perineum at least once daily to be certain that there is no inflammation or other indication of infection. She will also instruct you in postpartum perineal hygiene, which is important in preventing infection not only of the repair site but of the genital tract as well (puerperal fever). For this reason, the same precautions apply for those who were neither torn nor had an episiotomy. Follow this 10-day plan for the care of the perineum:

❖ Use a fresh sanitary pad at least every four to six hours. Secure snugly so that it doesn't slide back and forth.

❖ Remove the pad front to back to avoid dragging germs from the rectum to the vagina.

❖ Pour or squirt warm water (or an antiseptic solution, if one was recommended by your practitioner) over the perineum after urinating or defecating. Pat dry with gauze pads, or with the paper wipes which may come with hospital-provided sanitary pads, always from front to back.

❖ Keep your hands off the area until healing is complete.

Though discomfort is likely to be greater if you've had a repair (with itchiness around the stitches possibly accompanying soreness), suggestions for relief are usually welcomed by all recently delivered mothers:

❖ Warm sitz baths, hot compresses, or heat lamp exposure.[1]

---

1. Use a heat lamp only under supervision in the hospital, or at home with instructions from your practitioner on how to avoid burns.

❖ Chilled witch hazel on a sterile gauze pad or a glove filled with crushed ice applied to the site.

❖ Local anesthetics in the form of sprays, creams, or pads; mild pain relievers may be prescribed by your physician.

❖ Lying on your side; avoiding long periods of standing or sitting, to decrease strain on the area. Sitting on a pillow or inflated tube may help, as may tightening your buttocks before sitting.

❖ Doing Kegel exercises (see pages 162, 318) as frequently as possible after delivery, and right through the postpartum period, to stimulate circulation to the area, which will promote healing and improve muscle tone. (Don't be alarmed if you can't feel yourself doing them; the area will be numb right after delivery. Feeling will return to the perineum gradually over the next few weeks.)

DIFFICULTY WITH URINATION

"It's been several hours since I gave birth, and I haven't been able to urinate yet."

Difficulty in passing urine during the first 24 postpartum hours is common. Some women feel no urge at all; others feel the urge but are unable to fulfill it. Still others do urinate, but with accompanying pain and burning. There are a host of reasons why bladder function often becomes such an effort after delivery:

❖ The holding capacity of the bladder increases because it suddenly has more room to expand—thus the need for urination may be less frequent.

❖ The bladder may have been traumatized or bruised during delivery due to pressure created by the fetus, and become temporarily paralyzed. Even when it's full, it may not send the necessary signals of urgency.

❖ Drugs or anesthesia may decrease the sensitivity of the bladder or the alertness of the mother to signals.

❖ Pain in the perineal area may cause reflex spasms in the urethra, making urination difficult. Edema (swelling) of the perineum may also interfere with urination.

❖ Any number of psychological factors may inhibit urination—fear that voiding may prove painful, lack of privacy, embarrassment or discomfort over using a bedpan or needing assistance at the toilet.

❖ The sensitivity of the site of an episiotomy or laceration repair can cause burning and/or pain with urination. (Burning may be alleviated somewhat by standing astride the toilet while urinating so that the flow comes straight down, without touching sore spots.)

As difficult as urination may be after delivery, it's essential that the bladder be emptied within six to eight hours—to avoid urinary tract infection, loss of muscle tone in the bladder from overdistension, and bleeding due to the bladder hindering the proper descent of the uterus. You can expect, therefore, that the nurse will ask you frequently after delivery if you've urinated. She may request that you void for the first time postpartum into a container, so that she can measure your output, and may palpate your bladder to make sure it's not distended.

If you haven't urinated within eight hours or so, your physician may have you catheterized (a tube is inserted into your urethra) to empty the bladder of urine. You may be able to avoid this with the following:

❖ Take a walk. Getting up from bed and going for a stroll as soon after delivery as you're allowed will help get your bladder (and your bowels) moving.

❖ If you're uncomfortable with an audience, have the nurse wait outside the room while you urinate. She can come back in when you've finished, to give you a demonstration of perineal hygiene.

❖ If you're too weak to walk to the bathroom and must use a bedpan, ask for privacy; have the nurse warm the pan (if it's metal) and give you warm water to pour over the perineal area (which may stimulate the urge); and sit on the pan instead of lying on it.

❖ Warm the area in a sitz bath or chill it with ice packs, whichever seems to induce urgency for you.

❖ Turn the water on while you try. Running the water in the sink really does help encourage your own faucet to flow.

After 24 hours, the problem of too little becomes one of too much. Postpartum women begin urinating frequently and copiously as the excess body fluids of pregnancy are excreted. If urinating is still difficult, or if output is scant during the next few days, it's possible you have a urinary tract infection. The symptoms of simple cystitis (bladder infection) include: pain and/or burning with urination (which continues even after the sensitivity of the episiotomy or laceration repair has lessened); frequency and urgency with little urine passed; and, sometimes, a low-grade fever. Symptoms of a kidney infection are more severe, and may include a fever of 101 to 104 degrees, back pain on one or both sides—usually in addition to the symptoms of cystitis. Your physician will want to begin antibiotic treatment specific to the infection-causing organism, if infection is confirmed. You can help speed recovery by drinking plenty of extra fluids. (Also see page 175.)

HAVING A BOWEL MOVEMENT

"I delivered almost a week ago and I haven't had a bowel movement yet. Although I've felt the urge, I've been too afraid that straining would open my episiotomy."

The passage of the first bowel movement after childbirth is a milestone in the postpartum period. Every day that precedes it is fraught with increasing emotional and physical discomfort.

Several physiological factors may interfere with the return of normal bowel function after delivery. For one thing, the abdominal muscles that assist in elimination have been stretched during childbirth, making them flaccid and ineffective. For another, the bowel itself may have been traumatized by delivery, leaving it sluggish. And, of course, it may have been emptied before or during delivery, and probably remained empty because no solid food was taken for the duration of labor.

But perhaps the most potent inhibitors of postpartum bowel activity are psychological: the unfounded fear of splitting open the stitches; the natural embarrassment over the lack of privacy in the hospital; and the pressure to perform, which often makes performance all the more elusive.

Although reregulating your system is rarely effortless, it isn't necessary to suffer endlessly. There are several steps you can take to resolve the problem:

Don't Worry. Nothing keeps you from moving your bowels more effectively than worrying about moving your bowels. Don't worry about opening the stitches—you won't. And don't worry if it takes a few days to get things moving; that's okay, too.

Request Roughage. Select whole grains and fresh fruits and vegetables from the hospital menu, if possible. Supplement the hospital diet, which many patients find constipating, with bowel-stimulating food brought in from outside. Apples, raisins and other dried fruit, nuts, bran muffins, and small boxes of bran cereal will help. Chocolate—so often a gift to hospital patients—will only worsen constipation.

Keep the Liquids Coming. Not only must you compensate for fluids lost during labor and delivery, you must take in additional liquids—especially water and fruit juices—to help soften stool if you're constipated.

Get Off Your Bottom. You won't be running marathons the day after delivery, but you should be able to take short strolls through the corridors. An inactive body encourages inactive bowels. Kegel exercises, which can be practiced in your bed almost immediately after delivery, will help tone up not only the perineum, but also the rectum.

Don't Strain. Straining won't break your stitches open, but it can lead to hemorrhoids. If you do have hemorrhoids, you may find relief with sitz baths, topical anesthetics, suppositories, hot or cold compresses.

The first few bowel movements may pass with great discomfort. But as stools soften and you become more regular, the discomfort will ease.

EXCESSIVE PERSPIRATION

"I've been waking up at night soaked with perspiration. Is this normal?"

W hat your doctor probably calls diaphoresis (but is more commonly referred to as perspiration or sweating) is one of the ways your body rids itself of pregnancy-accumulated fluids during the week following delivery. Often perspiration continues to be a problem for several weeks, because of the postpartum hormonal adjustments. Don't worry about it; but do make sure essential fluids are replaced—particularly if you're breast-feeding—by taking extra liquids. An absorbent towel over your pillow may help make you more comfortable if you do most of your perspiring during the night.

As a precaution, it's a good idea to take your temperature, and to report it to your doctor if it's over 100 degrees.

ADEQUACY OF YOUR MILK SUPPLY

"It's been two days since I delivered, and nothing comes out of my breasts when I squeeze them, not even colostrum. I'm worried that my baby is starving."

N ot only is your baby not starving, he or she isn't even hungry yet. Babies aren't born with an appetite, or with immediate nutritional needs. And by the time your baby begins to hunger for a breast full of milk (on the third or fourth postpartum day), you will undoubtedly be able to oblige.

Which isn't to say that your breasts are empty now. Colostrum (which provides your baby with enough nourishment and with important antibodies his or her own body can't yet produce, while helping to empty the digestive system of excess mucus and the bowels of meconium) is definitely present in the tiny amounts necessary. (A teaspoon or so is all your baby needs at this point.) But until the third or fourth postpartum day, when your breasts begin to swell and feel full, it's not that easy to express manually. Even a day-old baby, with no previous experience, is better equipped to extract this premilk than you are.

ENGORGED BREASTS

"My milk finally came in, leaving my breasts swollen to three times their normal size—and so hard, engorged, and painful that I can't bear to put on a bra. Is this what I have to look forward to until I wean my baby?"

If painfully tender, granite-hard breasts, the size of an exotic dancer's, were indeed what mothers had to look forward to for the duration of the breastfeeding experience, most babies would be weaned before they entered their second week of life. The engorgement, caused by the milk's arrival, can make nursing agonizing for the mother and, because the nipples are flattened by the swelling, frustrating for the baby. The condition can be aggravated when the initial feeding doesn't begin until 24 to 36 hours after birth, as is common in some hospitals.

Happily, the engorgement and its distressing effects gradually diminish once a well-coordinated milk supply-and-demand system is established—within a matter of days. Nipple soreness, too—which usually peaks at about the 20th feeding—generally disappears rapidly as the nipples toughen up from frequent nursing. Some women, particularly those with fair skin, may also experience nipple cracking and bleeding. This, with proper care, is also only temporary. Until nursing becomes as gratifying and fulfilling as you had hoped it would be—and, believe it or not, painless—there are some steps you can take to reduce the discomfort and speed the establishment of a good milk supply (see Getting Started Breastfeeding, page 294).

ENGORGEMENT IF YOU'RE NOT BREASTFEEDING

"I'm not nursing. I understand that drying up the milk can be painful."

Whether you nurse or not, your breasts will become engorged (overfilled) with milk on the third or fourth postpartum day. This can be uncomfortable, even painful. However, it is blessedly temporary.

Some physicians rely on hormones to suppress lactation. But since the drugs sometimes fail to relieve engorgement (and, if they do, it often returns a week or two after the medication is discontinued), most practitioners prefer the natural course, letting the body itself take care of suppressing milk production. The breasts are designed to produce milk only as needed. If the milk isn't used, production ceases. Though sporadic leaking may continue for several days, or even weeks, severe engorgement shouldn't last more than 12 to 24 hours. During this time, ice packs and mild pain relievers may be prescribed. Wearing a well-fitting, supportive bra is important until your breasts return to normal.

BONDING

"My new son was premature and I won't get to hold him for at least two weeks. Will it be too late for good bonding?"

Bonding, the process of attachment between a mother and her newborn child, has in recent years become a *cause célèbre* in childbirth circles. The term originated in the 1970s, when some studies began to show that the separation of an infant from its mother immediately after birth posed a threat both to their lifelong relationship and to the infant's future relationships with others. Some very positive changes in postchildbirth procedure have come about because of this work. Today, many hospitals permit new mothers to hold their babies moments after birth, and to cuddle and nurse them for anywhere from 10 minutes to an hour or more, instead of whisking the newborns off to the nursery the moment the cord is cut.

But as sometimes happens with the popularization of a good idea, the concept of bonding became misunderstood and abused (one of the doctors who published the first book on the subject now says: "I wish we'd never written the statement"), with some unfortunate results. Mothers who have surgical deliveries and are unable to see their babies at birth worry that their parent-child relationship will be forever tarnished. The same worry haunts parents whose babies must be in neonatal intensive care for several days or weeks, giving them little bonding opportunity. So frantic have some parents become about the necessity for instant bonding that they are demanding it even at risk to their infants.

Of course, initial bonding in the delivery room is nice. This early meeting of mother and baby gives them a chance to make contact, skin to skin, eye to eye. It's the first step in the development of a lasting parent-child bond. But only the *first* step. And it doesn't have to take place at the moment of birth. It can take place later in a hospital bed, or through the portholes of an incubator, or even weeks later at home. When your parents were born, they probably saw little of their mothers and even less of their fathers until they went home—usually 10 days after birth—and the vast majority of this "deprived" generation grew up with strong, loving family ties. Mothers who had the chance to bond at birth with one child and not with another usually report no difference in their feelings toward the children. And adoptive parents, who often don't meet their babies until hospital discharge (or even much later) manage to foster strong bonds. Some experts believe, in fact, that bonding doesn't really take place until somewhere in the second half of the baby's first year. Certainly it is a complex process that isn't accomplished in minutes.

It's never too late to tie the bonds that bind. So, instead of wasting energy regretting the time you've lost, prepare to make the most of the lifetime of mothering you have ahead.

"I've been told that bonding brings mother and child closer together, but every time I hold my baby, she seems like a stranger to me."

Love at first sight is a concept that flourishes in romantic books and movies, but rarely materializes in real life. The kind of love that lasts a lifetime usually requires time, nurturing, and plenty of patience to develop and deepen. And that's as true for the love between a newborn and its parents as it is between a man and a woman.

Physical closeness between mother and child immediately after birth does not guarantee instant emotional closeness. Feelings of affection don't flow as quickly and surely as lochia; those first few postpartum seconds aren't automatically bathed in the glow of maternal love. In fact, the first sensation a woman experiences after birth is far more likely to be relief than love—relief that the baby is normal and, especially if her labor was difficult, that the ordeal is over. It's not at all unusual to see that squalling and unsociable infant as a stranger—with very little connection to the cozy, idealized little fetus you carried for nine months—and to feel little more than neutral toward him or her. One study found that it took an average of over two weeks (and often as long

as nine weeks) for mothers to begin having positive feelings toward their newborns.

Just how a woman reacts to her newborn at their first meeting may depend on a variety of factors: the length and intensity of her labor; whether she received tranquilizers and/or anesthetics during labor; her previous experience (or lack of it) with infants; her feelings about having a child; her relationship with her husband; extraneous worries that may preoccupy her; her general health; and, probably most important of all, her personality. *Your* reaction is normal for *you*.

And as long as you feel an increasing sense of comfort and attachment as the days go by, you can relax. Some of the best relationships get off to the slowest starts. Give yourself and your baby a chance to get to know and appreciate each other, and let the love grow unhurriedly.

If you don't feel a growing closeness after a few weeks, or if you feel anger or antipathy toward your baby, discuss these feelings with your pediatrician. It's important to work them out early on, to prevent lasting damage to your relationship.

ROOMING-IN

"In childbirth class, having the baby room-in with me sounded like heaven. Since I gave birth, it's been more like hell. I can't get the baby to stop crying—yet what kind of mother would I be if I asked the nurse to take her?"

You would be a very human mother. You've just completed

the more-than-Herculean task (Hercules couldn't have done it) of giving birth, and are about to embark on an even greater challenge: child rearing. Needing a few days' rest in between is nothing to feel guilty about.

Of course, some women handle rooming-in with ease. They may have had easy deliveries that left them feeling exhilarated instead of exhausted. Or they may have had experience caring for newborns, their own or other people's. For these women, an inconsolable infant at 3 A.M. may not be a joy, but it's not a nightmare, either. For a woman who's been without sleep for 48 hours, however, whose body has been left limp from an enervating labor, and who's never been closer to a baby than a diaper ad, such predawn bouts can leave her wondering tearfully: "Why did I ever decide to become a mother?"

Playing the martyr can raise motherly resentments against the baby, feelings the baby will be likely to sense. If, instead, the baby is sent back to the nursery between feedings at night, mother and child, both well rested, may have a better chance to get acquainted when morning comes.

Full-time rooming-in is a wonderful new option in family-centered maternity care—but it's not for everyone. You are *not* a failure or a bad mother if you don't enjoy, or feel too tired for, rooming-in. Don't be pushed into it if you don't think you want it; and once you've committed yourself, don't feel you can't change your mind. Partial rooming-in (during the day but not at night) may be a good solution for you. Or you might prefer to get a good night's sleep the first night and start rooming-in on the second.

Be flexible. Be more concerned with the quality of the time you spend with your baby in the hospital than the quantity. Round-the-clock rooming-in will begin soon enough at home. And by then, if you are sensible now, you should be emotionally and physically ready to deal with it.

GOING HOME

"My labor was almost effortless, and I feel great. Why should I have to stay in the hospital if I have nothing to recover from?"

Chances are *you* don't have to stay in the hospital. Though 10-day hospital stays were once considered a necessary precaution after giving birth, it's now recognized that a woman who's had an uncomplicated delivery really doesn't need any hospitalization. Your baby, on the other hand, generally does. A minimum of two, but an average of three, days of observation is fairly standard in most hospitals, although that standard may be adjusted at the discretion of your pediatrician—and occasionally a pediatrician will allow for discharge within 24 hours after birth. The major reason for a delay in discharge is to watch for jaundice (a yellowing of the skin), which develops in more than 50% of newborns within the first 24 to 36 hours after birth. Though jaundice is rarely a major complication, many pediatricians prefer to keep the newborn in the hospital an extra day or two, or until it clears up. Others allow for early discharge in mild cases, assuming the infant is otherwise in good health, and providing that the doctor will be able to see him or her within a few days.

Of course, no one can hold you or your baby hostage in the hospital against your will. You have the right to sign yourself and your baby out of the hospital A.M.A. (against medical advice) at any time—if you take full legal, written responsibility for the consequences. But unless you have a degree in medicine, it would be extremely unwise to play doctor. If either your pediatrician or obstetrician recommends a prolonged stay, ask for an explanation—but do follow their professional advice. And try to make the best of your longer sojourn, getting as much rest as you can while you still have the chance.

Even if your doctors authorize your early release, you'd be smart to veto it if you don't have full-time help (either hired or volunteer) waiting for you. It's important to rest postpartum—in the hospital or at home.

RECOVERY FROM A CESAREAN SECTION

"How different will my recuperation be from that of a woman with a vaginal delivery?"

Recovery from a cesarean section is similar to recovery from any major abdominal surgery—with a delightful difference: Instead of losing an old gall bladder or appendix,

you've gained a brand new baby.

Of course, there's another difference, slightly less delightful. In addition to recovering from surgery, you'll also be recovering from childbirth. Except for a neatly intact perineum, you'll experience all the same postpartum discomforts you would have had if you'd delivered vaginally—afterpains, lochia, breast engorgement, fatigue, hormonal changes, hair loss, excessive perspiration, and the baby blues. (See this chapter and the next for tips on how to deal with all of these.)

As for your surgical recovery, you can expect the following in the recovery room:

A Wearing Off of Anesthesia. Until your general anesthesia wears off, you will be observed carefully in the recovery room. Your memory of this time may later be fuzzy or totally absent. Since everyone responds differently to drugs—and each drug is different—whether you are clearheaded and alert in a few hours or not for a day or two will depend upon you and upon the medications you were given. If you feel disoriented, or have hallucinations or bad dreams when you awaken, your husband or an understanding nurse can help you get back to reality quickly. You will also stay in the recovery room if you've had a spinal or epidural block. It will take longer for these to wear off—which they usually do from the toes up. You will be encouraged to wiggle your toes and move your feet as soon as you can. If you've had a spinal block, you will have to stay flat on your back for about 8 to 12 hours. You may be allowed to have both your husband and your baby visit with you in the recovery room.

Pain Around Your Incision. Once the anesthesia wears off, your wound, like any wound, is going to hurt—though just how much depends on many factors, including your personal pain threshold and how many cesareans you've had. (The first is usually the most uncomfortable.) You will probably be given pain relief medication as needed, which may give you a woozy or drugged feeling. It will also allow you to get some needed sleep. You needn't be concerned if you're nursing; the medication won't get into your colostrum, and by the time your milk comes in, you probably won't need any medication.

Possible Nausea, and Maybe Vomiting. This doesn't always happen, but if it does, you may be given an antiemetic preparation to prevent vomiting. (If you vomit easily, you might want to talk to your doctor about giving you such a medication before the symptoms appear.)

Breathing and Coughing Exercises. These help rid your system of any leftover general anesthetic, and help to expand your lungs and keep them clear to prevent pneumonia. Such necessary lung calisthenics may be very uncomfortable if you do them correctly. You may be able to minimize this discomfort by "splinting" your incision with a pillow.

Regular Evaluations of Your Condition. A nurse will check your vital signs (temperature, blood pressure, pulse, respiration), your urinary output and vaginal flow, the dressing on your incision, and the firmness and level of your uterus (as it shrinks in size and makes its way back into the pelvis). She will also check your IV and urinary catheter.

Once you have been moved to your hospital room, you can expect:

Continuing Evaluation of Your Condition. Your vital signs, your urinary output and vaginal flow, your dressing, and your uterus, as well as your IV and catheter (as long as they remain in place) will be checked regularly.

Removal of the Catheter After 24 Hours. Urination may be difficult, so try the tips on page 284. If they don't work, the catheter may be reinserted until you can urinate by yourself.

Afterpains. These start about 12 to 24 hours after delivery. See page 282 for more about these occasional contractions.

Removal of the IV. About 24 hours after surgery, or when your bowels begin to show signs of activity (by producing gas), your IV will be discontinued and you will be allowed some fluids by mouth. Over the next few days, you will probably progress to soft foods, and then to a normal diet. Even if you feel as though you are starving, don't try to circumvent doctor's orders by having someone sneak in a Big Mac. Take it easy getting back to your normal diet. If you are breastfeeding, be sure to get plenty of fluids.

Referred Shoulder Pain. Irritation of the diaphragm following surgery can cause a few hours of sharp shoulder pain. An analgesic may help.

Possible Constipation. It may be a few days until you have a bowel movement, and that's all right. A stool softener may be prescribed to help move things along. Try some of the tips given on page 285, but exclude the roughage for the first few days. If you haven't had a movement by the fifth or sixth day, you may be given a laxative, an enema, or a suppository.

Encouragement to Exercise. Before you are out of bed, you will be encouraged to wiggle your toes, flex your calves, bend your feet up at the ankles, push against the end of the bed with your feet, and turn from side to side. You can also try these: (1) Lie flat on your back, bend one knee, then extend the other leg, while tightening your abdomen slightly. Slide the bent leg slowly back down; repeat with the other leg. (2) Lie on your back, knees pulled up, feet flat on the bed, and raise your head for about 30 seconds. (3) On your back, knees bent, tighten your abdomen, and reach with one arm across your body to the other side of the bed, at about waist level. Reverse. These exercises will improve circulation, especially in your legs, and prevent the development of blood clots. (But be prepared for some of these to be quite painful, at least for the first 24 hours or so.)

To Get Up Between 8 and 24 Hours After Surgery. With the help of the nurse, you'll sit up first, supported by the raised head of the bed. Then, using your hands for support, you will slide your legs over the side of the bed and dangle them for a few minutes. Then, slowly, you'll be helped to step down on the floor, your hands still on the bed. If you feel dizzy (which is normal), sit right back down. Steady yourself for a few more minutes before taking a couple of steps. Those steps may be extremely painful. Stand as straight as you can, though the temptation to hunch over to ease the discomfort may be great. (This difficulty in getting around is temporary; in fact, you may soon find yourself more mobile than the vaginal deliveree next door—and you will certainly have the edge in sitting.)

To Wear Elastic Stockings. These improve circulation and help prevent blood clots in the legs.

Abdominal Discomfort. As your digestive tract (temporarily put out of business by surgery) begins to function again, trapped gas can cause considerable pain, especially when it presses against your incision line. The discomfort may be worse when you laugh, cough, or sneeze. Tell the nurse or doctor about your problem and they will suggest some remedies. Narcotics are not usually recommended because they can prolong the difficulties, which ordinarily last just a day or two. You may get a small enema or a suppository to release the gas. Or you may be advised to walk up and down the corridor. Lying on your left side or on your back, your knees drawn up, taking deep breaths while holding your incision, may help. If the pain remains severe, a tube may be inserted in your rectum to help the gas escape.

Time with Your Baby. You can't lift the baby yet, but you can cuddle and feed him or her. (If you're nursing, place the baby on a pillow over your incision.) Depending on how you feel, and on hospital regulations, you may be able to have modified rooming-in. Some hospitals even allow full rooming-in.

Sponge Baths. Until the stitches are removed (or absorbed), you probably won't be allowed a real bath or shower.

Removal of Stitches. If your stitches aren't self-absorbing, they will be removed about five or six days after delivery. And although the procedure isn't very painful, you may find it uncomfortable. When the dressing is off, look at the incision with the nurse or doctor; ask how soon you can expect the area to heal, which changes will be normal, which might require medical care.

You can expect to go home about five to seven days postpartum.

WHAT IT'S IMPORTANT TO KNOW
GETTING STARTED BREASTFEEDING

E ver since Eve put Cain to suckle for the first time, breastfeeding has been coming naturally to mothers and newborns. Right?

Well, not always—at least not immediately. Though nursing does come naturally, it comes naturally a little later for some mothers and babies than for others. Sometimes there are physical factors which foil those first few attempts; at other times it's just a simple lack of experience on the part of both participants. But whatever might be keeping your baby and your breasts apart, it won't be long before they're in perfect synch—as long as you don't give up first. Some of the most

mutually satisfying breast-baby relationships begin with several days of fumbling, of bungled efforts, and of tears on both sides.

Knowing just what to expect and how to deal with setbacks can help ease the mutual adjustment:

❖ Start as soon as possible after birth. Right in the delivery room is best, when that's feasible. (See Breastfeeding Basics, page 296.) But sometimes mother's not in any condition to nurse, sometimes baby isn't—neither of which means they won't be able to start successfully later. (That's not to say that if you feel well and the baby does, too, this first nursing experience will necessarily go smoothly. You both have a lot to learn.)

❖ Don't let hospital bureaucracy break your tentative connection with insensitivity, ignorance, and unnecessary rules. Enlist the support of your doctor in advance to be sure that you will be allowed to nurse in the delivery room if all goes normally. Also, arrange for full or partial rooming-in, or for a demand-feeding schedule (having the nursery bring the baby when he or she is hungry) if the staff will oblige. If the baby is with you all day, this may mean limiting visiting privileges to just your husband, which is probably for the best anyway since it allows the three of you to get to know each other, while maintaining the relaxed atmosphere needed for nursing.

❖ Don't let sleeping babies lie, if it means that they'll sleep through a feeding. If you have rooming-in, you're not likely to have a problem with this. You'll be able to demand-feed the baby when he or she is hungry and let the baby sleep when he or she's sleepy. If you're dependent on the nursery staff to bring the baby—on their schedule, not junior's—you may find that the allotted feeding period will be up before the baby wakes, and that someone will come to collect him or her unfed. Don't let this happen. If the baby isn't awake on arrival at your room, wake him or her. This sounds crueler than it actually is. Gently set the baby on the bed in a sitting position, one hand holding up the chin, the other supporting the back. Next, bend the baby forward at the waist. The moment he or she stirs, quickly adopt the nursing position. If your baby is swaddled, loosen the blanket so he or she can be close to you.

❖ Be patient if your baby is still recovering from your labor. If you received anesthesia or had a prolonged, difficult labor, you can expect your baby to be drowsy and sluggish at the breast for a few days. This is no reflection on you, your nursing ability, or your baby. There's no danger the baby will starve in the meantime, since newborns have little need for nourishment during the first days of life. What they do need, though, is nurturing. Cuddling at the breast is just as important as suckling.

❖ Make sure your baby's appetite and sucking instinct aren't sabotaged between feedings. It's routine in some hospital nurseries to quiet a crying baby between mother's feedings with a bottle of sugar water. This can have a twofold detrimental effect. Firstly, it satisfies the baby's still-delicate appetite for hours. Later, when brought to you for feeding, your baby won't want to nurse, and your breasts won't be stimulated to produce milk—a vicious cycle is begun. Second, because the rubber nipple requires less effort, the baby's sucking reflex becomes lazy. Faced with the greater challenge of tackling the breast, he or

Breastfeeding Basics

1. Get into a comfortable position.

2. Use your thumb and index finger to pull the nipple erect.

3. Tilt the nipple slightly upward, toward the roof of the baby's mouth.

4. Bring the nipple toward the baby's cheek so that it brushes the corner of his or her mouth. This will stimulate the rooting reflex (or you can use a spare finger to do this) which makes the baby turn its mouth toward the touch.

5. Repeat steps 3 and 4 several times; the baby should eventually take the nipple in his or her mouth. (Let the baby take the initiative; don't stuff the nipple into an unwilling mouth.)

6. Be sure the areola and the nipple, and not just the nipple, are in the baby's mouth. Sucking on just the nipple won't compress the milk glands and can cause soreness and cracking. Also be sure that it is the nipple that the baby is busily milking. Some infants are eager to suck (even if no milk is forthcoming) and can give you a painful bruise by gumming sensitive breast tissue.

7. Use your finger to press the breast away from the baby's nose to prevent interference with breathing.

8. You can assure yourself that your baby is suckling if there is a strong steady rhythmic motion in his or her cheek.

9. If your baby has finished suckling but is still holding on to the breast, pulling it out abruptly can cause injury to the nipple. Instead, break the suction first by depressing the breast or by putting your finger into the corner of the baby's mouth to admit some air.

Whatever is comfortable for you and the baby is a good position; prop with pillows as necessary. And be sure not to block the baby's tiny nose with your breast.

she may just give up. *Don't let anyone talk you into the sugar water.* Give strict orders—through your pediatrician—that supplementary feedings are not to be given to your baby in the nursery unless medically necessary.[2]

❖ Don't try to feed a screaming baby. It's hard enough for an inexperienced suckler to find the nipple when calm. When your baby is overexcited, it may be impossible. Rock and soothe him or her before you start nursing.

❖ If you're having trouble establishing breastfeeding, ask for assistance from hospital personnel or from your practitioner. If you are lucky, a nursery nurse will join you at your first baby feeding to provide hands-on instruction, helpful hints and, perhaps, literature. If this is not a policy in your hospital (or you are somehow bypassed), you can find empathy and advice by calling your local La Leche League chapter.

❖ No matter how frustrating nursing becomes, try to stay calm. Start out as relaxed as you can. Clear out the visitors 15 minutes before feeding time, and don't look at your hospital bill or anything else that might upset you. Then remain cool throughout the nursing period, no matter how badly it's going. Tension not only hampers your ability to give milk, it can cause anxiety in your baby. An infant is extremely sensitive to your moods, and reacts accordingly.

WHEN THE MILK COMES IN

Just when you and your baby seem to be getting the hang of it, your milk comes in. Up until now, your baby has been getting tiny amounts of colostrum (premilk), and your breasts have been quite comfortable. Then, within a few hours, your breasts become swollen, hard, and painful. Nursing is difficult for the baby and agonizing for you.[3] Fortunately, this period of engorement is brief. While it lasts, there are a variety of ways of relieving it and the accompanying discomfort:

❖ Nurse more often, for shorter periods—a four-hour schedule can lead to engorement, and 20-minute nursing periods to sore nipples; both make nursing difficult in the long run for mother and baby. Start off with 5 minutes on each breast, gradually building up to 15 minutes each by the third or fourth day.

❖ Don't be tempted to skip or skimp on a feeding because of pain. The less your baby sucks, the more engorged you will be-

---

2. You may also want to discuss with your pediatrician the pros and cons of a pacifier being given to your baby in the nursery. On the one hand, it could get him or her hooked on a rubber nipple; on the other, it may be comforting when there's no one to cuddle with in the middle of the night.

3. A few lucky new mothers don't experience engorement when their milk comes in, possibly because their babies were vigorous nursers from birth; there is also less engorement with subsequent babies.

Baby and Breast—A Perfect Feeding Team

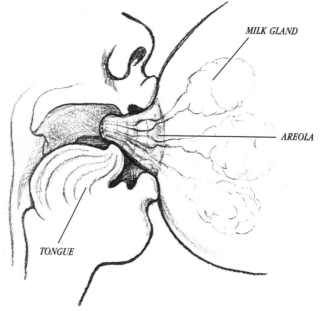

MILK GLAND

AREOLA

TONGUE

Just be sure that the nursing baby has the areola and not just the nipple in his or her mouth. This way the milk can be efficiently and, eventually, painlessly extracted.

come. Don't favor one breast because it is less sore or because the nipple isn't cracked; the only way to toughen up nipples is to use them. Use both breasts at every feeding, even if only for a few minutes—but nurse from the less sore one first, since the baby will suck more vigorously when hungry. If both nipples are equally sore (or not sore at all), start off the next feeding with the breast you used last.

❖ Use a breast pump on each breast before nursing to lessen the engorgement so that your baby can get a better hold on the nipple, and to get milk flow started. After nursing, empty the second breast

if the baby hasn't already done so.

❖ Use ice packs to reduce engorgement. Or a hot shower or hot soaks, if you find them more soothing.

❖ Support is important in a nursing bra, but pressure against your sore and engorged breasts can be painful. Whenever leaking isn't a problem—and especially after nursing—leave the flaps of your nursing bra open.

SORE NIPPLES

Tender nipples sometimes compound the difficulties of early nursing. Most toughen up quickly.

But in some women, particularly those who are fair skinned, the nipples become sore and cracked. To relieve the discomfort:

❖ Expose sore or cracked nipples to the air as much as possible.

❖ Let nature—and not the cosmetic companies—take care of your nipples. Nipples are naturally protected and lubricated by sweat glands and skin oils. A commercial preparation should be used only when nipple cracking is severe, and then should be as pure as possible. Unmedicated lanolin is effective; petroleum-based ointments are not. Wash only with water—never with soap, alcohol, tincture of benzoin, or premoistened towelettes—whether your nipples are sore or not: Your baby is already protected from your germs, and the milk itself is clean.

❖ Vary your nursing position so a different part of the nipple will be compressed at each feeding.

❖ Relax for 15 minutes or so before feeding, occasionally with a small glass of wine or beer. Relaxation will enhance the let-down of milk, whereas tension will only hinder it.

OCCASIONAL COMPLICATIONS

Once nursing is established, it generally continues uneventfully until weaning. But once in a while, complications occur, among them:

Clogged Milk Ducts. Sometimes a milk duct clogs, causing milk to back up. Since this condition (characterized by a small, red, and tender lump on the breast) can lead to infection, it's important to try to remedy it quickly. The best way to do this is to offer the affected breast first at each feeding, and let your baby empty it as completely as possible. If he or she doesn't do the job, any remaining milk should be expressed by hand or with a breast pump. Keep pressure off the duct by being sure your bra is not too tight, and by varying your nursing positions to put pressure on different ducts. Also, check to see if dried milk is blocking the nipple after nursing. If so, clean it off with sterile cotton dipped in boiled and cooled water. Do not use this time to wean the baby; discontinuing nursing now will only compound your problem.

Breast Infection. A more serious complication of breastfeeding is mastitis, or breast infection, which usually occurs in one or both breasts between the 10th and 28th postpartum day, in about 1% of mothers— usually first-timers. A crack or fissure in the skin of the nipple occurs and allows the passage of germs into the milk ducts.

Symptoms of mastitis are severe soreness, hardness, redness, heat, and swelling of the breast, with generalized chills and a fever of about 101 to 102 degrees. If you develop some of these symptoms, contact your doctor. Prompt medical treatment is necessary, and may include bed rest, antibiotics, pain relievers, and ice or heat applications. During

Best-Odds Nursing Diet

The levels of protein, fat, and carbohydrates in your breast milk aren't usually affected by the levels of these nutrients in your diet; however, levels of some vitamins are (A and B$_{12}$, for example). But though the quality of your milk isn't always directly related to the quality of your diet, the quantity of milk usually is. Women whose diets are deficient in protein and/or calories, for example, will produce milk of good composition but in smaller amounts. To make good breast milk, and plenty of it, continue taking your pregnancy (or pregnancy/lactation) vitamin-mineral supplement, and adhere closely to the Best-Odds Diet on page 75, with the following modifications:

❖ Increase your caloric intake to about 500 calories per day over your pre-pregnancy requirements. This is flexible, and as during pregnancy, you can let your scale be your guide. If you have a lot of fat stored from pregnancy (or before), you can take fewer calories, as the fat will be burned to produce milk (and you will lose weight). If you are underweight, you will probably need more than 500 additional calories daily (the recommended daily allowance assumes some use of fat stores, which you don't have). No matter what your weight, you may find that you need more calories as the baby grows and demands more milk. Again, you will be able to determine this by checking your scale. If your weight starts dipping below the ideal, increase your daily intake.

❖ Increase your calcium requirement by one serving per day.

❖ Reduce your protein intake by one serving per day.

❖ Drink at least eight glasses of fluids (milk, water, broths or soups, and juices); take more if it's very hot, and if you've been losing a lot through perspiration. (Though it's all right to drink moderate amounts of tea or coffee, and an occasional alcoholic beverage, you can't count them in your fluid allowance, since they have a dehydrating effect.) Excess is not best, however; flooding yourself with too much fluid (more than 12 glasses per day) can paradoxically *slow* milk production. Thirst and urinary output can help gauge your needs.

❖ Splurge occasionally. You've served your nine-month sentence of abstinence; you're entitled to your just desserts, at least once in a while. The key is moderation. Small amounts of sugar won't interfere with milk production, but a steady diet of sweets will, by cutting down on your appetite for necessary nutrients. Ditto for other nutritionally superfluous foods, such as potato chips, french fries, white bread; eat them only *after* you've fulfilled your nutritional obligations.

---

treatment you should continue to nurse. Since germs from the baby probably gave you the infection, it won't harm him or her. And emptying the breast will help to prevent clogged milk ducts. Nurse first on the infected breast and empty it with a pump if the baby doesn't.

Delay in treating mastitis could lead to the development of a breast abscess, the symptoms of which include: excruciating, throbbing pain; localized swelling, tenderness, and heat in the area of the abscess; and temperature swings between 100 and 103 degrees. Treatment includes antibiotics and, generally, surgical drainage under anesthesia. Breastfeeding with the affected breast must be halted, and a breast pump should be used regularly to empty it until healing is complete and breastfeeding can be resumed. In the meantime, nursing can continue on the unaffected breast.

Don't let breast and nursing problems with your first baby discourage you from nursing future babies. Engorgement and nipple soreness are far less common with subsequent births.

BREASTFEEDING TWINS

B reastfeeding, like just about every aspect of caring for newborn twins, seems impossible until you get into the rhythm of it. Once you have a routine, it is not only possible, but very rewarding. To successfully nurse twins, you should:

❖ Fulfill all the dietary recommendations for lactating mothers (see the Best-Odds Nursing Diet), with these additions: take 400 to 500 calories above your prepregnancy needs for *each* baby you are nursing (you may need to increase your caloric intake as the babies grow bigger and hungrier, or decrease it if you supplement nursing with formula and/or solids, or if you have considerable fat reserves you would like to burn); an additional serving of protein (four total) and an additional serving of calcium (six total) or a calcium supplement.

❖ Drink 8 to 12 cups of fluid a day, but not more, because too much may suppress milk production.

❖ Get as much help as you can with housework, meal preparation, and infant care, to conserve your energy.

❖ Explore the various feeding options: nurse one baby, bottle feed the other; alternate feedings of bottle and breast with each baby; or nurse each separately (which can take 10 hours or more a day just for feeding), or both together. Combining individual and group feedings, and giving each infant one private feeding a day, is a good compromise which encourages mother-baby closeness. Father might give a bottle to the other baby at these feedings. Such relief bottles, given by the father or another helper, can be formula or expressed milk.

❖ Recognize that the twins have different needs, personalities, and nursing patterns, and don't try to treat them identically. Keep records to be sure both are fed at each feeding.

16
Postpartum: The First Six Weeks

WHAT YOU CAN EXPECT AT YOUR SIX-WEEK CHECKUP

Most practitioners will schedule the mother for a five- or six-week postpartum visit.[1] During that visit, you can expect the following to be checked, though the exact content of the visit will vary depending upon your particular needs and your practitioner's style of practice.

❖ Blood pressure

❖ Weight, which should be down by 17 to 20 pounds or more

❖ Shape, size, and location of uterus, to see if it has returned to prepregnant condition and location

❖ Condition of cervix, which will be on its way back to its prepregnant state, but will still be somewhat engorged, and the surface possibly eroded

❖ Condition of vagina, which will have contracted and regained much of its muscle tone

❖ The episiotomy or laceration repair site, if any; or, if you had a cesarean delivery, the site of your incision

❖ Your breasts, for any abnormalities

❖ Hemorrhoids or varicose veins, if they developed during pregnancy

❖ Questions or problems you want to discuss—have a list ready

At this visit, the practitioner will

---

1. If you had a cesarean, your physician may also check your incision at about three weeks postpartum.

also discuss with you the method of birth control that you will be using. (See page 314.) If you plan on using a diaphragm and your cervix has recovered sufficiently, you will be fitted for one; if not, you may have to use condoms until you can be fitted. If you're not breastfeeding and plan to take birth control pills, they may be prescribed now.

WHAT YOU MAY BE FEELING

PHYSICALLY:

❖ Continued vaginal discharge (lochia), turned brownish, then yellowish-white

❖ Fatigue

❖ Some pain, discomfort, and numbness in the perineum, if you had a vaginal delivery (especially if you had stitches)

❖ Diminishing incisional pain; continuing numbness, if you had a cesarean delivery (especially if it was your first)

❖ Continued constipation (although this should be easing up)

❖ Gradual flattening of your abdomen as your uterus recedes into the pelvis (but only exercise will bring you back to prepregnancy shape)

❖ Gradual loss of weight

❖ Breast discomfort and nipple soreness until breastfeeding is well established

❖ Achiness in arms and neck (from carrying the baby)

❖ Hair loss

EMOTIONALLY:

❖ Elation, depression, or swings between the two

❖ A sense of being overwhelmed, a growing feeling of confidence, or swings between the two

❖ Lowered libido

❖ Decreased sexual desire

WHAT YOU MAY BE CONCERNED ABOUT

FEVER

"I've just returned home from the hospital and I'm running a fever of about 101 degrees. Could it be related to childbirth?"

Thanks to Dr. Ignaz Semmelweiss, the chances of a new mother developing childbirth (or puerperal) fever today are extremely slight. It was in 1847 that this young Viennese physician discovered that if birth attendants washed their hands before delivering babies, the risk of childbirth-related infection could be greatly reduced (though at the time, his theory was considered so outlandish that he was driven from his post, ostracized, and later died a broken man). And thanks to Sir Alexander Fleming, the British scientist who developed the first infection-fighting antibiotics, the occasional case that does occur is easily cured.

The most severe cases of infection usually begin within 24 hours of delivery. A fever on the third or fourth day, when you are already at home, could possibly be a sign of postpartum infection—but it could also be caused by a virus or other minor problem. A low-grade fever (of about 100 degrees) can occasionally accompany engorgement when your milk first comes in, or even result from the excitement of coming home with your baby.

In postpartum infection, the symptoms will vary according to the site of origin. A slight fever, vague lower abdominal pain, and perhaps a foul-smelling vaginal discharge characterize endometritis, an infection of the endometrium (the lining of the uterus), vulnerable because of detachment of the placenta. Infection is even more likely to occur here if a fragment of the placenta has been retained. With infection of a laceration to the cervix, vagina, or vulva, there will usually be pain and tenderness in the area; sometimes a foul-smelling, thick discharge; abdominal or flank pain; or difficult urination. In certain types of infection, the fever spikes as high as 105 degrees, and there are chills, headache, malaise. On occasion, there are no obvious symptoms but fever.

Treatment with antibiotics is very effective, but it should begin quickly. Report any fever during the first three postpartum weeks to the doctor—even if it's accompanied by obvious cold or flu symptoms—so that its cause can be diagnosed and any necessary treatment started.

DEPRESSION

"I have everything I have always wanted: a wonderful husband, a beautiful new baby—why do I feel so blue?"

Why should roughly one half of all new mothers be so miserable during one of the happiest times of their lives? That's the paradox of postpartum depression, for which experts have yet to provide any definitive explanations or solutions.

Hormones, so often the culprit fingered in the case of a woman's mood swings, may offer some rationale. Levels of estrogen and progesterone drop precipitously after childbirth and may trigger depression, just as hormonal fluctuations prior to menstruation may do. The fact that sensitivity to hormonal fluctuations varies from woman to woman is believed to explain at least partially why, though all women experience the same shift in hormone levels after delivery, only about 50% suffer from postpartum depression.

But there are a host of other factors that probably contribute to the postpartum blues—which are most common around the third day after delivery, but which can strike at anytime during the first year, and which afflict second-time mothers more often than first-timers:

The Shift from Center Stage to Backstage. Your baby is now the star of the show. Visitors would rather run to the nursery than sit at your bedside inquiring after your health. This change in status will accompany you home; the pregnant princess is now the postpartum Cinderella.

Hospitalization. When you're eager to get home and begin mothering, you may be frustrated by the lack of control you have over your life and your baby's in the hospital.

Going Home. It's not unusual to feel overwhelmed and overworked by the responsibilities that greet you (particularly if you have other children and no help).

Exhaustion. Fatigue from a strenuous labor and from too little sleep in the hospital is compounded by the rigors of caring for a newborn, and often leads to the feeling that you aren't equal to the demands of motherhood.

A Sense of Disappointment in the Baby. He or she's so small, so red, so puffy, so unresponsive—not quite the all-smiles Ivory Snow baby you'd pictured. Resultant guilt adds to depression.

A Sense of Disappointment in the Birth and/or in Yourself. If unrealistic expectations of an idealized childbirth experience weren't realized, you may feel (unnecessarily) that you're a failure.

A Feeling of Anticlimax. Childbirth—the big event you'd schooled for and looked forward to—is over.

Feelings of Inadequacy. A novice mother may wonder, "Why did I have a baby if I can't take care of it?"

A Sense of Mourning for the Old You. Your carefree, possibly career-oriented self, has died (at least temporarily) with your baby's birth.

Unhappiness over Your Looks. Before you were fat and pregnant, now you're just fat. You can't stand wearing maternity clothes, but nothing else fits.

Probably the only good thing that can be said about postpartum depression is that it doesn't last very long—about 48 hours for most women. And though there's no cure other than the passage of time, there are ways of fading those baby blues:

❖ If the blues arrive at the hospital, try to have your husband bring in dinner for the two of you; limit visitors if their chattering grates on your nerves, have more of them if they cheer you up. If it's the hospital that's getting you down, inquire about early discharge. (See Going Home, page 290.)

❖ Fight fatigue by accepting help from others, by being less compulsive about doing things that can wait, by trying to squeeze in a nap or rest period when your baby is sleeping. Use feeding times as rest periods, nursing or bottle-feeding in bed or in a comfortable chair with your feet up.

❖ Follow the Best-Odds Nursing Diet (see page 300) to keep your strength up (minus 500 calories and three calcium servings if you're not breastfeeding). Avoid sugar (especially combined with chocolate), which can act as a depressant.

❖ Unwind with your husband over a cocktail during the baby's evening feeding, but be careful not to overdo—too much can lead to morning-after depression.

❖ Treat yourself to dinner out, if possible. If not, make believe. Order dinner in (or let your husband cook), dress up, create a restaurant ambiance with candlelight and soft music, open a bottle of wine. And keep your sense of humor handy, in case the baby decides to interrupt your romantic interlude.

❖ Look good so you'll feel good. Walking around in a robe all day with unkempt hair would depress anyone. Shower before your husband leaves in the morning (or you may not have a chance again); comb your hair; put on makeup if you ordinarily wear it.

❖ Get out of the house. Go for a walk with the baby or, if someone volunteers to stay with him or her, without the baby. Exercise helps chase away the baby blues and will help you get rid of any postpartum flab that might be adding to your depression.

❖ If you think your misery might like some company, get together with any new mothers you know, and share your feelings with them. If you don't have any newly delivered friends, make some.

Ask your pediatrician for names of new mothers in your neighborhood, or contact women who were in your childbirth class, possibly organizing a weekly after-birth reunion. Or join a postpartum exercise class.

❖ If yours is the kind of misery that would rather be by itself, indulge in some solitude. Though depression usually feeds on itself, some experts believe that this is not true of the postpartum variety. If going out with cheerful people, or having cheerful people visit, makes you feel worse—don't do it. Don't, however, leave your husband out in the cold. Communication in the immediate postpartum period is vital for you both. (Husbands, too, are susceptible to postpartum depression, and yours may need you as much as you need him.)

Severe postpartum depression, which requires professional therapy, is extremely rare—less than 1 in 1,000. If your depression persists for more than two weeks and is accompanied by sleeplessness, lack of appetite, a feeling of hopelessness and helplessness—even suicidal urges—seek counseling promptly.

"I feel terrific, and have since the moment I delivered three weeks ago. Is all this good feeling building up to one terrific case of letdown?"

It's an unfortunate fact that feeling good doesn't get the kind of attention that feeling bad does. There's no shortage of articles in magazines and newspapers, or chapters in books, about the 50% of newly delivered women who suffer from postpartum depression; but there's little or nothing written about the other 50% who feel terrific after giving birth.

Baby blues are common, but they're by no means an absolute requirement of the postpartum period. And there's no reason to believe that you're in for an emotional crash because you've been feeling buoyant. Since the majority of baby blues cases occur within the first postpartum week, it's pretty safe to assume you've escaped them. If you'd like to play it even safer (or if you'd like to prevent a case next pregnancy around), see the tips for fading those baby blues, in the previous section.

RETURNING TO PREPREGNANCY WEIGHT AND SHAPE

"I knew I wouldn't be ready for a bikini right after delivery, but I still look six months pregnant a week later."

Though childbearing produces more rapid weight loss than the Scarsdale, Stillman, and Mayo Clinic diets combined (an average of 12 pounds at delivery), most women don't find it quite rapid enough. Particularly after they catch a glimpse of their postpartum silhouettes in the mirror—which can still look distressingly pregnant. But happily, most will be able to pack away their pregnancy jeans within the month.

Of course, how quickly you return to your prepregnant shape and weight will depend on how many pounds and inches you put on during pregnancy. Women who gained 25 pounds or less should be able, without dieting, to shed the weight by the end of the second month. Others will find that delivery won't make thighs and hips thickened by over-indulgence during pregnancy magically disappear. But sticking to the Best-Odds Nursing Diet (see page 300) if they are breastfeeding (or to the Diet minus the 500 extra nursing calories and three of the calcium servings[2] if they are not) should start them on the way to slow, steady weight loss. Non-nursers can, after the first six weeks, go on a good, well-balanced reducing diet, such as Weight Watchers. Nursing mothers with considerable amounts of excess body fat can cut their caloric intake somewhat without cutting into milk production and also lose weight. They will usually take off any remaining excess poundage when they wean their babies.

Unlike weight loss, getting back into shape is a problem even for those women who didn't gain excess weight. No one comes out of the delivery room looking much slimmer than when they went in. Part of the reason for that protruding postpartum abdomen is the still-enlarged uterus, which will be reduced to prepregnancy size by the end of six weeks, reducing your ab-

---

2. Though you won't need the calories and other nutrients of milk after pregnancy and/or lactation, it is now recommended that *all* women take a calcium supplement to bring their daily intake to 1,200 mg.

domen in the process. (You can follow the progress of your uterus by asking the nurse or your practitioner to show you how to palpate it in your abdomen. When you can no longer feel it, it has slipped back into the pelvis.) Another reason for your bloated belly is leftover fluids, 5 pounds or so of which will flush out within a few days. But the rest of the problem is stretched out abdominal muscles and skin, which will sag for a lifetime unless a concerted exercise effort is made. (See Getting Back into Shape, page 317.)

BREAST MILK

"Does everything I eat, drink, or take get into my breast milk? Could any of it harm my baby?"

Feeding your baby outside the womb doesn't demand quite as Spartan an existence as feeding him or her inside did. But as long as you're breastfeeding, a certain amount of restraint in what goes into you will ensure that everything that goes into your baby is safe.

The basic fat-protein-carbohydrate composition of human milk isn't dependent on what a mother eats. If a mother doesn't eat enough calories and protein to produce milk, her body's stores will be tapped and the baby will be fed—until the stores run out. Some vitamin deficiencies in the mother's diet will, however, affect the vitamin content of her breast milk. So will excesses of some vitamins. A wide variety of substances, from medications to seasonings, can also show

up in milk, with varying results.

To keep breast milk safe and healthful:

❖ Follow the Best-Odds Nursing Diet (page 300).

❖ Avoid foods to which your baby seems sensitive. Garlic, onion, cabbage, and chocolate are common offenders, causing bothersome gas in some, though by no means all, babies. Infants with discriminating palates may also be displeased by the taste a strong seasoning may impart.

❖ Take a vitamin supplement especially formulated for pregnant and/or lactating mothers. Do not take any other vitamins without the advice of your physician.

❖ Do not smoke. Many of the toxic substances in tobacco enter the bloodstream, and eventually your milk. (Besides, smoking near the baby can cause respiratory problems for him or her and may even be associated with sudden infant death syndrome, or crib death.)

❖ Do not take any medications or recreational drugs (other than moderate quantities of alcohol) without consulting your physician. Most drugs pass into the breast milk, and even in small doses can be harmful to a tiny infant. (Particularly dangerous are: antithyroid, antihypertensive, anticancer drugs; penicillin;[3] narcotic drugs, including heroin, methadone, and prescrip-

---

3. Exposure to penicillin at this early age could lead to a baby developing a sensitivity, or allergy, to the drug.

tion painkillers; marijuana and cocaine; tranquilizers, barbiturates and sedatives; lithium; hormones, such as birth control pills; radioactive iodine; bromides.) Often, safe substitutes can be found for a medication you must take; or perhaps a particular medication can be discontinued for the duration of nursing. (Do make sure that any doctor who prescribes a medication for you is aware that you are breastfeeding.)

❖ Drink alcoholic beverages only occasionally. Daily imbibing or binge drinking can make baby drowsy, depress the nervous system, and may slow motor development.

❖ Restrict your intake of caffeine. One cup of coffee or tea a day probably won't affect your baby. Six cups could make him or her jittery.

❖ Don't take laxatives (some of them will have a laxative effect on your baby); increase your fiber intake instead.

❖ Take aspirin or aspirin substitutes only with your practitioner's approval, but don't take more than the recommended dose, and don't take the drugs frequently.

❖ Avoid excessive amounts of chemicals in the foods you eat. An occasional diet soda won't hurt, but frequent use of saccharine or aspartame isn't a good idea. Read labels to steer clear of foods composed largely of synthetic chemicals—the possible effects of which are unknown.

❖ Minimize the incidental pesticides in your diet. A certain amount of pesticide residue in your diet (from produce, for example), and thus in your milk, is inevitable—and not proven to be harmful to a nursing infant. But though hysteria about breast milk contamination is unwarranted, it's prudent to keep your baby's exposure to pesticides from affected foods as low as you can without giving up eating. Scrub vegetable and fruit skins with detergent and water; eat low-fat milk products, lean meats, white-meat poultry with the skin removed, and limited amounts of organ meats. (The pesticides ingested by animals are stored in fat and skin.)

❖ Avoid eating freshwater fish, which might be contaminated. (The same rules for safe fish and seafood consumption that apply to pregnant women apply to lactating women; see pages 116-117.)

LONG-TERM CESAREAN RECOVERY

"I am just now going home, a week after a cesarean. What can I expect?"

A Need for Plenty of Help. Paid help is best for the first week, but if that's not possible, ask your husband, mother, or another relative to lend a hand. It's best not to do any lifting (including the baby), or any housework, at least for the first week. If you must lift the baby, lift from waist level, so you use your arms, not your abdomen. Bend at the knees, not at the waist.

Little or No Pain. But if you do hurt, a mild pain reliever will help. Don't take medication, however, if you are breastfeeding, unless approved by your doctor.

Progressive Improvement. The scar will be sore and sensitive for a few weeks, but will improve steadily. A light dressing may protect it from irritation. Wearing loose clothing will be more comfortable. Occasional pulling, twitching, and other brief pains in the region of the scar are a normal part of healing and will eventually subside. Itchiness may follow. The numbness of the abdomen around the scar will last longer, possibly several months. Lumpiness in the scar tissue will probably diminish (unless you tend to get that kind of scar), and the scar may turn pink or purple before it finally fades.

If pain becomes persistent, if the area around the incision turns an angry red, or if a brown, gray, green, or yellow discharge oozes from the wound, call your doctor. The incision may have become infected. (A small amount of clear fluid discharge may be normal, but report it to your physician anyway.)

To Wait at Least Four Weeks Before Resuming Sexual Intercourse. Depending on how your incision is healing and when your cervix returns to normal, your doctor may recommend that you wait anywhere from four to six weeks for actual intercourse (though other kinds of lovemaking are certainly permissible). See page 312 for tips on making postpartum intercourse more successful. Also see Postpartum Contraception, page 314. You are, incidentally, much more likely to find early postpartum intercourse comfortable than are women who delivered vaginally.

To Be Able to Start Exercising Once You Are Free of Pain. Since the muscle tone of your perineum probably hasn't been compromised, you may not need to do Kegel exercises. Concentrate instead on those that tighten the abdominal muscles. (See Getting Back into Shape, page 317.) Make "slow and steady" your motto; get into the program gradually and continue it daily. Expect it to take several months before you're back to your old self.

RESUMING SEXUAL RELATIONS

"My doctor says I have to wait six weeks before having sex. Friends say that isn't necessary."

It's fairly safe to assume that your doctor is more familiar with your medical condition than your friends are. And his or her restriction is probably based on what's best for you, taking into consideration the kind of labor and delivery you had, whether or not you had an episiotomy or laceration, and the speed of healing and recovery. Some practitioners, of course, apply the six-week rule routinely to all their postpartum patients, regardless of condition. If you think that's the case with your doctor, and you're feeling up to making love, ask if he or she will consider bending the rule for you. This will be possible only if your cervix has healed and the lochia has stopped. And, for your own comfort, you probably will also want to wait until intercourse no longer causes pain in your perineal area.

Should your plea be denied, however, it's wise to follow your doctor's orders. Waiting the full six weeks can't hurt (at least not physically), while not waiting might.

LACK OF INTEREST IN MAKING LOVE

"Ever since the baby was born I just don't feel very interested in sex."

Sex takes energy, concentration, and time—all of which are in particularly short supply in the lives of new parents. Your libido—and your husband's—must regularly compete with sleepless nights, exhausting days, dirty diapers, and an endlessly demanding baby. Your body is still recuperating from the trauma of childbearing; your hormones are readjusting. Fears (of pain, of doing some damage internally, of not being the same, of becoming pregnant again too soon) may plague you. If you are breastfeeding, you may unconsciously be letting it satisfy your sexual needs. Or making love may stimulate uncomfortable leakage of milk. All in all, it's not surprising—and perfectly normal—if your sexual appetite, no matter how voracious it once was, is temporarily suppressed. (On the other hand, some women have strong sexual drives now, particularly in the immediate postpartum period, when there is engorgement of the genital region.

If your problem is lack of interest, there are many ways to make making love good again. Which ones will work for you will depend on you, your husband, and on your problems:

Make Time Your Ally. It takes at least six weeks for your body to heal, and sometimes much longer—especially if you had a difficult delivery or a cesarean. Your hormonal balance won't be back to normal until you start menstruating, which, if you are breastfeeding, may not be for many months. Don't feel obligated to make love because the doctor's given you the go-ahead, if it doesn't feel good, emotionally or physically. And when you do, start slowly, possibly with cuddling and petting but no penetration.

Don't Be Discouraged by Pain. Many women are surprised and disheartened to find that postpartum intercourse can really hurt. If you've had an episiotomy or a laceration, there may be discomfort (ranging from slight to severe) for weeks, even months, after the stitches have healed. You may also have pain with intercourse, although possibly less, if you delivered with the perineum intact—and even if you've had a cesarean. Until the pain disappears, you can minimize it in the ways described in Easing Back into Sex, page 312.

Easing Back into Sex

Lubricate. Lowered hormone levels during the postpartum period (which may not rise in the nursing mother until her baby is either partially or totally weaned) can make the vagina uncomfortably dry. Use a lubricating cream, like K-Y Jelly, until your own natural secretions return.

Medicate, If Necessary. Your practitioner may prescribe an estrogen cream to lessen pain and tenderness.

Inebriate. Don't get drunk, of course (since too much alcohol can interfere with sexual enjoyment and performance), but do enjoy a glass of wine with your husband before making love, to help both of you relax physically and emotionally. It will also numb some of your pain, lessen the fear of it in you, and the fear of causing it in him.

Vary Positions. Side-to-side or woman-on-top positions allow more control of penetration and less pressure on the episiotomy site. Experiment to find what works best for you.

Find Alternate Means of Gratification.

If intercourse isn't pleasurable yet, seek sexual satisfaction through mutual masturbation. Or, if you're both too pooped to pop, find pleasure in just being together. There's absolutely nothing wrong (and everything right) about lying in bed together, cuddling, kissing, and swapping baby stories.

Keep Your Expectations Realistic.

Don't insist on simultaneous orgasms the first time you make love after delivery. Some usually orgasmic women don't have orgasms at all for several weeks, or even longer. With love and patience, sex will eventually be as satisfying as ever—or more so.

Readjust Your Sex Life to Dovetail with Your Life with the Baby.

When your companionable two becomes a crowded three, you can no longer make love when and where you want to. Instead you'll have to either grab it when you can (if the baby is napping at 3 o'clock on Saturday afternoon, drop everything) or make a point of planning ahead. Don't feel that unspontaneous sex can't be fun. Instead, think of the advance planning as giving you the opportunity to look forward to making love (the baby will be asleep at 8—can't wait!). Accept interruptions—there will be many—with a sense of humor, and try to start again where you left off as soon as possible. And, should sex turn out to be less frequent than before, strive for quality, not quantity.

Don't Be a Perfectionist.

A lot of postpartum exhaustion is natural; learning to become parents is certainly taxing. But some of it is unnecessary, often due to trying to do too much too soon. Pack away your white gloves and forgo the dusting sometimes. Use frozen vegetables instead of fresh. Cut some dispensable corners, so that you occasionally have energy left for loving.

Communicate. A really good sexual relationship must be built on trust, understanding, and communication. If, for instance, you're too wrapped up in motherhood one night to feel sexy, don't beg off with a headache. Be honest. A husband who's been included in parenting since conception is most likely to understand. If intercourse is painful, don't be a martyr. Explain to your spouse what hurts, what feels good, what you'd rather put off until another time.

Don't Worry. Despite what you may be feeling now, you will live to love again, with as much passion and pleasure as ever. (And because shared parenthood can often bring couples closer together, you may find the flame not only rekindled, but burning brighter than before.) Worry now can only put an unnecessary damper on your sexual relationship.

BECOMING PREGNANT AGAIN

"I thought that breastfeeding was a form of birth control. Now I hear you can get pregnant while nursing, even before you start menstruating again."

How completely you can rely on nursing as a means of birth control depends on how completely devastated you would be if you became pregnant again now. If you're like most brand-new parents, tummy-to-tummy pregnancies just months apart are not your idea of perfect family planning. And if that is indeed the case, breastfeeding by itself shouldn't be relied on for contraception.

It's true that women who nurse, on the average, resume normal menstrual cycles later than those who don't. Menstruation usually begins in non-lactating mothers somewhere between four and eight weeks after delivery, whereas in lactating women the average is somewhere between three and four months. As usual, however, averages are deceptive. Nursing women have been known to begin menstruating as early as 6 weeks and as late as 18 months postpartum. The problem is, there's no sure way to predict when you will again begin menstruating, though several variables influence the timing. For example, frequency of feeding (more than three times a day seems to suppress ovulation better), duration of nursing (the longer you nurse, the greater the delay in ovulation), and whether or not feedings are being supplemented (your baby's taking bottles, solids, even water, can interfere with the ovulation-suppressing effect of nursing).

Why worry about birth control before that first menstrual period? Because the point at which you ovulate for the first time after delivery is as unpredictable as when you menstruate. Some women have a sterile first period; that is, they don't ovulate during that cycle. Others ovulate before the period, and therefore can go from pregnancy to pregnancy without ever having had a menstrual period. Since you don't know which will come first, the period or the egg, caution in the form of contraception is highly advisable.

POSTPARTUM CONTRACEPTION

Oral Contraceptives. The Pill is the most effective, and most popular, form of birth control—but it also presents many health risks, particularly for women over 35. Though it causes unpleasant side effects in some women, it is convenient (if one remembers to take it as prescribed) and doesn't interfere with intercourse. It is not usually prescribed during the first six weeks of lactation, because it can interfere with the production of milk. But because the effects of the hormones on a suckling infant aren't known, it is probably unwise to take birth control pills at all while breastfeeding. The Pill is also contraindicated if you have a history of coronary artery, gall bladder, or liver disease; diabetes; high blood pressure; thrombosis; epilepsy; menstrual irregularity; diagnosed or suspected cancer of the reproductive organs; or if you smoke. If you are interested in using oral contraceptives, discuss their possible side effects and risks with your doctor, and weigh them against the benefits before having it prescribed. Also ask that the type of oral contraceptive prescribed be the one that is most appropriate for your individual needs.

Diaphragm. The diaphragm, a dome-shaped rubber cap that fits over the cervix, is an effective birth control method when used properly with a spermicidal gel. It is also safe and without any side effects, and in no way affects lactation. But it must be prescribed and fitted by a medical professional. *It is very important to be refitted after childbirth,* as the size and shape of the cervix may have changed. The diaphragm has the disadvantages of having to be inserted before each intercourse and of having to be left in for six to eight hours afterward.

The IUD. This intrauterine device (it is not strictly speaking a contraceptive, since it interferes with implantation rather than conception) has lost some favor in recent years because of the associated risks of infection and ectopic pregnancy—conditions that could lead to infertility. Many physicians refuse to insert IUDs for fear of later lawsuits; all but one company have stopped making them, for the same reason. Because of the risks, the IUD is not recommended for women who want to have more children, are exposed to multiple partners, have a history of PID (pelvic inflammatory disease or infection), are unusually susceptible to infection, or have a known or suspected uterine or cervical malignancy or premalignancy, or menstrual or other bleeding irregularities. The main advantage of the IUD is that after your doctor inserts it, you can forget about it for at least a year except to check periodically for the string. The IUD has no effect on lactation or on the nursing infant.

Rhythm Method. This approach, which depends on knowing exactly when you ovulate and avoiding intercourse at that time, is impossible to use during lactation. It is the least effective of the various popular methods, though when based on a combination of steadfast timing, temperature taking, and vaginal mucus samples, it has only about a 24% failure rate.[4] It is completely harmless, except for the risk of pregnancy, and has the additional advantage for some religious groups of being morally acceptable.

The Sponge. The most recent addition to the birth control arsenal, the sponge, like the diaphragm, is a barrier method of contraception, one that blocks the entrance to the cervix. It appears to be less effective than the diaphragm or condom (studies have been done on relatively small numbers of women so far), and its safety is still under question because it contains chemicals that can cause cancer in animals, and because it's been linked tentatively to cases of toxic shock syndrome. The sponge is relatively easy to use (you insert it yourself, like a diaphragm), allows for greater spontaneity (it provides protection for 24 hours after insertion and allows for unlimited sexual activity during that time), is available without a prescription, and is not believed to have any effect on the nursing infant. The contraceptive sponge should not be used in the postpartum period (or directly after a miscarriage or abortion), however, without a physician's approval.

Condom. Very effective if used conscientiously (but somewhat less foolproof than the Pill), the condom (or rubber) is totally harmless. Its effectiveness is enhanced if it is used with a spermicidal foam or jelly. It has the advantages of not requiring a doctor's prescription, of being easily available and easy to carry. It in no way interferes with breastfeeding. Some find, however, that because it must be put on before intercourse (and not until erection), it interferes with spontaneity. Others claim it reduces sensation. Care should be taken when sheathing the penis to leave a small reservoir at the tip of the condom to hold the semen. The penis should be withdrawn before the erection is totally lost and while the condom is held on. The use of lubricated condoms or of a separate lubricating cream will help make insertion more comfortable when the vagina is dry after pregnancy.

Surgical Sterilization. Tubal ligation for women and vasectomy for men must be considered permanent, though occasionally it is possible to reverse them. They are also increasingly safer and virtually foolproof, though you do hear an occasional story of failure.[5] Sterilization is the frequent choice of couples who feel their family units are complete. Sterilization in women is often performed immediately after delivery.

Of course, accidents can happen. Medical science has yet to develop a method of contraception (with the possible exception of sterilization)

---

4. This rate is for the typical user. The theoretical rate is much lower, possibly 5%.

5. This isn't generally a failure of the method, but due to a slip-up in the surgery, or carelessness on the part of a man who fails to use other birth control methods until all viable sperm have been ejaculated.

that is 100% effective. So even if you've been using contraception—and especially if you haven't been—pregnancy is still a possibility. Unfortunately, the first symptom of pregnancy you would ordinarily look for (absence of menstruation) will not be apparent if you've been nursing and not menstruating. But because of hormonal changes (there are different sets of hormones in operation during pregnancy and lactation), your milk supply will diminish noticeably soon after the new pregnancy is established. You might, in addition, experience any or all of the other symptoms of pregnancy. (See Signs of Pregnancy, page 18.) Of course, if you do have any suspicion that you might be pregnant, the best thing to do is to visit your practitioner as soon as possible. Because it is virtually impossible to do a good job of nourishing both a breastfed infant and a developing fetus at the same time, it is highly inadvisable to continue nursing during a new pregnancy.

HAIR LOSS

"My hair seems to be falling out suddenly."

D on't order a hairpiece. Hair fall is normal, and will stop well in advance of baldness. Ordinarily, the average head sheds 100 hairs a day, which are being continually replaced. During pregnancy (as when you're taking oral contraceptives), the change in hormone levels keeps those hairs from falling out. But the reprieve is only temporary. Those hairs are slated to go, and they will—within three to six months of delivery (or after you stop taking the pill).

TAKING TUB BATHS

"I seem to be getting a lot of contradictory advice about whether or not tub baths are all right in the postpartum period. Are they?"

A t one time, new mothers weren't permitted to set a foot in a tub until at least one month after delivery, because of fear of infection from the bath water. Today, because it's known that still bath water does not enter the vagina, infection from bathing is no longer considered a threat. Some physicians, in fact, recommend tub baths in the hospital (when a tub is available) because they believe bathing removes lochia from the perineum—and from between the folds of the labia—more efficiently than showering. In addition, the warm water is comforting to the episiotomy site, relieves soreness and edema in the area, and soothes hemorrhoids.

Still, your doctor may prefer you to hold off on bathing until you are home, or even later. If you're anxious to bathe (especially if you have no shower at home), discuss the issue with him or her. You may be able to get a dispensation.

If you do bathe during the first week or two following delivery, be sure the tub is scrubbed meticulously before it's filled. (But be sure you're not the one who does the scrubbing.) And get help getting into and out of the tub during the first few postpartum days, when you're still likely to be shaky.

EXHAUSTION

"It's nearly two months since I had the baby, but I feel more tired than ever. Could I be sick?"

Many a new mother has dragged herself into her doctor's office and complained of overwhelming chronic fatigue—convinced that she's fallen victim to some fatal malady. The nearly invariable diagnosis? A classic case of motherhood.

Rare is the mother who escapes this maternal fatigue syndrome, characterized by tiredness that never seems to ease up and an almost total lack of energy. And it's not surprising. There's no other job as emotionally and physically taxing as that of being a mother. The strain and pressures are not, as in most other jobs, limited to eight hours a day or five days a week. (And mothers don't get lunch hours or coffee breaks, either.) Motherhood for first-timers also adds the stress inherent in any new job: there's always something new to learn, mistakes to be made, problems to solve. If all this isn't enough to produce symptoms, add the energy that goes into breastfeeding, the strength sapped by toting around a rapidly growing infant and accompanying paraphernalia, and night after night of broken sleep.

Check with your doctor to be sure there is no physical cause for your exhaustion. If you get a clean bill of health, be assured that time, experience, and your baby sleeping through the night will gradually help relieve much of your fatigue. And once your body adjusts to the new demands, your energy level should pick up a bit, too. In the meantime, try the tips for relieving postpartum depression (page 304), which is closely tied to fatigue.

WHAT IT'S IMPORTANT TO KNOW: GETTING BACK INTO SHAPE

It's one thing to look six months pregnant when you *are* six months pregnant, and quite another to look it when you've already delivered. Yet most women can expect to be wheeled out of the delivery room not much trimmer than when they were wheeled in—with a little bundle in their arms and several still around their middles. As for the pencil-thin skirts optimistically packed for the going-home trip, they're likely to stay packed, with maternity jeans the depressing substitute.

How soon after you become a new mother will you stop looking like a mother-to-be? With active exercise, that old prepregnancy figure (or a newly slender one) is only a couple of months away.

"Who needs exercise?" you may wonder. "I've been in perpetual motion since I got home from the hospital. Doesn't that count?"

Unfortunately, not much. Exhausting as it is, that kind of general activity won't tighten up the perineal and abdominal muscles that have been left saggy by pregnancy. Only an exercise program will.

You can start a postpartum exercise program as early as 24 hours after delivery. But be careful not to overdo it. The following is geared for women who've had uncomplicated vaginal deliveries. If you've had a surgical or a traumatic one, check with your doctor before beginning:

GROUND RULES

❖ Always start each session with the least strenuous exercise, as a warm-up.

❖ Keep your exercise sessions brief and frequent, rather than doing one long session a day (this tones muscles better).

❖ If you have the time and really enjoy exercise, take a class for new mothers or buy a postpartum exercise book and develop an extensive program. If that prospect is unappealing, doing just a few simple routines regularly can also get you back into shape, especially if you gear them directly to problem areas, such as abdomen, thighs, buttocks, and so on.

❖ Do exercises slowly, and don't do a rapid series of repetitions with inadequate recovery time between each.

❖ Rest briefly between exercises (the muscle buildup occurs then, not while you are in motion).

❖ Don't do more than recommended, even if you feel you can.

❖ Quit before you feel tired: If you overdo it, you usually won't feel it until the next day—by which time you may be unable to exercise at all.

❖ Don't let mothering stop you from mothering yourself—your baby will love lying on your chest as you exercise.

❖ Do not do knee-chest exercises, full sit-ups, or double leg lifts during the six-week postpartum period.

All the following exercises are done in the basic position, though Kegels can be done in any comfortable position. The early exercises can be done in bed; the others are best done on a harder surface, such as the floor. (An exercise mat is a good investment because the baby can try his or her first tentative crawls on it later.)

PHASE ONE: 24 HOURS AFTER DELIVERY

Kegel Exercises. You can begin these immediately after delivery, though you won't be able to feel yourself doing them at first. (See page 162 for directions.) This exercise can also be performed in bed or in a sitz bath. Or while you're urinating—contract to stop, then relax to release the flow of urine. Repeat several times. As the muscles regain tone, you will be able to allow just a few drops of urine to pass between repetitions.

Deep Diaphragmatic Breathing. In the basic position, place your hands on your abdomen so you can feel it rise as you inhale slowly through your nose; tighten the abdominal muscles as you exhale slowly through your mouth. Start with just two or three deep breaths at a time to prevent hyperventilating. (Signs that you've overdone it are dizziness or faintness, tingling, or blurred vision. See page 262 for dealing with hyperventilation.)

PHASE TWO: THREE DAYS AFTER DELIVERY

Three days after you deliver, you can begin doing more serious exercises. But only if you are sure that the pair of vertical muscles of your abdominal wall (called the recti abdominis) have not separated during pregnancy. Fairly common, especially in women who have had several children, this separation (or diastasis) will get worse if you do anything even mildly strenuous before it heals. Ask your nurse or doctor about the condition of these muscles, or examine them yourself this way: As you lie in the basic position, raise your head slightly with your arms extended; then feel for a soft lump below your navel. Such a lump indicates a separation.

You can help correct a diastasis, if you have one, with this exercise: Assume the basic position, inhale. Now cross your hands over your abdomen, using your fingers to draw the sides of your abdominal muscles together as you breathe out while raising your head slowly. Inhale as you lower your head slowly. Repeat 3 or 4 times, twice a day. When the separation has closed, or if you've never had one, move on to the following exercises.

HEAD LIFTS

Assume the basic position (see page 162). Take a deep breath, then raise your head very slightly, exhaling as you do. Lower your head slowly, and inhale. Raise your head a little more each day, gradually working up to lifting your shoulders slightly off the floor. Don't try full sit-ups for at least three or four weeks—and then only if you have always had very good abdominal muscle tone.

Leg Slides

Assume the basic position (see page 162). Slowly extend both legs until they are flat on the floor. Slide your right foot, sole flat on the floor, back toward your buttocks. Keep the small of your back against the floor. Slide your leg back down. Repeat with your left foot. Start with three or four slides per side, and increase gradually until you can do a dozen or more comfortably. After three weeks, move to a modified leg lift (lifting one leg at a time slightly off the floor and lowering it again very slowly), if it is comfortable.

The Pelvic Tilt (see illustration, page 162). Lie on your back, with your knees bent and your feet about 12 inches apart, soles flat on the floor. Inhale as you press the small of your back against the floor. Then exhale, and relax. Repeat 3 or 4 times to start; increasing gradually to 12, and then 24.

A postpartum exercise program will do more than flatten your tummy and tighten your perineum. The perineal exercises will help you avoid stress incontinence (difficulty holding urine), a dropping (prolapse) of pelvic organs, and sexual difficulties. Abdominal exercises will reduce the risk of backache, varicose veins, leg cramps, edema, and the formation of clots in the veins (thrombi), as well as improve circulation. Regular exercise will also promote healing of your traumatized uterine, abdominal, and pelvic muscles, hasten their return to normal tone, and lessen the further weakening that inactivity could encourage. Planned activity will also help the pregnancy- and delivery-loosened joints to return to normal, and prevent further weakening and strain. Finally, exercise can have a psychological benefit (ask any runner), improving your ability to handle stress and to relax—and minimizing the chance of postpartum blues.

17
Fathers Are Expectant, Too

Mothers- and fathers-to-be today share not only the joys of pregnancy, childbirth, and childrearing, but the worries as well; and the chances are good that there is considerable overlap in what concerns each member of your expectant (or newly delivered) team. Yet fathers are entitled to a few worries of their own—and to some very special reassurance, not only during the pregnancy and the birth, but in the postpartum period as well.

And so this chapter—dedicated to the equal, but often neglected, partner-in-reproduction. But it isn't intended for fathers' eyes only—any more than the rest of the book is intended only for mothers'. An expectant mother can gain some valuable insights into what her husband is feeling, fearing, and hoping by reading this chapter; an expectant father can gain a better understanding of the physical and emotional changes his wife will undergo during pregnancy, and after, by reading the rest of the book (while also better preparing himself for his own role in the unfolding drama).

WHAT YOU MAY BE CONCERNED ABOUT

FEELING LEFT OUT

"So much attention has been focused on my wife since she became pregnant that I hardly feel I have anything to do with it."

In generations past, the father's involvement in the reproductive process ended once his sperm had fertilized his wife's ovum. Fathers watched pregnancy from afar, and childbirth not at all.

Great strides have undeniably

been made in the past decade for fathers' rights. But social re-education hasn't changed the fact that pregnancy takes place within a woman's body. Or the fact that some fathers are lost in what is still largely a woman's shuffle. Or that they end up feeling forgotten, left out—even jealous of their wives.

Sometimes the woman is unwittingly responsible, sometimes the man is. Either way, it's vital that the father's feelings are resolved before resentment grows and is allowed to spoil what should be one of the most wonderful experiences of *both* parents' lives. The best way to accomplish this is for you to get involved in as many aspects of your wife's pregnancy as you can:

See an Obstetrician (or Midwife). Your wife's—as often as she does, if possible. Most practitioners will allow the husband to attend the monthly appointment, and many will encourage him to do so. If your schedule won't permit a monthly visit, perhaps you can arrange to attend the landmark appointments—when the heartbeat will first be heard, for instance. Also try to schedule prenatal tests when you'll be able to be there.

Act Pregnant. You don't have to show up for work in maternity clothes or start drinking a quart of milk a day. But you can do your wife's pregnancy exercise routine with her; give up junk food for nine months; quit smoking, if you're a smoker. And when someone offers you a drink, tell them, "No thanks, we're pregnant."

Get an Education. Even Harvard Ph.D.s have a lot to learn when it comes to pregnancy and childbirth. Read as many books and articles as you can. Attend childbirth classes with your wife. Talk to friends who've been through it recently.

Shop for a Layette. And a crib, and a stroller. Help your wife decorate the nursery. In general, become active in picking out, planning, and preparing for the baby's arrival.

Talk It Out. Your wife may be leaving you out unintentionally—she may not even be aware that you'd like to be more involved. It's very likely that she'd be as happy to make you a part of her pregnancy as you would to be a part of it.

FEAR OF SEX

"Even though the doctor has assured us that sex is safe throughout pregnancy, I often have trouble following through for fear of hurting my wife or the baby."

Never is sex more a mind-over-matter situation—for both partners—than during pregnancy. This is true particularly as gestation advances and the mind (and libido) must confront a very sizable matter: the expanding pregnant belly and its precious contents.

Fortunately, you can put your mind to rest and enjoy the matter. As vulnerable as mother and baby may seem to an anxious father contemplating intercourse, in a normally progressing low-risk pregnancy, neither one is. (There are a few caveats, particularly in the last two months, detailed in Making Love During Pregnancy, page 139.)

Not only can making love to your wife not do her any harm (assuming the caveats are observed), but because pregnancy is a time for emotional and physical closeness, it can do her a world of good. And as for your baby, though basically oblivious to the whole event, he or she may be pacified by the gentle rocking motion of intercourse and of the contracting uterus during orgasm.

IMPATIENCE WITH YOUR WIFE'S MOOD SWINGS

"I know it's my wife's hormonal changes that are making her so weepy and volatile. But I don't know how much longer I can be patient."

If patience is a virtue, you're going to have to be very virtuous for the rest of your wife's pregnancy. Although the stabilization of hormone levels by the fourth month eases the pronounced premenstrual-like weepiness and moodiness of early pregnancy, the stresses of being pregnant continue. And many women continue to be subject to sudden bursts of emotion and attacks of vulnerability right up to delivery. It doubtless won't be easy, and at times you may find it close to impossible. But there's also little doubt that your efforts will pay off. Touchiness met with understanding will dissipate faster than touchiness met with anger and frustration; shoulders offered to your wife for a

15-minute cry won't have to carry around the weight of her unvented anxiety for days at a time.

Try to keep in mind that pregnancy is *not* a permanent condition, and that the changes in your wife's emotional status are as transient as the changes in her figure.

SYMPATHY SYMPTOMS

"If it's my wife who's pregnant, why am I having morning sickness?"

You may well be among the estimated 11% to 65% (depending on the study) of expectant fathers who suffer from the couvade syndrome during their wives' pregnancies. The symptoms of couvade (which comes from the French for "to hatch") most often appear in the third month and again at delivery, and can mimic in a man virtually all the normal symptoms of pregnancy in a woman—including nausea and vomiting, abdominal pain, appetite changes, weight gain, food cravings, constipation, leg cramps, dizziness, fatigue, and mood swings.

Many theories have been suggested to explain couvade—all, some, or none of which may be appropriate to you: sympathy for and identification with the pregnant wife; jealousy over being left out, and a resultant desire for attention; guilt over being responsible for putting the wife in such an uncomfortable situation; stress from living with a woman who's become irritable, moody, and possibly off-limits sexually; and anxiety over the impending addition to the family.

Of course your symptoms could also indicate illness, so it's a good idea to see a doctor. But should an examination show no physical cause, couvade is a likely diagnosis. The cause, if you can identify it, may be a clue to the cure. For instance, if the cause is jealousy, becoming more involved in your wife's pregnancy may relieve your morning sickness. Or if it's anxiety over handling a newborn for the first time, taking a course in infant care, reading a copy of Dr. Spock, or even spending some time with a friend's baby might prove helpful.

Even if you can't put your finger on any one cause for your symptoms, talking out all your feelings about pregnancy, childbirth, and parenthood with your wife may alleviate your sympathy pains. So might discussing them with other expectant parents in your childbirth class. Should none of this help, be assured that your reactions are normal, and that all symptoms which don't go away during pregnancy will disappear soon after delivery.

Equally normal, of course, is the father who doesn't have a sick day during his wife's pregnancy. Not suffering from morning sickness or not putting on weight doesn't mean an expectant father doesn't empathize and identify with his wife.

ANXIETY OVER YOUR WIFE'S HEALTH

"I know pregnancy and childbirth are safe today, yet I still can't stop worrying that something will happen to my wife."

There's something undeniably vulnerable about a pregnant woman—and something very natural about your desire, as a loving husband, to want to protect your wife from any possible harm. But you can relax. Your wife is in virtually no danger. Women very, very rarely die as a result of pregnancy or childbirth anymore—and the vast majority of those who do are from crowded inner cities or remote rural areas and haven't had the benefits of prenatal care or adequate nourishment. (See page 75.)

But even though pregnancy doesn't pose a serious physical threat to your wife, you can still help make it an even safer and more comfortable experience for her: by making sure she gets the best medical care possible and that she eats the best possible diet; by letting her get extra rest while you do the laundry, make dinner, or clean the house; and by giving her the kind of emotional support she can't get from any other source (no matter how far obstetrical science advances, pregnant women will always be *emotionally* vulnerable).

ANXIETY OVER THE BABY'S HEALTH

"I'm so afraid that something will be wrong with the baby, I can't even sleep at night."

Mothers-to-be by no means hold a corner on the worry market. And like almost every expectant mother, virtually every expectant father worries about his unborn baby's health and well-being. Happily, nearly all worry is needless. The odds that your baby will be born both alive and completely normal are overwhelming—far better than in previous generations.

Of course, even the most reassuring statistics probably won't be able to banish all your worries; only the birth of a healthy baby will. But sharing your fears with your wife, and letting her share hers with you, may serve to unburden you both and will make the waiting—and sleeping—a little easier.

YOUR WIFE'S LOOKS

"As petty as this might seem, I'm afraid my wife's going to get fat and flabby with pregnancy, and stay that way afterward."

If it were in your wife's obstetrical interest to gain 50 pounds with pregnancy, you (and the countless other expectant husbands who share your "petty" concern) would have no option, of course, but to accept fat and flab as the price of a healthy baby. But though such calories-are-no-object weight gains are the current vogue, they just aren't medically justifiable—and can, in fact, lead to unnecessary complications during both pregnancy and delivery. A moderate, steady, carefully monitored weight increase of between 20 and 30 pounds, gained through a diet of highly nutritious food and no junk food, gives your baby the best odds for healthy development and safe delivery—and your wife the speediest return to slenderness after

childbirth. (See the Best-Odds Diet, page 75; Weight Gain, page 127).

Sticking to a rigid diet even for two weeks isn't easy. Sticking to one for nine months can be close to impossible, unless the dieter has the support, understanding, and assistance of those close to her. In the case of your wife, that's you. Not only do many husbands fail to provide their wives with that help, they may unwittingly sabotage their efforts. Husbands have probably done more to undermine their wives' diets than Carvel, Cadbury's, and Sara Lee put together—either by bringing temptation into the house, ordering it in restaurants, or even offering it directly to their wives ("Come on—one bite won't hurt!").

With the following tips, you'll be able to become your wife's best ally in her campaign to gain weight moderately and eat sensibly during pregnancy—while protecting your own selfish interests (a thin wife):

Lead Your Wife Not into Temptation. If you must indulge in dietary indiscretion, do so out of your home and away from your wife. You can't expect her to live happily on broiled meats, steamed vegetables, and fresh fruit while you gorge on burgers, fries, and Heavenly Hash ice cream beside her.

Practice What You Preach to Her. What's good for the goose and the gosling is good for the gander, too. Your staying close to the Best-Odds Diet (recognizing that you don't need all that protein or calcium) will not only support your wife, but will improve your health as well.

Don't Be Too Preachy. If she slips, nagging will only help her to fall faster and farther. Remind, don't remonstrate. Prod her conscience, don't try to become it. Signal her quietly when in public, rather than making a pointed announcement to all within earshot about her ordering her chicken breaded and fried. Most important, do it with a sense of humor and a lot of love.

Accentuate the Positive. Nothing will undermine her willpower like a faltering ego. So make a point of building her up, admiring her new pregnant shape, commenting often on how pregnancy becomes her.

Exercise with Her. It's much more fun for two to tango—or to follow a pregnancy exercise program. Proper exercise during pregnancy is important not only for keeping your wife (and you) trim, but also for getting her in good shape for labor and delivery.

FALLING APART DURING LABOR

"I'm afraid I'll faint or become ill during the delivery."

F ew fathers enter the delivery room without fear. Even obstetricians who've assisted at births of thousands of other people's babies can experience a sudden loss of self-confidence when confronted with their own baby's delivery.

Yet very few of these fears—of freezing, falling apart, fainting, or becoming sick to the stomach while watching the delivery—are ever realized. And though being prepared for the birth (by taking childbirth education classes, for instance) generally makes the experience more satisfying, even most unprepared fathers come through labor and delivery better than they'd thought they would. One study of fathers who attended their babies' births with no previous preparation found that though 70% expected that the delivery would be a frightening, unpleasant, and negative experience, all described it afterwards in highly positive terms.

But like anything new and unfamiliar, childbirth becomes less frightening and intimidating if you know what to expect. So become an expert on the subject. Read the entire chapter on labor and delivery, beginning on page 238. Attend childbirth education classes, watching the labor and delivery films with your eyes open. Visit the hospital ahead of time so that you'll be acquainted with the technology that's used in labor and delivery rooms. Talk to friends who have recently gone through the experience. You will probably find they had the same anxieties beforehand but came through feeling terrific.

Though it's important to get an education, it's also important to remember that childbirth isn't the final exam in your childbirth education course. Don't feel that you must perform perfectly (as some women feel obligated to) at the delivery. Nurses and doctors won't be evaluating your every move or comparing you to the husband next door. More important, neither will your wife.

She won't care if you forget every coaching technique you learned in class. Your being beside her, holding her hand, urging her on, giving her the comfort of a familiar face and touch, will do her more good than having Drs. Lamaze, Bradley, and Dick-Reade themselves at her bedside.

"I would really rather not be at the birth, but I feel pressured to be there."

Just because it's currently de rigueur in the birthing business for fathers to attend births doesn't mean it's mandatory. Studies have shown that fathers who attend births don't have more meaningful relationships with their offspring than fathers who don't attend; just as fathers who bond with their babies immediately after birth don't seem automatically to become better, more loving fathers. What's important is that you do what's right for you and your wife. If it doesn't feel right for you to attend the delivery, for whatever reason, you would probably do more harm than good to all concerned by being there. Ignore those who try to pressure you into a decision that would be wrong for you. Remember, more generations of fathers *haven't* seen their babies born than *have*—with no ill effects.

However, that's not to say that attending the birth of your child is not a worthwhile experience, or one you should abandon without careful consideration. Though it's important that you not let anyone else make up your mind for you, it's equally important that you not make up—and close—your mind until the last minute. Go through all the preparations: accompany your wife on her prenatal visits, take childbirth classes, do extensive reading. Many once-hesitant fathers find that familiarity with labor and delivery breeds a new perspective, which allows them to feel comfortable enough with childbirth to attend and participate fully.

Others, however, still end up deciding that being at the birth would be counterproductive for themselves and their spouses. Still others decide to give labor a try but find, sometime before or during delivery, that they'd rather step outside. All should feel free to follow their instincts, with the reassurance that doing so won't reflect in any way on their capacity for fathering.

"My wife is having a planned cesarean. Hospital regulations won't allow me to be there, and I'm afraid that our new family won't get off to the best start."

If you made the decision to be at the birth only to discover that the decision wasn't yours to make (as in the case of a cesarean, in a hospital that doesn't permit husbands to attend), don't give up without a civilized fight. With the support of your wife's obstetrician (if such support is forthcoming), try first to persuade hospital officials to bend—or even change—the regulations. (It may help to remind them that a majority of hospitals now allow fathers to be present at non-emergency surgical deliveries.) If your campaign is unsuccessful (or if a hasty delivery precludes your presence), you have every right to be disappointed. But you have no right to let that disappointment taint the joy that should surround the birth of your child. Your not being at the birth can threaten your relationship with your baby only if you let it, by harboring feelings of guilt, resentment, or frustration.

BONDING

"My wife had a last-minute cesarean and I wasn't allowed to be with her. I didn't hold the baby for 24 hours and I'm afraid I didn't bond with him."

Until this decade, few fathers ever witnessed the birth of their children, and since the word "bonding" originated only in the 1970s, none were ever even aware of the possibility of bonding with their offspring. But such a lack of enlightenment didn't stop generations of loving father-son and father-daughter relationships from developing. Conversely, every father who attends his child's birth and is allowed to bond with him or her isn't automatically guaranteed a lifetime of closeness with his offspring.

Being with your wife during delivery is ideal, and being deprived of that opportunity is reason for disappointment—particularly if you spent months training together for childbirth. But it's no reason for a less than fulfilling relationship with your baby. What really bonds you with your baby is daily loving contact—changing diapers, giving baths, feeding, cuddling, lullabying. He or she will never know that you didn't share in the moment of birth, but your child will know if you aren't there when he or she needs you from then on.

EXCLUSION DURING BREASTFEEDING

"My wife is breastfeeding our baby. There's a closeness between them that I can't seem to share, and I feel left out."

There are certain immutable biological aspects of parenting that exclude the father: he can't be pregnant, he can't labor and deliver, and he can't breastfeed. But, as millions of new fathers discover each year, a man's natural physical limitations don't have to relegate him to spectator status. You can share in nearly all the joys, expectations, trials, and tribulations of your wife's pregnancy, labor, and delivery—from the first kick to the last push—as an active, supportive participant. And though you'll never be able to put your baby to the breast (at least not with the kind of results the baby's looking for), you *can* share in the feeding process:

Be Your Baby's Supplementary Feeder. There's more than one way to feed a baby. And though you can't nurse, you can be the one to give any supplementary bottles. Not only will it give your wife a break (whether in the middle of the night or in the middle of dinner), it will give you opportunities for closeness with your baby. Don't waste the opportunity by propping the bottle up to the baby's mouth. Strike a nursing position, with the bottle where your wife's breast would be and your baby snuggled close to you.

Don't Sleep Through the Night Until Your Baby Does. Sharing in the joys of feeding also means sharing in the sleepless nights. Even if you're not giving supplementary bottles, you can become a part of nighttime feeding rituals. You can be the one to take the baby out of the crib, do any necessary diaper changing, and put him or her back to bed once he or she has fallen asleep again.

Watch in Wonder, and Appreciate. There can be enormous satisfaction in simply watching the miracle of breastfeeding—as there is in watching the miracle of birth. Instead of feeling left out, feel privileged to be a witness to the love that passes between your wife and your baby as they nurse.

Participate in All Other Daily Rituals. Nursing is the *only* daily chore limited to mothers. And chances are that if you make at least one other chore your responsibility (and as many as possible), you'll be too busy to be jealous.

FEELING UNSEXY AFTER DELIVERY

"The delivery was absolutely miraculous to watch. But seeing our baby come out of my wife's vagina seems to have turned me off sexually."

H uman sexual response, compared to that of other animals, is extremely delicate. It's at the mercy not only of the body but of the mind as well. And the mind can, at times, play merciless havoc with it. One of those times, as you probably already know, is during pregnancy. Another, as you seem to be discovering, is during the postpartum period.

It's very possible that the cause of your sudden sexual ambivalence has nothing to do with having seen your baby delivered. Most brand new fathers find both the spirit and the flesh somewhat less willing after delivery (although there's nothing abnormal about those who don't), for many very understandable reasons: fatigue, especially if the baby still isn't sleeping through the night; uneasiness about having a third person in your home; fear that he or she will awake crying at the first caress (particularly if the baby is sharing your room); concern that you may hurt your wife by having intercourse before her body is thoroughly healed; and finally, a general physical and mental preoccupation with your newborn, which sensibly concentrates your energies where they are most needed at this stage of your lives.

In other words, it's probably just as well that you aren't feeling sexually motivated, particularly if your wife (like many women in the immediate postpartum period) isn't feeling emotionally or physically up to it either. Just how long it will take for your interest, and hers, to return is impossible to predict. As with all matters sexual, there is a wide range of what is "normal." For some couples, the urge will precede even the doctor's go-ahead at six weeks. For others, six months can pass before l'amour and le bébé begin to coexist harmoniously in the same home. (Some women find desire lacking until they stop breastfeeding.)

Some fathers, even if they've been prepared for the childbirth experience, do come out of it feeling that their "territory" has been "violated," that the special place that had been meant for loving has suddenly taken on a practical purpose. But as the days pass, that feeling usually does too. The father begins to realize that the vagina has two functions, equally important and miraculous. Neither excludes the other, and in fact they are very much interconnected. He also comes to recognize that the vagina is a vehicle for childbirth only briefly, while it is a source of pleasure for himself and his wife for a lifetime.

If the sexual urge doesn't return and its absence begins to cause tension, professional counseling is probably needed.

"Before the baby, my wife's breasts were a center of sexual pleasure—for both of us. Now that she's breastfeeding, they seem too functional to be sexy."

Like the vagina, breasts were designed to serve both a practical and a sexual purpose (which, from a strictly procreative standpoint, is also practical). And though these purposes aren't mutually exclusive in the long run, they can conflict temporarily during lactation.

Some couples find breastfeeding a sexual turn-on. Others, for esthetic reasons (leaking milk, for instance) or because they feel uncomfortable about using the baby's source of nourishment for their sexual pleasure, find it a very definite turn-off.

Whatever turns you on—or off— is what is normal for you. If you feel that your wife's breasts are too functional to be sexy now, don't try to force yourself to feel otherwise. Leave them out of sexual foreplay for now, with the reassurance that you will feel differently once the baby has been weaned. Be sure, however, to be open and honest with your wife; taking a sudden, unexplained hands-off approach to her breasts could leave her feeling unappealing. Be careful, also, not to harbor any resentment against the baby for using "your" breasts; try to think of nursing as a temporary "loan" instead.

18
Preparing for the Next Baby

I n the best of all possible worlds, we would be able to plan life to our precise specifications. In the real world, where most of us live, the best-laid plans often give way to the unexpected twists and turns of fate, over which we have precious little control—leaving us to accept, and to make the best of, what comes our way.

In the best of all possible pregnancies, we would know in advance when we would conceive and could make all the changes and adjustments in our lifestyle to help ensure our baby the best of all possible odds of being born alive and well. Such advance planning is a rare luxury, which many women (because of menstrual irregularity and/or the frailties of contraception) may never indulge in. And as has been stressed throughout this book, what a woman does before she realizes she's pregnant (a few drinks, a few dietary indiscretions, a dental x-ray) does little to affect her baby's odds. Few women act pregnant from the moment of conception, and yet the vast majority give birth to normal, healthy babies.

But it would be remiss not to outline a plan for the best of all possible pregnancies—simply because the possibility does, for many women, exist. The plan is appropriate whether you're already in the process of trying to conceive or if you're thinking ahead. Although it's never too late to start taking care of your body, it's also never too early. And, in fact, your good prepregnancy care will benefit not only your own children but your children's children. Act now, and:

Get a Thorough Physical. Both you and your husband should see your internist or family doctor. An exam will pick up any potential problems that need to be corrected beforehand, or that will need to be monitored during pregnancy. Update your immunizations; especially be sure you're immune to rubella. Also take care of allergy shots, minor elective surgery, and anything else medical—major or minor—that you've been putting off. (If you start allergy desensitization now, you will probably be able to continue once you conceive.)

See Your Dentist. Make an appointment for a thorough examination and cleaning. Have any necessary work, including x-rays, fillings, dental or periodontal surgery completed now.

Select a Practitioner—and Have a Prepregnancy Exam. It's easier to choose a practitioner now, in an unhurried manner, than when that first prenatal checkup is hanging over your head. If you think you might like to use a certified nurse-midwife, have a gynecologist or family physician whose medical opinion you respect perform this examination to make certain that your next pregnancy won't fall into a high-risk category. If you know, or suspect that, your mother took diethylstilbestrol (DES) when she was pregnant with you, tell the doctor, so your reproductive organs can be carefully examined—with colposcopy, if necessary. If you've had a previous pregnancy problem, such as a miscarriage or premature delivery, discuss the measures that can be taken to head off a repeat. Even if you're sure you couldn't have a sexually transmitted disease, ask for tests for syphilis, gonorrhea, chlamydia, and herpes. Get treatment, if needed.

Have Genetic Screening. If either of you has any genetic problem in your personal or family history, see a genetic counselor.

Evaluate Your Birth Control Method. If you are using a method of birth control that might present some risk (however slight) to a future pregnancy, change it before you start trying to conceive. Birth control pills should be discontinued several months before conception, if possible, to allow your reproductive system to go through at least two normal cycles before you start making babies. The IUD should be removed before you begin trying. Since the risks of spermicides are as yet unclear, playing it extra safe means discontinuing their use (alone or with a diaphragm) one month to six weeks before you want to become pregnant. The birth control method to switch to for the interim: the condom (used with care, as described on page 315).

Improve Your Diet. Start eliminating junk food and refined sugars from your diet, and increase whole grains and fiber. Since it's best to embark on your pregnancy as close to normal weight as possible, try to get there before conceiving. Add or cut calories as necessary. (Use the Best-Odds Diet, page 75, for a good basic food plan; but you will only need 2 calcium and 2 protein servings daily until you conceive.) Don't go on a crash diet.

Improve Your Husband's Diet. The better your husband's nutrition, the healthier his sperm. His diet should mirror your prepregnancy diet, with caloric intake adjusted to accommodate his weight and activity.

Take a Vitamin-Mineral Supplement Formulated for Pregnancy. Studies show that certain birth defects can be avoided by taking a supplement prior to conception. In addition, the supplement will ensure that you will be getting necessary vitamins, particularly folic acid, and minerals, particularly iron, when you conceive.

Shape Up. An exercise program will tone and strengthen your muscles in preparation for the challenging tasks of carrying and delivering your baby-to-be. It will also help you take off excess weight.

Avoid Unnecessary X-Rays and Chemical Exposure. Some (though far from all) kinds of exposure can be harmful to your husband's sperm or your ova before conception, and later to a developing embryo or fetus. Avoid potentially hazardous exposure on the job (OSHA, the Occupational Safety and Health Administration, can supply you with information; see page 71). If you're trying to conceive you may have already succeeded. Inform doctors who are treating you, or x-ray technicians taking x-rays, that you might be pregnant, and do not permit unneeded x-rays (see page 63). Don't inhale directly fumes from such materials as paints, insecticides, and cleaning products (see pages 66–69).

Cut Back on Caffeine. Moderating (and gradually cutting out, if possible) your intake of coffee, tea, and colas now will spare you the symptoms of withdrawal once you're pregnant. That means no more than two cups total of coffee, strong tea, or soft drinks containing caffeine before you conceive, and preferably none afterwards (see page 60).

Cut Down on Alcohol Consumption. Even a daily cocktail or glass of wine will not be harmful in your pregnancy-preparation phase, but avoid heavy drinking. Once you start trying to conceive, stop drinking altogether (see page 54).

Quit Smoking. Not only you: Recent studies indicate it would also be a good idea for your husband to quit, if he's a smoker. (See page 58 for tips on how to quit.)

Avoid Marijuana and Other "Recreational" Drugs. These can interfere with conception, and their effects on the fetus range from unknown to serious (see page 59).

Limit Prescription and Over-the-Counter Drugs. Discuss your plans with a doctor to see if any medication you are taking regularly may present a problem should you conceive. Are there alternatives? Can the dose be reduced? Avoid taking any non-prescription drugs without medical advice once you start trying to conceive.

Check for Immunity to Toxoplasmosis (if you have a cat or eat raw meat regularly). If you are immune, you needn't worry about this problem during pregnancy; if you're not, check your cat for the disease (have him treated if he has it), and stop eating raw or rare meats. (See page 62.)

Relax. This is perhaps the most important of all. Getting tense and uptight about conception could prevent you from conceiving at all.

Appendix

COMMON TESTS DURING PREGNANCY[1]

TEST AND WHEN PERFORMED	PROCEDURE	REASON
Blood type; first visit, unless already known from previous pregnancy or test	Examination of blood drawn from your arm.	To determine blood and Rh type in case blood transfusion is needed at some point, and to be prepared for the possibility of Rh incompatibility (see page 40).
Sugar (glucose) in the urine; at each visit	A specially treated stick, dipped in a specimen of your urine, shows presence of sugar.	While an occasional increase in sugar is normal in pregnancy (see page 132), persistent high levels could indicate hyperglycemia; further tests will determine if gestational diabetes is present, requiring special diet and care.
Albumin (protein) in the urine; at each visit	A special strip, dipped in a urine specimen, shows presence of albumin.	High albumin levels could be related to toxemia; if routine test shows increase, a 24-hour test may be ordered.
Bacteria in urine; first visit	Urine specimen is examined in lab.	Bacteria in urine could indicate susceptibility to infection; treatment may be initiated.

1. Your practitioner may omit some of these tests or add others, depending upon your condition and his or her professional opinion.

Blood pressure; at each visit	Blood pressure is measured with cuff and stethoscope, or with an electronic device.	A sudden rise in your normal blood pressure of more than 30 points in the upper (systolic) range, or 15 in the lower (diastolic) range, could be warning of complication such as preeclampsia (see pages 130, 176).
Hematocrit or hemoglobin; first visit and often fourth month (repeated if values are low or anemia diagnosed)	Blood drawn from arm or from pricked finger is examined.	Values are slightly reduced in pregnancy, but abnormally low levels require further examination and treatment.
Rubella titer; first visit	Blood drawn from your arm is tested for levels of antibodies to rubella.	High levels of rubella (German measles) antibodies in your blood indicate you are immune to the disease; if you aren't immune, it is important to avoid exposure to the disease—particularly in your first trimester—and to be immunized before another pregnancy.
VDRL; first visit, sometimes again in seventh or eighth month	Blood drawn from your arm is tested.	To test for syphilis infection; if present, prompt treatment will prevent harm to fetus.
Gonorrhea culture; first visit[2]	Vaginal secretions are collected on a swab and cultured in the lab.	If gonococcus is present, treatment will prevent eye infection in baby at birth.
Pap smear; first visit	Cervical secretions are collected on a swab and examined under a microscope for abnormal cells.	Abnormal cells could, on further study, turn out to be malignant, requiring treatment.

2. Tests for chlamydia and herpes may also be done at the first visit.

NON-DRUG TREATMENTS DURING PREGNANCY

SYMPTOMS	TREATMENT	PROCEDURE
Colds, flu, diarrhea	Additional fluids	Drink water, juices, soups—8 ounces every hour. (With diarrhea, use only diluted juices, avoid prune.) Take milk as recommended by your doctor.
Itchy abdomen	Baking soda and ammonia paste	Mix ½ cup of baking soda with enough household ammonia to make a paste (avoid breathing the fumes); apply to itchy skin. Check any persistent skin problems with your practitioner.
Swelling or bruises	Cold compresses	Dip a soft cloth in a basin of ice cubes and cold water, wring it out, and place over affected site. Re-chill when cold dissipates.
Sinusitis	Alternating hot and cold compresses	Dip a cloth in hot water, wring it out, and apply to the painful area until the heat dissipates, about 30 seconds; then apply a cold compress until the cold dissipates. Continue alternating heat and cold for 10 minutes 4 times daily.
Sore or scratchy throat	Gargle	Dissolve 1 teaspoon of salt in 8 ounces of hot water (the temperature of tea) and gargle for 5 minutes; repeat as needed, or every 2 hours.

Itchy eye discharge	Warm soaks	Use a cloth dipped in warm, not hot, water (test it for comfort on your inner forearm), and apply to your eye for 5 or 10 minutes every 3 hours.
Colds, coughs	Inhalation	Use a standard humidifier or vaporizer or a steaming kettle; prepare a tent by draping a sheet over an open umbrella which is resting on a chair back; place humidifier on chair. Spend 15 minutes 3 or 4 times a day under tent; extend the time to 30 minutes, if you aren't too uncomfortable. (Don't stay under tent if you become uncomfortably warm.) Keep the humidifier near your bedside when you are sleeping or resting.
Tight muscles, tension, bruises and sprains	Hot soaks	Twenty-four hours after injury, wet a towel thoroughly in warm water, then wring it out and place it over the affected site, covering all completely with a plastic bag. Place a heating pad over the plastic at a medium setting, being careful that it does not touch the wet towel. Apply for 1 hour twice daily.
Bruises, sprains, burns, on the hands, wrists, and feet	Cold soaks	Place a tray or two of ice cubes in a basin (a styrofoam bucket or cooler is best) of cold water and immerse the injured part for 30 minutes; repeat 30 minutes later if necessary.

Hemorrhoids	Sitz bath	Sit in enough hot water (hotter than your usual bath) to cover the affected area for 20 to 30 minutes, 2 or 3 times daily.
	Sponge bath	Using a plastic sheet to catch drips, apply cold towels soaked in 2 quarts of water, 1 pint of rubbing alcohol, and 1 quart of ice cubes to the skin. Stop if shivering begins.
Fever	Cooling bath	Use a tub of tepid water and gradually cool it by adding ice cubes— stopping immediately if shivering begins.

INDEX

P

AFTERWORD

Now that you have read *What to Expect When You're Expecting,* you can see that every pregnancy (like every expectant parent) is different, that there are few hard and fast rules about what you can (or should) expect. You have learned that today we can control much of what happens in our pregnancies and childbirths—through the way we utilize medical care, the way we eat, through our lifestyles—making our chances of having a healthy baby better than those of any generation of parents in history. And we hope you have benefited from the fact that, though all of us worry, accurate information can go a long way toward easing our anxieties.

We hope that this book will answer all of your questions, quiet your fears, help you sleep better at night. We hope that by knowing what you can *really* expect, both the expectation and the reality will become more manageable, more exciting, and more truly fulfilling.

In our preparation and research for this book, we strove to leave no question unanswered. We relied not only on our personal experiences but also on those of the hundreds of pregnant parents we surveyed and interviewed. But since the variations of what expectant couples worry about are great, we're likely to have missed a few questions. If we overlooked any of yours, we'd like to know. That way we'll be able to include your concerns (and reassurances for them) in our next edition—in plenty of time, we hope, for *your* next edition.

Wishing you the happiest of pregnancies and the most joyous of outcomes,

Arlene Eisenberg
Heidi Eisenberg Murkoff
Sandee Eisenberg Hathaway